Statistics in Nutrition
and Dietetics

Statistics in Nutrition and Dietetics

Michael Nelson

Emeritus Reader in Public Health Nutrition
King's College London
Public Health Nutrition Research Ltd
UK

WILEY Blackwell

Registered Office(s)
John Wiley & Sons, Inc., 111 River Street, Hoboken, NJ 07030, USA
John Wiley & Sons Ltd, The Atrium, Southern Gate, Chichester, West Sussex, PO19 8SQ, UK

Editorial Office
9600 Garsington Road, Oxford, OX4 2DQ, UK

For details of our global editorial offices, customer services, and more information about Wiley products visit us at www.wiley.com.
Wiley also publishes its books in a variety of electronic formats and by print-on-demand. Some content that appears in standard print versions of this book may not be available in other formats.

Library of Congress Cataloging-in-Publication Data
Names: Nelson, Michael (Nutritionist), author.
Title: Statistics in nutrition and dietetics / Michael Nelson.
Description: Hoboken, NJ : John Wiley & Sons, 2020. | Includes
    bibliographical references and index.
Identifiers: LCCN 2019030279 (print) | ISBN 9781118930649 (paperback) |
    ISBN 9781118930632 (adobe pdf) | ISBN 9781118930625 (epub)
Subjects: MESH: Nutritional Sciences–statistics & numerical data |
    Statistics as Topic | Research Design
Classification: LCC RM217 (print) | LCC RM217 (ebook) | NLM QU 16.1 |
    DDC 613.2072/7–dc23
LC record available at https://lccn.loc.gov/2019030279
LC ebook record available at https://lccn.loc.gov/2019030280

Cover Design: Laurence Parc | NimbleJack &Partners | www.nimblejack.co.uk
Cover Image: © filo/Getty Images; PHN Courtesy of Public Health Nutrition Research Ltd

Set in 10.5/13pt STIXTwoText by SPi Global, Pondicherry, India
Printed and bound by CPI Group (UK) Ltd, Croydon, CR0 4YY

10 9 8 7 6 5 4 3 2 1

To Stephanie

Contents

About the Author

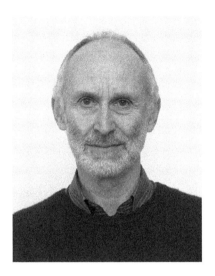

Dr. Michael Nelson is Emeritus Reader in Public Health Nutrition at King's College London, and former Director of Research and Nutrition at the Children's Food Trust. He is currently Director of Public Health Nutrition Research Ltd (http://www.phnresearch.org.uk/).

His early career with the Medical Research Council sparked a keen interest in nutritional epidemiology, statistics, and measurement validity. Research interests have included the diets of UK school children and links between diet and poverty, cognitive function, behaviour and attainment, and monitoring the impact of standards on school lunch take-up and consumption. He collaborates nationally and internationally to promote a strong evidence base for school food policy. He has published over 200 peer-reviewed articles and other publications in the public domain.

January 2020

Preface

WHY IS THIS BOOK NEEDED?

Worldwide, there is no basic statistics textbook that provides examples relevant to nutrition and dietetics. While it could be argued that general medical science statistics texts address the needs of nutrition and dietetics students, it is clear that students find it easier to take on board the concepts relating to statistical analysis and research if the examples are drawn from their own area of study. Many books also make basic assumptions about students' backgrounds that may not always be appropriate, and use statistical jargon that can be very off-putting for students who are coming to statistics for the first time.

WHO IS THIS BOOK FOR?

The book is aimed at undergraduate and postgraduate students studying nutrition and dietetics, as well as their tutors and lecturers. In addition, there are many researchers in nutrition and dietetics who apply basic statistical techniques in the analysis of their data, for whom a basic textbook provides useful guidance, and which helps to refresh their university learning in this area with examples relevant to their own field.

LEVEL AND PRE-REQUISITE

The level of the material is *basic*. It is based on a course that I taught at King's College London over many years to nutrition and dietetics students, physiotherapists, nurses, and medical students. One of the aims was to take the fear and boredom out of

statistics. I did away with exams, and assessed understanding through practical exercises and coursework.

This book takes you only to the foothills of statistical analysis. A reasonable competence with arithmetic and a little algebra are required. For the application of more demanding and complex statistical techniques, the help of a statistician will be needed. Once you have mastered the material in this book, you may want to attempt a more advanced course on statistics.

AIMS AND SCOPE

The aim of this book is to provide clear, uncomplicated explanations and examples of statistical concepts and techniques for data analysis relevant to learning and research in nutrition and dietetics. There are lots of short, practical exercises to work through. These support insight into why various tests work. There are also examples of SPSS[1] output for each test. This makes it is possible to marry up the outcomes computed manually with those produced by the computer. Examples are taken from around the globe relating to all aspects of nutrition, from biochemical experiments to public health nutrition, and from clinical and community practice

---

[1]SPSS stands for 'Statistical Package for the Social Sciences'. It was developed at Stamford University in California, and the first manual was authored by Norman Nie, Dale Bent, and Hadlai Hull in 1970. The package was bought in 2009 by IBM. The worked examples and syntax in this book are based on Version 24 (2016). It has come a long way since its first incarnation, in terms of ease of use, error trapping, and output. Be grateful.

in dietetics. All of this is complemented by material online, including data sets ready for analysis, so that students can begin to understand how to generate and interpret SPSS output more clearly.

The book focuses on quantitative analysis. Qualitative analysis is highly valuable, but uses different approaches to data collection, analysis, and interpretation. There is an element of overlap, for example when quantitative statistical approaches are used to assess opinion data collected using questionnaires. But the two approaches have different underlying principles regarding data collection and analysis. They complement one another, but cannot replace one another.

Two things this book is not. First, it is not a 'cookbook' with formulas. Learning to plug numbers in to formulas by rote does not provide insight into why and how statistical tests work. Such books are good for reminding readers of the formulas which underlie the tests, but useless at conveying the necessary understanding to analyze data properly or read the scientific literature intelligently. Second, it is not a course in SPSS or Excel. While SPSS and Excel are used to provide examples of output (with some supporting syntax for clarity), it is no substitute for a proper course in computer-based statistical analysis.

Scope

The book provides:

- a basic introduction to the scientific method
- an understanding of populations and samples, principles of measurement, and confidence intervals
- an understanding of the basic theory underlying basic statistical tests, including 'parametric' tests (those intended for use with data that follow mathematically defined distributions such as the so-called 'normal' distribution); and 'non-parametric' tests, for use with data distributions that are not parametric

- lots of worked examples and exercises that show how to compute the relevant outcome measures for each test, both by hand and using SPSS
- real examples from the nutrition and dietetics literature, including biochemical, clinical, and population-based examples
- principles of research design, transformations, the relevance of sample size, and the concept and calculation of Power

All of the exercises have worked solutions.

Some students say, 'Why do we have to do the exercises by hand when the computer can do the same computations in a fraction of a second?' The answer is: computers are stupid. The old adage 'garbage in, garbage out' means that if you don't have insight into why certain tests work the way they do, a computer will generate output that might be meaningless, but it won't tell you that you've made a mistake, or ask 'Is this really what you wanted to do?' So, the purpose of the textbook and supporting learning materials is to help ensure that when you do use a computer, what goes in isn't garbage, and what comes out is correct and provides meaningful answers to your research questions that you can interpret intelligently.

Finally, it is worth saying that some students will find this textbook providing welcome explanations about why things work the way they do. Others will find it annoyingly slow and detailed, with too much explanation for concepts and applications that seem readily apparent. If you are in the first group, I hope you enjoy the care with which explanations and examples are presented and that it helps to demystify what may at first seem a difficult topic. If you are in the second group, read quickly to get to the heart of the matter, and look for other references and resources for material that you feel is better suited to what you want to achieve. However hard or easy the text seems, students in both groups should seek to make friends with a local statistician or tutor experienced in statistical analysis and not try and do it alone.

Unique features

There are many unique features in this textbook and supporting material:

- Examples specific to nutrition and dietetics
- Clear simple language for students unfamiliar with statistical terms and approaches. For many students, the study of statistics is seen as either a burden or irrelevant to their decision to study nutrition and/or dietetics. But they will be required to pass a statistics module as part of their course. The aim is to make this as engaging and painless as possible.
- Lots of worked examples, with examples of SPSS output to help students with the interpretation of their analyses in the future.
- Putting statistics into context so that it is relevant to many undergraduate and postgraduate research projects.
- A website that provides complementary exercises, data sets, and learning and teaching tools and resources for both students and tutors.

CONTENTS

This textbook is based on over 20 years of teaching experience. There are four parts:

Part 1: Setting the statistical scene

This introduces concepts related to the scientific method and approaches to research; populations and samples; principles of measurement; probability and types of distribution of observations; and the notion of statistical testing.

Part 2: Statistical tests

This covers the basic statistical tests for data analysis. For each test, the underlying theory is explained,

and practical examples are worked through, complemented by interpretation of SPSS output.

Part 3: Doing research

Most undergraduate and postgraduate courses require students to collect data and/or interpret existing data sets. This section places the concepts in Part 1 and the learning in Part 2 into a framework to help you design studies, and determine sample size and the strength of a study to test your hypothesis ('Power'). A Flow Chart helps you select the appropriate statistical test for a given study design.

The last chapter explores briefly how to present findings to different audiences – what you say to a group of parents in a school should differ in language and visual aids from a presentation to a conference of your peers.

Part 4: Solutions to exercises

It would be desperately unfair of me to set exercises at the end of each chapter and not provide the solutions. Sometimes the solutions are obvious. Other times, you will find a commentary about why the solution is what it is, and not something else.

ONLINE

No textbook is complete these days without online resources that students and tutors can access. For this textbook, the online elements include:

- Teaching tools
  - Teaching notes
  - PowerPoint slides for each chapter
  - SPSS data, syntax, and output files
- Learning resources:
  - Links to online software and websites that support learning about statistics and use of statistical software

TEACHING TOOLS

Teaching notes

For lecturers delivering courses based on the text-book, I have prepared brief teaching notes. These outline the approach taken to teach the concepts set out in the textbook. I used traditional lecturing coupled with in-class work, practical exercises, home-work, and research protocol development. My current practice is to avoid exams for any of this material. Exams and formal tests tend to distract students from revision of study materials more central to their course. Some students get completely tied up in knots about learning stats, and they fret about not passing the exam, ultimately to their academic disadvantage.

PowerPoint slide sets

The principal aid for tutors and lecturers is slide sets in PowerPoint. These save hours of preparation, provide consistent format of presentation, and build on approaches that have worked well with literally thousands of students that have taken these courses. **When using the slides outside the context of teaching based on the text book, please ensure that you cite the source of the material.**

SPSS data, syntax, and output files

A complete set of SPSS files for the examples and exercises in the text book is provided.

Learning resources

The page on Learning Resources includes website links and reviews of the strengths of a number of sites that I like and find especially helpful.

Unsurprisingly, there is a wealth of websites that support learning about statistics. Some focus on the basics. These are mainly notes from University courses that have been made available to students online. Some are good, some are not so good. Many go beyond the basics presented in this text book. Diligent searching by the student (or tutor) will no doubt unearth useful material. This will be equivalent to perusing the reading that I outline in the Introduction to Chapter 1.

Flow Charts are useful to find the statistical test that best fits the data. Appendix A10 in this book shows one. There are more online. Two that I like are described in more detail on the Learning Resources page. I have also included links to sites for determining Power and sample size.

Finally, guidance on the use of Excel and SPSS in statistics is very helpful. There are many sites that offer support, but my favourites are listed on the Learning Resources page.

Acknowledgements

I would like to thank the hundreds of students who attended my classes on research methods and statistics. They gave me valuable feedback on what worked and what didn't in the teaching sessions, the notes, and exercises. Irja Haapala and Peter Emery at King's College London took over the reins when I was working on other projects and made helpful contributions to the notes and slides. Charles Zaiontz at Real Statistics kindly helped with the Wilcoxon U table, and Ellen Marshall at Sheffield Hallam University very helpfully made available the data on diet for the two-way analysis of variance. Mary Hickson at the University of Plymouth made helpful comments on the text. Mary Hickson, Sarah Berry, and Wendy Hall at King's College London, and Charlotte Evans at the University of Leeds kindly made data sets available. Thanks to the many colleagues who said, 'You should turn the notes into a book!' Stephanie, Rob, Tom, Cherie, and Cora all gave me great encouragement to keep going and get the book finished. Tom and Cora deserve a special thanks for the illustrations of statisticians. The Javamen supplied the coffee. Finally, I would like to thank Sandeep Kumar, Yogalakshmi Mohanakrishnan, Thaatcher Missier Glen, Mary Aswinee Anton, James Schultz, Madeleine Hurd, and Hayley Wood at Wiley's for bearing with me over the years, and for their support, patience and encouragement.

About the Companion Website

This book is accompanied by a companion Website:

www.wiley.com/go/nelson/statistics

The Website includes:

- Datasets
- Learning resources
- Teaching notes

PART 1

SETTING THE STATISTICAL SCENE

Learning Objectives

You should be reading this textbook because you want to:

- Learn how to design and analyze research projects
- Develop the skills to communicate the results and inferences from research
- Learn to evaluate the scientific literature

The ideas upon which these skills are founded – an understanding of the scientific method, an introduction to different models of scientific investigation, and the statistical tools to understand the significance of research findings – form the core of this book. Practical, worked examples are used throughout to facilitate an understanding of how research methods and statistics operate at their most fundamental level. Exercises are given at the end of each chapter (with detailed, worked solutions at the end of the book, with more examples and solutions online) to enable you to learn for yourself how to apply and interpret the statistical tools.

Approaching the Statistician

I have a grown-up son and a grand-daughter, age 6 and ¾. They are both very artistic. When I asked them to put their heads together and draw a picture of a statistician by way of illustration for this book, this is what they came up with (Figure 1):

'What's that!' I cried. 'He's hideous!'

'Well', they explained, 'the eyes are for peering into the dark recesses of the student's incompetence, the teeth for tearing apart their feeble attempts at research design and statistical analysis and reporting, and the tongue for lashing them for being so stupid'.

'No, no, no', I said. 'Statisticians are not like that'. So here was their second attempt (Figure 2):

'That's better', I said.

They interpreted the new drawing. 'Statisticians may appear a bit monstrous, but really they're quite cuddly. You just have to become familiar with their language, and then they will be very friendly and

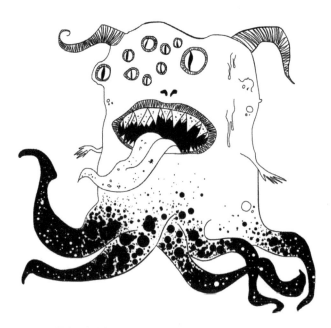

FIGURE 1 A SCARY STATISTICIAN.

helpful. Don't be put off if some of them look a bit flabby or scaly. This one can also recommend a great dentist and a very creative hair-stylist'.

Using Computers

Because computers can do in a few seconds what takes minutes or hours by hand, the use of computer statistical software is recommended and encouraged. However, computers are inherently stupid, and if they are not given the correct instructions, they will display on screen a result which is meaningless in relation to the problem being solved. It is vitally important, therefore, to learn how to enter relevant data and instructions correctly and interpret computer output to ensure that the computer has done what you wanted it to do. Throughout the book, examples of output from SPSS are used to show how computers can display the results of analyses, and how these results can be interpreted.

This text is unashamedly oriented toward experimental science and the idea that things can be *measured objectively or in controlled circumstances.*

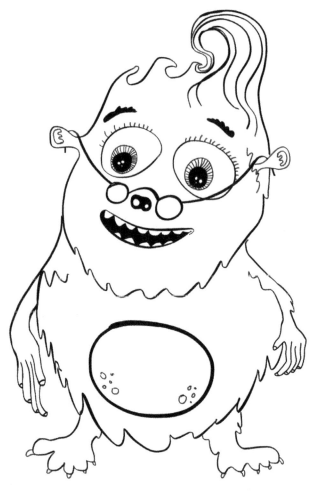

FIGURE 2 A FRIENDLY STATISTICIAN.

This is a different emphasis from books which are oriented toward qualitative science, where descriptions of how people feel or perceive themselves or others are of greater importance than quantitative measures such as nutrient intake or blood pressure. Both approaches have their strengths and weaknesses, and it is not my intention to argue their relative merits here.

The examples are taken mainly from studies in nutrition and dietetics. The aim is to provide material relevant to the reader's working life, be they students, researchers, tutors, or practicing nutrition scientists or dietitians.

CHAPTER 1

The Scientific Method

Learning Objectives

After studying this chapter you should be able to:

- Describe the process called the scientific method: the way scientists plan, design, and carry out research
- Define different types of logic hypotheses, and research designs
- Know the principles of presenting data and reporting the results of scientific research

1.1 KNOWING THINGS

What can I know?
—Immanuel Kant, philosopher

The need to know things is essential to our being in the world. Without learning we die. At the very least, we must learn how to find food and keep ourselves warm. Most people, of course, are interested in more than these basics, in developing lives which could be described as fulfilling. We endeavour to learn how to develop relationships, earn a livelihood, cope with illness, write poetry (most of it pretty terrible), and make sense of our existence. At the core of these endeavours is the belief that somewhere there is the 'truth' about how things 'really' are.

Much of the seeking after truth is based on feelings and intuition. We may 'believe' that all politicians are corrupt (based on one lot of evidence), and at the same time believe that people are inherently good (based on a different lot of evidence). Underlying these beliefs is a tacit conviction that there is truth in what we believe, even though all of our observations are not consistent. There are useful expressions like: 'It is the exception that proves the rule' to help us cope with observations that do not fit neatly into our belief systems. But fundamentally, we want to be able to 'prove' that what we believe is correct (i.e. true), and we busy ourselves collecting examples that support our point of view.

Some beliefs are easier to prove than others. Arguments rage about politics and religion, mainly because the evidence which is presented in favour of one position is often seen as biased and invalid by those who hold differing or opposing points of view. Some types of observations, however, are seen as more 'objective'. In science, it is these so-called objective measures, ostensibly free from bias, that are supposed to enable us to discover truths which will help us, in a systematic way, to make progress in improving our understanding of the world and how it works. This notion may be thought to apply not only to the physical and biological sciences but also the social sciences, and even disciplines such as economics. There are 'laws' which are meant to govern the ways in which things or people or economies behave or interact. These 'laws' are developed from careful observation of systems. They may even be derived from controlled experiments in which researchers try to hold constant the many factors which can vary from one setting to another, and allow only one or two factors to vary in ways which can be measured systematically.

It is clear, however, that most of the laws which are derived are soon superseded by other laws (or truths) which are meant to provide better understanding of the ways in which the world behaves. This process of old truths being supplanted by new truths is often a source of frustration to those who seek an absolute truth which is secure and immutable. It is also a source of frustration to those who believe that science provides us with objective facts, and who cannot therefore understand why one set of 'facts' is regularly replaced by another set of 'facts' which are somehow 'more true' than the last lot. It is possible, however, to view this process of continual replacement as a truth in itself: this law states that we are unlikely[1] ever to find absolute truths or wholly objective observations, but we can work to refine our understanding and observations so that they more nearly approximate the truth (the world 'as it is'). This assumes that there is in fact an underlying truth which (for reasons which we will discuss shortly) we are unable to observe directly.[2]

Karl Popper puts it this way:

We can learn from our mistakes. The way in which knowledge progresses, and especially our scientific knowledge, is by unjustified (and unjustifiable) anticipations, by guesses, by tentative solutions to our problems, by conjectures. These conjectures are controlled by criticism; that is, by attempted refutations, which include severely critical tests. Criticism of our conjectures is of decisive importance: by bringing out our mistakes it makes us understand the difficulties of the problems which we are trying to solve. This is how we become better acquainted with our problem, and able to propose more mature solutions: the very refutation of a theory – that is, of any serious tentative solution to our problem – is always a step forward that takes us nearer to the truth. And this is how we can learn from our mistakes.

From 'Conjectures and Refutations. The Growth of Scientific Knowledge' [1].

This is a very compassionate view of human scientific endeavour. It recognizes that even the simplest of measurements is likely to be flawed, and that it is only as we refine and improve our ability to make measurements that we will be able to develop laws which more closely approximate the truth. It also emphasizes a notion which the atomic physicist Heisenberg formulated in his Uncertainty Principle. The Uncertainty Principle states in general terms that as we stop a process to measure it, we change its characteristics. This is allied to the other argument which

[1]As you can see, I am already beginning to hedge my bets. I am not saying that we will never find absolute truths or wholly objective observations. I am saying that it is unlikely. *How* unlikely is the basis for another discussion.

[2]My favourite description of the world is Proposition 1 from Wittgenstein's *Tractatus Logico-Philosophicus*: 'The world is everything that is the case'. The Propositions get better and better. Have a look at: http://en.wikipedia.org/wiki/Tractatus_Logico-Philosophicus, or *Wittgenstein for Beginners* by John Heaton and Judy Groves (1994), Icon Books Ltd., if you want to get more serious.

states that the observer interacts with the measurement process. Heisenberg was talking in terms of subatomic particles, but the same problem applies when measuring diet, or blood pressure, or even more subjective things like pain or well-being. Asking someone to reflect on how they feel, and the interaction between the person doing the measuring and the subject, has the potential to change the subject's behaviour and responses. This is contrary to Newton's idea that measurement, if carried out properly, could be entirely objective. It helps to explain why the discovery of the 'truth' is a process under continual refinement and not something which can be achieved 'if only we could get the measurements right'.

Consider the question: 'What do you understand if someone says that something has been proven "scientifically"?' While we might like to apply to the demonstration of scientific proof words like 'objective', 'valid', 'reliable', 'measured', 'true', and so on, the common meanings of these words are very difficult to establish in relation to scientific investigation. For all practical purposes, *it is impossible to 'prove' that something is 'true'*. This does not allow you to go out and rob a bank, for example. An inability on the part of the prosecution to establish the precise moment of the robbery, for instance, would not excuse your action in a court of law. We cope in the world by recognizing that there is a substantial amount of inexactitude, or 'error', in all that we do and consider. This does not mean we accept a shop-keeper giving us the wrong change, or worry that a train timetable gives us information only to the nearest minute when the train might arrive before (or more commonly after) the advertised time. There are lots of 'gross' measurements that are good enough for us to plan our days without having to worry about the microdetail of all that we see and do.

For example, it is very difficult to describe an individual's 'usual' intake of vitamin C, or to relate that person's intake of vitamin C to risk of stroke. On the other hand, if we can accumulate sufficient evidence from many observations to show that increasing levels of usual vitamin C intake are associated with reduced risk of stroke (allowing for measurement error in assessing vitamin C intake

and the diagnosis of particular types of stroke), it helps us to understand that we can work with imprecise observations and laws which are not immutable. Moreover, it is important (for the sake of the growth of scientific knowledge) that *any belief which we hold is formulated in a statement in such a way as to make it possible to test whether or not that statement is true*. Statements which convey great certainty about the world but which cannot be tested will do nothing to improve our scientific understanding of the world. The purpose of this book, therefore, is to learn how to design studies which allow beliefs to be tested, and how to cope with the imprecision and variation inherent in all measurements when both collecting and analyzing data.

1.2 LOGIC

In science, we rely on logic to interpret our observations. Our aim is usually to draw a conclusion about the 'truth' according to how 'strong' we think our evidence is. The type of observations we choose to collect, and how we collect them, is the focus of *research design*: 'How are we going to collect the information we need to test our belief?' The decision about whether evidence is 'strong' or 'weak' is the province of *statistics*: 'Is there good evidence that our ideas are correct?' As Sherlock Holmes put it, 'It is a capital mistake to theorise before one has data'.[3]

There are two types of logic commonly applied to experience.

1.2.1 Inductive Logic

The aim with inductive logic is to infer a general law from particular instances: arguing from the particular to the general. This type of logic is good for generating new ideas about what we think *might be* true. It is less good for *testing* ideas about what we think *is* true.

---

[3]*Sherlock Holmes to Watson in: The Scandal in Bohemia*

Examples of Research Designs that Depend on Inductive Logic

Case studies provide a single example of what is believed to be true. The example is so compelling by itself that it is used to infer that the particular instance described may be generally true. For example:

> *A dietitian treating a severely underweight teenage girl worked with a psychotherapist and the girl's family to create an understanding of both the physiological and psychological basis and consequences of the disordered eating, resulting in a return to normal weight within six months. The approach contained unique elements not previously combined, and could be expected to have widespread benefit for similar patients.*

A case study can be interesting and provide a powerful example. But it provides very limited evidence of the general truth of the observation.

Descriptive studies bring together evidence from a number of related observations that demonstrate repeatability in the evidence. For example:

> *In four old peoples' homes, improved dining environments using baffles to reduce noise interference and allowing more time for staff to take orders and serve meals resulted in improved nutritional status among residents after one year.*

This type of cross-sectional evidence from numerous homes is better than evidence from a single home or a case study.

The generalizable conclusion, however, depends on a number of factors that might also need to be taken into account: what was the turnover among residents – did new residents have better nutritional status when they arrived, were they younger with better appetites, did they have better hearing so that they could understand more clearly what options were available on the menu for that day, etc.? One of the difficulties with descriptive studies is that we may not always be comparing like with like. We would have to collect information to demonstrate that apart from differences in noise levels and serving times, there were no other differences which could account for the change in nutritional status. We would also want to know if the circumstances in the four selected care homes were generalizable to other care homes with a similar population of residents.

Experimental studies are designed to assess the effect of a particular influence (exposure) on a particular outcome. Other variables which might affect the outcome are assumed to be held constant (or as constant as possible) during the period of evaluation.

> *Establish if a liquid iron preparation is effective in treating anaemia.*

If an influence produces consistent effects in a chosen group of subjects, we are tempted to conclude that the same influences would have similar effects in all subjects with similar characteristics. When we evaluated the results from our observations, we would try to ensure that other factors which might affect the outcome (age, sex, dietary iron intake, dietary inhibitors of iron absorption, etc.) were taken into account.

1.2.2 Deductive Logic

Deductive logic argues from the general to the particular. This type of logic involves *a priori* reasoning. This means that we think we know the outcome of our observations or experiment even before we start. What is true generally for the population[4] will be true for each individual within the population. Here is a simple example:

> *All animals die.*
> *My dog is an animal.*
> *My dog will die.*

---

[4]The term 'population' is defined in Chapter 2. It is not limited to the lay definition of all people living in a country. Instead, we can *define* our 'population'. In the example above, we are talking about the population of all animals (from yeast to elephants). But we could equally well define a population as all women between 35 and 54 years of age living in London, or all GP surgeries in Liverpool. More to come in Chapter 2.

This type of logic is very powerful for testing to see if our ideas are 'true'. The logic is: *if 'a' is true, then 'b' will be the outcome.* If the evidence is robust (i.e. as good a measure as we can get, given the limitations of our measuring instruments) and shows a clear relationship, it should stand up to criticism. And as we shall see, it provides the basis for the statistical inferences based on the tests described in later chapters.

There is a problem, however. The example above about my dog is relatively simple and straightforward. We can define and measure what we mean by an 'animal', and we can define and measure what we mean by 'death'. But suppose we want to understand the impact of vitamin A supplementation on risk of morbidity and blindness from measles in children aged 1 to 5 years living in areas where vitamin A deficiency is endemic. Defining and measuring variables in complex biological systems is much harder (particularly in the field of nutrition and dietetics). It becomes harder to argue that what is true generally for the population will necessarily be true for each individual within the population. This is for two reasons. First, we cannot measure all the factors that link 'a' (vitamin A deficiency) and 'b' (morbidity and blindness from measles) with perfect accuracy. Second, individuals within a population will vary from one to the next in terms of their susceptibility to infection (for a wide range of reasons) and the consequent impact of vitamin A supplementation.

For deductive logic to operate, we have to assume that the group of subjects in whom we are conducting our study is *representative* of the population in which we are interested. (The group is usually referred to as a 'sample'. Ideas about populations and samples are discussed in detail in Chapter 2.) If the group *is* representative, then we may reasonably assume that what is true in the population should be evident in the group we are studying. There are caveats to this around the size of the sample and the accuracy of our measurements, which will be covered in Chapters 2 and 12.

Examples of Research Designs that Depend on Deductive Logic

Intervention trials are designed to prove that phenomena which are true in the population are also true in a representative sample drawn from that population.

> *Compare the relative impact of two iron preparations in the treatment of anaemia.*

This may sound similar to the statement that was made under 'Experimental Studies'. The two statements are different, however. In the intervention trial, we would try to ensure that the two groups in which we were comparing treatments were similar to each other and similar to the population from which they were drawn. In the experimental study, we chose a group of subjects, measured the exposure and outcome and other characteristics of the group, and assumed that if the outcome was true in that group, it would be true in the population with similar characteristics. These differences in approach and logic are subtle but important.

In practice, the aim of most studies is to find evidence which is generalizable to the population (or a clearly defined subgroup). The relationship between the type of logic used and the generalizability of the findings is discussed below. The limitations of inductive logic and their resolution are discussed lucidly by Popper [1, pp 54–55].

1.3 EXPERIMENTATION AND RESEARCH DESIGN

Here is a quote from 'The Design of Experiments' by Sir Ronald Fisher [2]:

> *Men[5] have always been capable of some mental processes of the kind we call 'learning by experience'. Doubtless this experience was*

---

[5]I presume he means men and women. And children. Or 'humans'. Use of the term 'men' was common to his time of writing. Don't take offence. The point he is making is important.

often a very imperfect basis, and the reasoning processes used in interpreting it were very insecure; but there must have been in these processes a sort of embryology of knowledge, by which new knowledge was gradually produced.

Experimental observations are only experience carefully planned in advance, and designed to form a secure basis of new knowledge; that is, they are systematically related to the body of knowledge already acquired, and the results are deliberately observed, and put on record accurately.

Research usually has one of two main purposes: either to describe in as accurate and reliable a way as possible what one observes, or to test an idea about what one believes to be true. To undertake research, be it quantitative or qualitative, a systematic process of investigation is needed. This involves formulating clear ideas about the nature of the problem to be investigated, designing methods for collecting information, analyzing the data in an appropriate way, and interpreting the results.

1.3.1 A Children's Story

One of my favourite children's stories is *The Phantom Tollbooth* by Norton Juster [3], in which he brilliantly summarizes the purpose of research and statistics. This may seem unlikely, but read on.

The book tells the story of Milo, a young boy living in an apartment in New York. He is endlessly bored and someone for whom everything is a waste of time. He arrives home after school one day to find a large package sitting in the middle of the living room. (I don't know where his parents are.) He unpacks and assembles a tollbooth (he lives in America, don't forget), gets in his electric car, deposits his coin, and drives through the tollbooth into a land of fanciful characters and logical challenges.

The story is this. The princesses Rhyme and Reason have been banished, and it is his job to rescue

them and restore prosperity to the Kingdom of Wisdom. He drives from Dictionopolis (where only words are important) to Digitopolis (where – you guessed it – only numbers are important) to reach the Castle in the Air, where the princesses are held captive. He shares his journey with two companions: a Watchdog named Tock who is very vigilant about paying attention to *everything* (provided he keeps himself wound up); and the Humbug, 'a large beetle-like insect dressed in a lavish coat, striped trousers, checked waistcoat, spats and a derby hat', whose favourite word is BALDERDASH – the great sceptic.

On the way to Digitopolis, the road divides into three, with an enormous sign pointing in all three directions stating clearly:

> *DIGITOPOLIS*
> *5 miles*
> *1 600 rods*
> *8 800 Yards*
> *26 400 ft*
> *316 800 in*
> *633 600 half inches*

They argue about which road to take. The Humbug thinks miles are shorter, Milo thinks half-inches are quicker, and Tock is convinced that whichever road they take it will make a difference. Suddenly, from behind the sign appears an odd creature, the Dodecahedron, with a different face for each emotion for, as he says, 'here in Digitopolis everything is quite precise'. Milo asks the Dodecahedron if he can help them decide which road to take, and the Dodecahedron promptly sets them a hideous problem, the type that makes maths pupils have nightmares and makes grown men weep:

If a small car carrying three people at thirty miles an hour for ten minutes along a road five miles long at 11.35 in the morning starts at the same time as three people who have been travelling in a little automobile at twenty miles an hour for fifteen minutes on another road and exactly twice as long as one half the distance of the other, while a dog, a bug, and a boy travel an equal distance in the same time or the same distance in an equal time along a third road in mid-October, then which one arrives first and which is the best way to go?

They each struggle to solve the problem.

'I'm not very good at problems',
   admitted Milo.
'What a shame', sighed the Dodecahedron. 'They're so very useful. Why, did you know that if a beaver two feet long with a tail a foot and half long can build a dam twelve feet high and six feet wide in two days, all you would need to build the Kariba Dam is a beaver sixty-eight feet long with a fifty one foot tail?'
'Where would you find a beaver as big as that?' grumbled the Humbug as his pencil snapped.
'I'm sure I don't know', he replied, 'but if you did, you'd certainly know what to do with him'.
'That's absurd', objected Milo, whose head was spinning from all the numbers and questions.
'That may be true', he acknowledged, 'but it's completely accurate, and as long as the answer is right, who cares if the question is wrong? If you want sense, you'll have to make it yourself'.
'All three roads arrive at the same place at the same time', interrupted Tock, who had patiently been doing the first problem.
'Correct!' shouted the Dodecahedron. 'Now you can see how important problems are. If you hadn't done this one properly, you might have gone the wrong way'.
'But if all the roads arrive at the same place at the same time, then aren't they all the right way?' asked Milo.

'Certainly not', he shouted, glaring from his most upset face. 'They're all the wrong way. Just because you have a choice, it doesn't mean that any of them has to be right'.

That is research design and statistics in a nutshell. Let me elaborate.

1.4 THE BASICS OF RESEARCH DESIGN

According to the Dodecahedron, the basic elements of research are as shown in Box 1.1:

He may be a little confused, but trust me, all the elements are there.

1.4.1 Developing the Hypothesis

The Dodecahedron: 'As long as the answer is right, who cares if the question is wrong?'

The Dodecahedron has clearly lost the plot here. Formulating the question correctly is the key starting point. If the question is wrong, no amount of experimentation or measuring will provide you with an answer.

The purpose of most research is to try and provide evidence in support of a general statement of what one believes to be true. The first step in this process is to establish a *hypothesis*. A hypothesis is a clear statement of what one believes to be true. The way in which the hypothesis is stated will also have an impact on which measurements are needed. The formulation of a clear hypothesis is the critical first step in the development of research. Even if we can't make measurements that reflect the truth, the hypothesis should always be a statement of what

---

BOX 1.1

The four key elements of research

Hypothesis

Design   **Statistics**

Interpretation

you believe to be true. Coping with the difference between what the hypothesis says is true and what we can measure is at the heart of research design and statistics.

TIP

Your first attempts at formulating hypotheses may not be very good. Always discuss your ideas with fellow students or researchers, or your tutor, or your friendly neighbourhood statistician. Then be prepared to make changes until your hypothesis is a clear statement of what you believe to be true. It takes practice – and don't think you should be able to do it on your own, or get it right first time. The best research is collaborative, and developing a clear hypothesis is a group activity.

We can test a hypothesis using both inductive and deductive logic. Inductive logic says that if we can demonstrate that something is true in a particular individual or group, we might argue that it is true generally in the population from which the individual or group was drawn. The evidence will always be relatively weak, however, and the truth of the hypothesis hard to test. Because we started with the individual or group, rather than the population, we are less certain that the person or group that we studied is representative of the population with similar characteristics. Generalizability remains an issue.

Deductive logic requires us to draw a sample from a defined population. It argues that if the sample in which we carry out our measurements can be shown to be representative of the population, then we can generalize our findings from our sample to the population as a whole. This is a much more powerful model for testing hypotheses.

As we shall see, these distinctions become important when we consider the generalizability of our findings and how we go about testing our hypothesis.

1.4.2 Developing the 'Null' Hypothesis

In thinking about how to establish the 'truth'[6] of a hypothesis, Ronald Fisher considered a series of statements:

> **No amount of experimentation can 'prove' an *inexact* hypothesis.**

The first task is to get the question right! Formulating a hypothesis takes time. It needs to be a clear, concise statement of what we believe to be true,[7] with no ambiguity. If our aim is to evaluate the effect of a new diet on reducing cholesterol levels in serum, we need to say specifically that the new diet will 'lower' cholesterol, not simply that it will 'affect' or 'change' it. If we are comparing growth in two groups of children living in different circumstances, we need to say in which group we think growth will be better, not simply that it will be 'different' between the two groups.

The hypothesis that we formulate will determine what we choose to measure. If we take the time to discuss the formulation of our hypothesis with colleagues, we are more likely to develop a robust hypothesis and to choose the appropriate measurements. Failure to get the hypothesis right may result in the wrong measurements being taken, in which case all your efforts will be wasted. For example, if the hypothesis relates to the effect of diet on serum cholesterol, there may be a particular

---

[6]You will see that I keep putting the word 'truth' in single quotes. This is because although we want to test whether or not our hypothesis is true – it is, after all, a statement of what we *believe* to be true – we will never be able to collect measures that are wholly accurate. Hence, the truth is illusory, not an absolute. This is what the single quotes are intended to convey.

[7]'The term "belief" is taken to cover our critical acceptance of scientific theories – a *tentative* acceptance combined with an eagerness to revise the theory if we succeed in designing a test which it cannot pass' [1, p. 51]. It is important to get used to the idea that any 'truth' which we hope to observe is likely to be superseded by a more convincing 'truth' based on a more robust experiment or set of observations using better measuring instruments, and which takes into account some important details which we did not observe the first time.

cholesterol fraction that is altered. If this is stated clearly in the hypothesis, then we must measure the relevant cholesterol fraction in order to provide appropriate evidence to test the hypothesis.

No finite amount of experimentation can 'prove' an exact hypothesis.

Suppose that we carry out a series of four studies with different samples, and we find that in each case our hypothesis is 'proven' (our findings are consistent with our beliefs). But what do we do if in a fifth study we get a different result which does not support the hypothesis? Do we ignore the unusual finding? Do we say, 'It is the exception that proves the rule?' Do we abandon the hypothesis? What would we have done if the first study which was carried out appeared not to support our hypothesis? Would we have abandoned the hypothesis, when all the subsequent studies would have suggested that it was true?

There are no simple answers to these questions. We *can* conclude that any system that we use to evaluate a hypothesis must take into account the possibility that there may be times when our hypothesis *appears* to be false when in fact it is true (and conversely, that it may appear to be true when in fact it is false). These potentially contradictory results may arise because of sampling variations (every sample drawn from the population will be different from the next, and because of sampling variation, not every set of observations will necessarily support a true hypothesis), and because our measurements can never be 100% accurate.

A finite amount of experimentation can *disprove* an exact hypothesis.

It is easier to disprove something than prove it. If we can devise a hypothesis which is the *negation* of what we believe to be true (rather than its opposite), and then *disprove* it, we could reasonably conclude that our hypothesis was true (that what we observe, for the moment, seems to be consistent with what we believe).

This negation of the hypothesis is called the 'null' hypothesis. The ability to *refute* the null hypothesis

lies at the heart of our ability to develop knowledge. A good null hypothesis, therefore, is one which can be tested and refuted. If I can refute (disprove) my null hypothesis, then I will accept my hypothesis.

> *A theory which is not refutable by any conceivable event is non-scientific. Irrefutability is not a virtue of a theory (as people often think) but a vice. [1, p. 36]*

Let us take an example. Suppose we want to know whether giving a mixture of three anti-oxidant vitamins (β-carotene, vitamin C, and vitamin E) will improve walking distance in patients with Peripheral Artery Disease (PAD), an atherosclerotic disease of the lower limbs. The hypothesis (which we denote by the symbol H_1) would be:

H_1: Giving anti-oxidant vitamins A, C, and E as a dietary supplement will improve walking distance in patients with PAD.[8]

The null hypothesis (denoted by the symbol H_0) would be:

H_0: Giving anti-oxidant vitamins A, C, and E as a dietary supplement will *not* improve walking distance in patients with PAD.

H_0 is the *negation* of H_1, suggesting that the vitamin supplements will make no difference. It is not the opposite, which would state that giving supplements *reduces* walking distance.

It is easier, in statistical terms, to set about disproving H_0. If we can show that H_0 is probably *not* true, there is a reasonable chance that our hypothesis *is* true. Box 1.2 summarizes the necessary steps. The statistical basis for taking this apparently convoluted approach will become apparent in Chapter 5.

---

[8]This is the hypothesis – short and sweet. The study protocol will specify which subjects we choose, the dosage of the supplement, how often it is administered over what period, how walking distance is measured in a standardized way, what we mean by 'improve,' whether we measure blood parameters to confirm compliance with the protocol, etc.

BOX 1.2

Testing the hypothesis

1. Formulate the Hypothesis (H_1)
2. Formulate the Null Hypothesis (H_0)
3. Try to disprove the Null Hypothesis

1.4.3 Hypothesis Generating Versus Hypothesis Testing

Some studies are observational rather than experimental in nature. The purpose of these studies is often to help in the generation of hypotheses by looking in the data for relationships between different subgroups and between variables. Once the relationships have been described, it may be necessary to set up a new study which is designed to test a specific hypothesis and to establish causal relationships between the variables relating to exposure and outcome. For example, Ancel Keys observed that there was a strong association between the average amount of saturated fat consumed in a country and the rate of death from coronary heart disease: the more saturated fat consumed, the higher the death rate. Numerous studies were carried out subsequently to test the hypothesis that saturated fat causes heart disease. Some repeated Ancel Keys' original design comparing values between countries, but with better use of the available data, including more countries. Other studies compared changes in saturated fat consumption over time with changes in coronary heart disease mortality. Yet other studies looked at the relationship between saturated fat consumption and risk of heart disease in individuals. Not all of the studies came to the same conclusions or supported the hypothesis. It took some time to understand why that was the case.

1.4.4 Design

The Dodecahedron: 'If you hadn't done this one properly, you might have gone the wrong way'.

When designing an experiment, you should do it in such a way that *allows* the null hypothesis to be disproved. The key is to **introduce** and **protect** a random element in the design.

Consider some research options for the study to test whether anti-oxidant vitamins supplements improve walking distance in peripheral arterial disease (PAD). In the sequence below, each of the designs has a weakness, which can be improved upon by introducing and protecting further elements of randomization.

a. Choose the first 100 patients with PAD coming into the clinic, give them the treatment, observe the outcome.
   *Patients may naturally improve with time, without any intervention at all. Alternatively, there may be a **placebo** effect (patients show improvement simply as a result of having taken part in the study because they believe they are taking something that is beneficial and alter their behaviour accordingly), even if the treatment itself is ineffective.*

   This is a weak observational study. Introduce a control group which receives a placebo.

b. Allocate the first 50 patients to the treatment group, the next 50 to the placebo group.
   If the two groups differ by age, sex, or disease severity, this could account for apparent differences in improvement between the groups.

   This is a weak experimental study. Introduce matching.

c. *Match patients in pairs for age, sex, disease severity; assign the first patient in each pair to receive treatment, the second patient to receive a placebo. The person assigning patients may have a subconscious preference for putting one patient first in each pair. Does the patient know which treatment they are getting?*

   This is a weak placebo-controlled intervention trial. Introduce randomization and blinding.

d. Allocate patients to treatment or placebo randomly within pairs. Make sure that the researcher does not know which patient is to receive which treatment (the researcher is then said to be 'blind' to the allocation of treatment). Make sure that the patient does not know which treatment they are receiving (keep the patient 'blind' as well). This makes the study 'double blind'.

e. Conduct a placebo-controlled randomized double-blind intervention trial.

'Randomization properly carried out is the key to success.' (Sir Ronald Fisher)

Intervention studies of this type are often regarded as the most robust for testing a hypothesis. But sometimes randomized controlled trials are not ethical, especially if the exposure may be harmful (e.g. smoking, or increasing someone's saturated fatty acid intake), or it is not possible to blind either the subjects or the researchers because the treatment being given is so obviously different from the placebo. In these cases, it is possible to mimic intervention studies in samples that are measured at baseline and then followed up over months or years. These types of studies raise issues about how to deal with factors that cannot be controlled for but which might affect the outcome (e.g. in a study looking at the impact of diet on risk of cardiovascular disease, the influence of smoking and diabetes) and changes in the general environment (e.g. indoor smoking bans) that have the potential to affect all the subjects in the study. Complex statistical analysis can be used to cope with some of these design issues. The ability to test the hypothesis in a robust way remains.

1.4.5 Statistics

The Dodecahedron: 'Just because you have a choice, it doesn't mean that any of them has to be right'.

Statistical tests enable you to analyze data in order to decide whether or not it is sensible to accept your hypothesis. There are literally thousands of values that can be calculated from hundreds of tests, but unless you know which test to choose, the values that you calculate may not be appropriate or meaningful. One of the main aims of this book is to help you learn to choose the test which is right for the given research problem. Once you have decided which test is appropriate for your data, the calculation is a straightforward manipulation of numbers. It is vitally important, however, to learn which data to use, how the manipulation is carried out, and how it relates to the theoretical basis which will enable you to make the decision about the truth of your hypothesis.

Most of the time it is better to use a computer to do the computation for you. Even if you enter the values correctly and generate a meaningful outcome, the computer will not tell you if your hypothesis is true. For that, you need to know how to interpret the results of the tests.

1.4.6 Interpretation

The Dodecahedron: 'If you want sense, you'll have to make it yourself'.

Every statistical test will produce a number (the *test statistic)* which you then need to interpret. This is the last stage and often the most difficult part of statistical analysis. The final emphasis in every chapter that deals with statistical tests will be on how to interpret the test statistic. We will also look at the SPSS output to verify that the right set of values has been entered for statistical analysis.

Two concepts deserve mention here: 'Inference' and 'Acceptance'. 'Inference' implies greater or lesser strength of fact. It is usually expressed as a probability of a given result being observed. If there is a high probability that the result which you have observed is associated with the hypothesis being true, we talk about 'strong' evidence. If the observed outcome is little different from what we would expect to see if the null hypothesis were true, we talk about 'weak' or 'no' evidence.

At some point, we need to make a decision about whether to accept or reject the null hypothesis, that is, to make a statement about whether or not we *believe* that the hypothesis is true. 'Acceptance' implies a cut-off point upon which action will be taken. We will discuss cut-off points in Chapter 5. It is important not to confuse political expediency (acceptance) with scientific validity (inference).

1.5 NEXT STEPS

Every year, at least one student shows up at my door, holds out an open notebook with a page full of numbers, and says, 'I've collected all this data[9] and now I don't know what to do with it'. I strongly resist the temptation to tell them to go away, or to ask why they didn't come to see me months ago. I usher them in and see what we can salvage. Usually, it is a debacle. The data collected are not suitable for testing the hypothesis; their sample is poorly defined; they don't have enough of the right types of observations; they have used different methods for collecting data at baseline and follow-up; the list goes on and on.

Box 1.3 summarizes the steps that *should* be undertaken when conducting research. Although Steps 1 and 2 are essential ('Getting the question right'), probably the most important step is Step 3, the point at which you design the research project. It is vital at this stage that you consult a statistician (as well as others who have done similar research). Be prepared to accept that your hypothesis may need modifying, and that the design that you first thought of is not perfect and would benefit from improvements. It is very unlikely that you will have got it right at your first attempt. *Be prepared to listen and to learn from your mistakes.* As I said in the Introduction to this book, statisticians may be perceived as monstrous, inhuman creatures intent only on humiliating those who come to consult them. In reality, the statistician is there to advise you concerning the likelihood of being able to prove your hypothesis, guide you in the design of the study, the choice of measurements which you intend to make, and the

type of analyses you plan to undertake. Months or years of effort can be wasted if you embark on a study which is flawed in its design. Do not take the chance! Be brave! Be thick-skinned! Talk with statisticians and accept their advice. Even get a second opinion if you feel very uncertain about the advice you are given.

1.6 RESEARCH DESIGN

There is a wide variety of research designs which can be used to address the many research questions that you are likely to ask. There is no strictly right or wrong answer concerning which design to use. You should recognize, however, that some designs are stronger when it comes to arguing the truth of your hypothesis. The aim in carrying out any research will always be to obtain the maximum information from a given design in relation to a particular research question, given the time and financial resources that are available.

1.6.1 Project Aims

Coming up with an interesting and useful research question will always involve reading the relevant literature (both books and journals) to explore how other people have tackled similar problems, and discussing with colleagues how best to investigate the problem at hand. Once you have done that, you can think about what it is you want to achieve in your research.

Projects have different aims. An undergraduate student project with 15 subjects carried out part-time over two months may not have much chance of establishing new findings that are statistically significant, but it will introduce the student to hypothesis formulation, designing a study, writing a research protocol, sampling, subject recruitment, data entry, computer analysis, and writing up the results. On the other hand, an MSc project carried out full-time over four months will require the same skills as the undergraduate project, but will usually involve a more detailed

---

[9]The word 'data' is plural, by the way – she should have said 'I have collected all *these* data' – but we will come to that later.

BOX 1.3

Steps in undertaking research

- **Step 1**. Make observations about the world. Science doesn't happen in a vacuum.
- **Step 2**. Construct a Hypothesis. State clearly the aims and objectives of your study.

Formulate the Null Hypothesis.

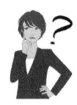

- **Step 3**. Design the experiment.

This is the stage at which you should seek the advice of a statistician

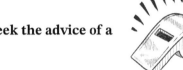

regarding the hypothesis, sample selection, sample bias, choice of measurements, and the type of analyses and statistical tests to be used. Failure to consult properly at this stage may mean that any work that you do may be a waste of time. Do not take that chance!
- **Step 4**. Conduct the research.
- **Step 5**. Analyze the data both observationally (do the numbers make sense?) and statistically.
- **Step 6**. Interpret the results (draw inferences) and write your report (for marking or for publication). Work that is not marked or published may just as well never have been completed.
- **Step 7**.Bask in the glory of a job well done.

Images © Fotosearch.com

---

consideration of design, sample size, and study power (see Chapter 12). It will also provide an opportunity to write a detailed report and to make a presentation of the findings (both for assessment), usually to an audience of postgraduate peers and their tutors. More demanding undergraduate projects may include some or all of these additional elements. For a PhD, or for funded research, all of these elements will be present, plus the requirement to write paper(s) for submission to a peer-reviewed journal and to present findings to a public audience at scientific meetings. As a professor of mine once said, 'If you haven't published the paper, you haven't done the work'.

1.6.2 Demonstrating Causality

The underlying purpose of most research is to find evidence in support of causality of the type: 'If A, then B'. Of course, we may just be interested in describing what is going on in physiological systems (what dietary factors are associated with low serum total cholesterol levels?) or in the population (are women aged 75 years and older at greater risk of osteoporosis-related fracture of the hip if they have low levels of physical activity?) More often, we want to know if there is a causal relationship between these factors (does an increased level of physical activity protect against osteoporosis-related hip fracture in women aged 75 and

BOX 1.4

Bradford Hill hierarchy of causality

- Strength of association — Is the evidence linking exposure and outcome strong? We shall see what we mean by 'strong' as we explore the different statistical tests used to evaluate associations.
- Consistency of association across studies — Are the same associations seen repeatedly in different groups or across different populations in different places and times?
- Specificity — Is there a specific link between exposure and outcome?
- Temporal association — Does A precede B? Evidence needs to show that cause (A) is followed by consequence (B). As we shall see, A and B may be associated in a cross-sectional analysis of data, but unless a clear time-sequence can be established, the evidence for causality is weak.
- Dose-response — Does increased exposure result in increased likelihood of the outcome? If fruit and vegetable consumption is protective against heart disease, can it be shown that the more fruit and vegetables are eaten, the lower the risk of disease?
- Plausible mechanism and coherence — Is there a clear physiological explanation for the observed link between A and B? What is it in fruit and vegetables that affect the factors that determine risk of heart disease? Does the new evidence fit in with what is already known? If not, why not? Are there any animal models that support evidence in humans?
- Experimental evidence — Does experimental evidence based on intervention studies support the argument for causation? Is the experimental evidence consistent across studies?
- Analogy — Are there related exposures or conditions that offer insight into the observed association?

older?). Public health recommendations to improve nutrition and nutrition-related outcomes need strong evidence of causality before they can be promoted to the general public. Confusion in the mind of the public is often caused by the media promoting a 'miracle cure' based on a single study (it makes good press but bad science). Food manufactures are often guilty of using weak evidence of causality or vague terms about 'healthiness' to promote sales of their products.[10]

We have seen earlier that the logic used to support notions of causality may be inductive or deductive. Whichever logical model is used, no single study in nutrition will provide conclusive evidence of the relationship between A and B. There is a hierarchy of evidence, first set out clearly

by Bradford Hill [4, 5], which suggests that a clear picture of causality can only be built from multiple pieces of evidence (Box 1.4). Published over 50 years ago, these criteria have withstood the test of time [6].

1.6.3 Types of Study Design

The summary below provides a brief overview of some of the types of study designs available. There are many more designs, of course, that address complex issues of multiple factors influencing multiple outcomes, with corresponding statistical analysis, but these are dealt with in more advanced textbooks on research design and analysis. The list below repeats some of the material covered in Section 1.2 on logic, but goes into more detail in relation to study design.

The principle aim is to conduct studies that are free from bias and based on relevant measures of exposure and outcome so that the hypothesis can be tested effectively.

[10]The UK rules governing labelling and packaging can be found here: https://www.gov.uk/food-labelling-and-packaging/nutrition-health-claims-and-supplement-labelling. Two things are immediately apparent: there are lots of exceptions; and the EU has a lot to say.

Observational Studies

Observational studies usually focus on the characteristics or distribution of phenomena in the population that you are investigating. Such studies may analyze data at one point in time or explore time trends in the relevant variables. They may be based on observations of individuals within a sample, or they may consider the relationship between variables observed in *groups* of subjects (for example, differences in diet and disease rate between countries). They are often the basis for *hypothesis generating*, rather than *hypothesis testing*.

Case studies are reports of potentially generalizable or particularly interesting phenomena. Individually, a case study cannot provide evidence that will help you to establish the truth of your hypothesis. Consistent findings across several case studies may provide support for an idea, but cannot be used in themselves to test a hypothesis.

Descriptive studies are careful analyses of the distribution of phenomena within or between groups, or a study of relationships existing between two or more variables within a sample. Descriptive studies are often well suited to qualitative examination of a problem (e.g. examining the coping strategies used by families on low income to ensure an adequate diet for their children when other demands [like the gas bill] are competing for limited cash). But of course they also provide descriptions of quantitative observations for single variables (e.g. how much money is spent on food, fuel, etc. in families on low income), or multiple variables (e.g. how money is spent on food in relation to total income or family size). Many epidemiological studies fall into this category (see below). They are useful for understanding the possible links between phenomena, but cannot in themselves demonstrate cause and effect.

Diagnostic studies establishing the extent of variation in disease states. They are helpful when selecting subjects for a study and deciding on which endpoints may be relevant when designing a study to explore cause and effect.

Experimental and Intervention Studies

These studies are designed to create differences in exposure to a factor which is believed to influence a particular outcome, for example, the effect of consuming oat bran on serum cholesterol levels, or the effect on birth weight of introducing an energy supplement during pregnancy. The aim is usually to analyze the differences in outcome associated with the variations in exposure which have been introduced, holding constant other factors which could also affect the outcome.

These types of studies are usually prospective or longitudinal in design. Alternatively, they may make use of existing data. Depending on how subjects are selected, they may use inductive or deductive logic to draw their conclusions (see Section 1.2)

Pre-test–post-test (Figure 1.1). This is the simplest (and weakest) of the prospective experimental designs. There is one sample. It may be 'adventitious' – subjects are selected as they become available (for example, a series of patients coming into a diabetic clinic, or a series of customers using a particular food shop); or it may be 'purposive' (the sample is drawn systematically from a population using techniques that support generalization of the findings). Each individual is measured at the start of the study (the 'baseline' or 'time zero'). There is then an intervention. Each subject is measured again at the end of the study.

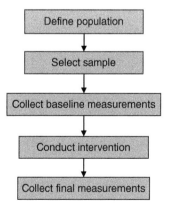

FIGURE 1.1   Pre-test–post-test design.

The weakness of this design is that there may have been a number of factors influencing the outcome of the study, but you may be aware of only some of them. An example is a study on the influence on growth of food supplements given to children. Was there bias in the way the children were recruited into the study? Did the supplement contain enough of the relevant energy or nutrients to have an impact on growth? Were the children at the right age for the supplement to have an impact? Was follow-up long enough to observe the impact of the supplement on growth? Participation in the study may in itself benefit growth (more social interaction, more stimulation from adults and peers, more food sharing, changing dietary patterns at home as a result of parental involvement in the study, etc.). It is possible that the direct effect of the supplement may represent only one of several factors that can have in impact on growth.

One sample (Figure 1.2). Here, two or more treatments are compared in one group of subjects. Each subject acts as their own control. There may be a placebo being compared with an active treatment.

The danger here is that the order of administration may have an effect on the outcome. It is therefore desirable to randomize the order of administration of the treatment and placebo (making the design more like a cross-over clinical trial – see below). Thus, for one subject, Intervention 1 will be the active treatment, and Intervention 2 the placebo; for another subject, Intervention 1 will be the placebo, and Intervention 2 the active treatment. A 'wash out' period may be required, so that any residual effect of the first treatment has time to disappear and not appear as an influence on the second treatment. This may not be possible where a psychological or attitudinal variable is being measured, because the views of a subject may be permanently influenced once they have started to participate in the study.

Two or more samples, unmatched (Figure 1.3). Similar experimental groups are given different treatments. One group acts as a control (or placebo) group.

This is a stronger experimental design than the pre-test–post-test or one-sample designs. However, the groups may differ in some characteristic which is important to the outcome (for example they may differ in age). Even if the groups are not 'matched' exactly, some attempt should be made to ensure that the groups are similar regarding variables which may be related to the outcome. For example, in a study to see if the administration of oral zinc supplements improves taste sensitivity in cancer patients, the type, degree, and severity of disease would need to be similar in both the treatment and placebo groups.

Two or more samples, matched (Figure 1.4). The participants in the study groups are matched in pairs on a subject-by-subject basis for variables such as age and gender (so-called 'confounding' variables). One group is then the control (or placebo) group, and the other group is given the active treatment(s).

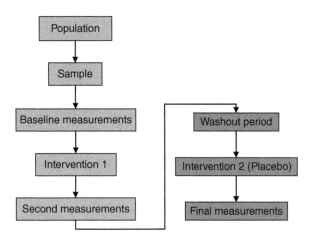

FIGURE 1.2   One-sample design.

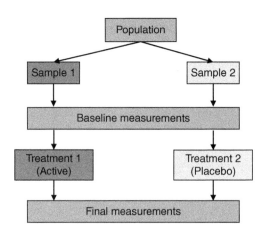

FIGURE 1.3   Two-sample (parallel) design.

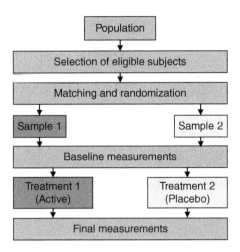

FIGURE 1.4 Two-sample (matched) design.

For example, if the aim was to test the effect of a nutrition education programme to persuade urban mothers to breast feed their infants (versus no education programme), it would be important to match on age of mother and parity (number of births). Matching could be carried out by first grouping mothers according to the number of children. Then, within each parity group, mothers could be ranked according to age. Starting with the two youngest mothers in the group with one child, one mother would be *randomly* assigned to the treatment group (the education programme), and the other would be assigned to the control group (no education programme).[11] The next two mothers would be assigned randomly to treatment or control, and so on, by parity group and age, until all the subjects have been assigned. In this way, the possible effects of age and parity would be controlled for. If there were three groups (Treatment A, Treatment B, and a control group), mothers would be matched in *triplets* according to parity and age and randomly assigned to Treatment A, Treatment B, or the control

group. Using this technique, all the groups should have very similar age and parity structures, and it could be argued that age and parity therefore have a similar influence in each group. Of course, other factors such as maternal education, income, or social class might also influence outcome. The difficulty with including too many factors as matching variables is that it becomes increasingly difficult to find adequate matches for everyone in the study. Use the two or three factors that you think will be the most powerful influence on the outcome as the matching variables. Then measure all the other factors that you think might be associated with the outcome so that they can be taken into account in the final analyses (see Chapters 10 and 11).

Clinical trials. These involve the assessment of the effects of clinical interventions such as drugs or feeding programmes. They are usually carried out in a controlled setting (that is, where the subject will be unable to obtain other supplies of the drug or where all aspects of diet are controlled). The intervention is compared with a placebo.

The design and analysis of clinical trials is a science in itself [7], and there are a great many variations in design which can be adopted. The so-called Rolls Royce of clinical trials, the randomized double-blind placebo-controlled cross over clinical trial (Figure 1.5), requires careful thought in its planning, implementation, and analysis.

Randomized controlled trials should not be embarked upon lightly! It is very demanding of time, staff, and money. Moreover, there are important limitations.

In recent years, it has been recognized that while clinical trials may be appropriate for providing proof of causality in some circumstances (e.g. understanding the impact of a new drug on disease outcomes, or a specific nutritional intervention), there may not always be equivalent, controlled circumstances that exist in the real world (e.g. promotion of five-a-day consumption in a sample versus a control group). The generalizability of findings may therefore be limited when it comes to saying whether or not a particular intervention is likely to be of benefit to individuals or

---

[11]Randomization is usually carried out by computer. You could do it equally well by simply tossing a coin, but if the coin is not tossed in exactly the same way for every pair, the randomization may be biased by the way in which the coin was tossed from one matched pair to the next. This introduces additional 'noise' in the system and is easily avoided by using the computer to generate the random numbers needed.

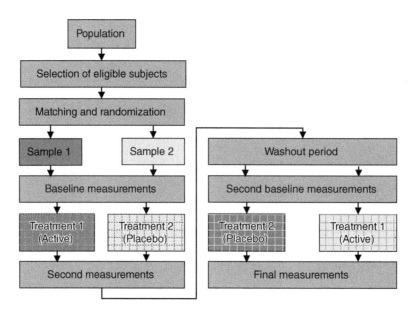

FIGURE 1.5   Randomized placebo controlled cross-over trial.

the population as a whole. To address these circumstances, alternate designs and analytical approaches have been developed in the last decade or more that aim to take complex, real-world circumstances into account [8]. The existing guidance is due to be updated in 2019.

1.6.4 Epidemiological Studies

Epidemiological studies examine relationships between exposures and health-related outcomes in populations. In the context of nutritional epidemiology, exposures might include individual diet, community health intervention programmes, supplementation, food advertising, dietary advice, or other nutrition-related variables. Outcomes can include changes in nutrition-related blood biochemistry (e.g. cholesterol levels, haemoglobin), clinical outcomes (e.g. xerophthalmia, obesity), or morbidity or mortality statistics relating to nutrition.

Epidemiological studies fall into three categories.

Descriptive Studies

Descriptive studies in epidemiology include ecological studies, cross-sectional studies, and time trend analysis. They are useful for generating hypotheses. Measurements can be made in individuals at a given point in time (cross-sectional studies) or accumulated over time in groups of people (ecological studies). They are used to relate measures of exposure and outcome in groups of people that share common characteristics (e.g. vegetarians versus omnivores) or to compare regions or countries. For example, they might compare diet and disease patterns between countries (are heart disease rates lower in countries where people eat lots of oily fish?) or between subgroups (do vegetarians have lower risk of heart disease compared to non-vegetarians?).

There are two main problems with this type of study. First, there may be other factors that could explain an observed association or changes in the population over time. For example, populations with higher oily fish consumption may be more active or less obese. Second, not everyone in the population or subgroup is exposed at the same level: some individuals in the population may eat lots of oily fish, while others may eat very little. Are the people with low oily fish consumption the ones that have higher rates of heart disease?

Analytical Studies

These include cohort and case-control studies. Their primary characteristic is that they relate exposures in individuals (factors that are likely to influence the occurrence of disease or mortality within the population) to outcomes (disease or mortality rates). Analytical studies are usually based on observations relating to large numbers of people in the population (hundreds or thousands). They provide much stronger evidence of diet–disease relationships than descriptive studies. In terms of the Bradford Hill model of causality (Box 1.4), they provide evidence of temporal association and dose-response. If blood or urine samples are collected, they may also provide evidence of a plausible physiological mechanism for causation. Detailed descriptions of these designs and their statistical analysis are given in epidemiological texts such as Rothman [9] or Margetts and Nelson [10].

Cohort studies are prospective in nature; they look *forward* in time, following a group of people who are free from the disease of interest at baseline. Relevant exposures are measured at baseline or time zero. Over time (usually years), the appearance of disease (morbidity), or relevant changes in blood or urine biochemistry, or nutrition-related mortality, is monitored (Figure 1.6).

The risk of developing disease (or related outcomes) in the exposed group is compared with the risk of developing disease in the unexposed group. This is known as the Relative Risk.

In nutritional epidemiology, the meanings of 'Exposed' and 'Unexposed' are different from the meanings in infectious disease or occupational epidemiology. In infectious disease epidemiology, for example, a subject either is or is not exposed to a particular bacterium that can cause illness. In occupational epidemiology, a subject may be classified either as exposed or not exposed to a potential risk factor (e.g. asbestos dust). In nutritional epidemiology, in contrast, variables are usually continuous – no one has a diet that does not contain energy or iron, for example. Subjects are therefore classified into bands of exposure. 'Exposed' might mean someone in the top half of the distribution of intake, and 'Unexposed' might mean someone in the bottom half. Of course, degrees of exposure may also be ascertained in other spheres of epidemiology, but in nutritional epidemiology it is the norm and forms the basis for most analysis of risk.

In cohort studies, the time sequence of cause and effect is not in question. There may be other factors, however, which over time, explain the apparent associations between the measures at baseline and the outcome measures collected years later (e.g. some individuals may gain more weight than others, or their socio-economic status at follow-up may not be the same as it was at baseline). The strength of cohort studies is that if these factors are measured at baseline and again at follow-up, they can be taken into account in the analysis. The main disadvantage of cohort studies is the length of time it takes to accumulate relevant outcome measures in

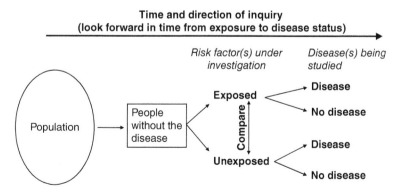

FIGURE 1.6 Cohort study design.

sufficient numbers of individuals, and the cost of collecting the measurements in hundreds or thousands of individuals over long periods of time.

Case-control studies, in contrast, start by identifying a group of subjects with a given disease or condition. Controls are subjects who do not have the disease or outcome being investigated. They are matched individually with the cases for age and sex, and often for other variables such as smoking or BMI or income or occupation. The study then looks *backward* in time to measure exposures that are potentially causal (Figure 1.7).

Measures of exposure in the past are usually determined by asking cases and controls about their habits in the past using a questionnaire (although sometimes there are records of exposure, for example the type of work someone did, or hospital records of birth weight). The past exposures of the cases are then compared with the past exposures of the controls. The relevant statistical outcome is the Odds Ratio: what are the chances of being exposed and in the disease group compared with being exposed and in the non-disease group. This is the best estimate of the Relative Risk, which cannot be measured directly in case-control studies [9, 10].

Case-control studies are much cheaper to carry out than cohort studies, but accurate measurements of past exposure are often difficult to collect. For example, asking someone what their diet was like 10 or 15 years ago is likely to be heavily influenced by the type of diet they consume now.

Experimental Studies

In epidemiology, experimental studies take two forms: clinical trials and community trials. The aim is to compare the impact of the active treatment on the relevant outcomes with the impact of a placebo.

Clinical trials in epidemiology usually take the form of randomized controlled trials. The aim is to see if an intervention to alter exposure results, over time, in a change in outcomes. In epidemiology, clinical trials can involve thousands of subjects followed over many years, whereas studies relating to drug treatments or food interventions relating to changes in blood or urine biochemistry may involve only tens of subjects. The purpose in having such large studies in epidemiology is to be able to generalize to the population with confidence, and to take into account the many confounders (see below) that may operate in the real world.

Researchers usually strive to achieve 'double blind' status in their study designs, but in nutritional interventions this may not always be possible. If the intervention involves changing diet, for example, or providing nutritional advice to increase fruit and vegetable consumption, the subject may be aware of the changes and is therefore no longer 'blind'. Similarly, the researcher involved in administering the changes may be aware of which subjects are in the treatment group and which are in the placebo group. If this is the case, it is important to ensure that the person undertaking the statistical analysis is blinded

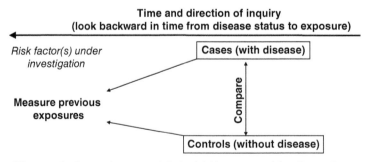

FIGURE 1.7   Case-control study design.

to the identity of the groups being compared. This can be done through the coding of results for computer analysis so that the comparison is simply between group A and group B. Only at the end of the analysis is the identity of the group revealed. Even here, it may not always be possible to blind the analyst. In that case, the procedures for carrying out the statistical analyses should be described in advance so as to avoid a 'fishing expedition', hunting for statistically significant findings.

Community trials are intervention studies carried out in whole communities to see if some change in exposure is associated with a subsequent change in disease or mortality rates. Again, the study will involve a treatment community and a placebo community. The communities are matched (e.g. age and sex structure of the population, percentage of the population not in work). There may be more than one community in each group.

Community trials are pragmatic in nature. The aim is to see if community-based interventions have sufficient penetration and impact to bring about changes in nutrition-related outcomes (e.g. the percentage of adults over the age of 45 who are overweight or obese). The identity of the individuals in the community who make the desired changes and their individual outcomes may not be known. A questionnaire can be used to find out the proportion of the population who were aware of the intervention (for example, advice on healthy eating provided in a GP surgery by the community dietitian), and height and weight data could be taken from the routine 'healthy man' or 'healthy woman' screening programmes being run in the same groups of GP surgeries.

Community trials are much cheaper to run than clinical trials. They do not, however, provide the same wealth of detail about individual behaviours and outcomes and, as a consequence, provide less insight into causal mechanisms.

Confounding and Bias

A key feature of epidemiological studies is the attention paid to *confounding factors* and *bias*.

Confounding factors are associated with both the exposure and the outcome. Suppose that we were comparing a group of cases who had recently had their first heart attack with a group of controls who had never had a heart attack. Say that we were interested in knowing if higher oily fish consumption was associated with lower rates of heart attack. We could measure oily fish consumption using a food frequency questionnaire that asked about usual diet. Suppose we found that it was lower among the cases. Is this good evidence that higher oily fish consumption is protective against having a heart attack? What if the cases, on average, were 10 years older than the controls, and that younger people tended to have higher levels of oily fish in their diet? This could explain the apparent association of higher oily fish consumption with decreased risk of heart attack. In this case, age would be referred to as a confounding factor. Confounding factors need to be associated with both the exposure and the outcome that we are interested in. We could match our cases with controls of the same age. Alternatively, we could use a statistical approach that took age into account in the analysis. The most common confounding factors – things like age, gender, social class, and education – need to be controlled for when comparing one group with another. Other factors such as smoking, disease status (e.g. diabetes), or body mass index (BMI) may also be taken into account, but these may be explanatory factors or factors in the causal pathway rather than true confounders.

Bias is a problem associated with measuring instruments or interviewers. *Systematic bias* occurs when everyone is measured with an instrument that always gives an answer that is too high or too low (like an inaccurate weighing machine). Bias can be *constant* (every measurement is inaccurate by the same amount) and or *proportional* (the size of the error is proportional to the size of the measurement, e.g. the more you weigh the greater the inaccuracy in the measurement). Bias is a factor that can affect any study and should be carefully controlled.

Some types of bias may simply reduce our ability to detect associations between exposure and outcome. This is 'noise in the system'. It means that there may be an association between exposure and outcome, but our data are too 'noisy' for us to be able to detect it. For example, we know that there is day-to-day and week-to-week variation in food and drink consumption. We need to try and collect sufficient information to be able to classify subjects according to their 'usual' consumption.

Other types of bias mean that the information that we obtain is influenced by the respondent's ability to give us accurate information. Subjects who are overweight or obese, for example, or who have higher levels of dietary restraint, tend to under-report their overall food consumption, especially things like confectionery or foods perceived as 'fatty'. Subjects who are more health-conscious may over-report their fruit and vegetable consumption because they regard these foods as 'healthy' and want to make a good impression on the interviewer. In these instances, making comparisons between groups becomes problematic because the amount of bias is related to the type of individual which may in turn be related to their disease risk.

Dealing with issues such as confounding, residual confounding, factors in the causal pathway, and different types of bias are fully addressed in epidemiological textbooks [9, 10].

1.7 DATA, RESULTS, AND PRESENTATION

First of all, a few definitions are needed:

- Statistic – a numerical observation
- Statistics – numerical facts systematically collected (also the science of the analysis of data)
- Data – what you collect (the word 'data' is plural – the singular is 'datum' – so we say 'the data are...' not 'the data is...')
- Results – a summary of your data

1.7.1 Data Are What You Collect, Results Are What You Report

No one else is as interested in your data as you are. You must love your data, look after them carefully (think of the cuddly statistician), and cherish each

observation. You must make sure that every observation collected is accurate, and that when the data are entered into a spreadsheet, they do not contain any errors. When you have entered all your data, you need to 'clean' your data, making sure that there are no rogue values, and that the mean and the distribution of values is roughly what you were expecting. Trapping the errors at this stage is essential. There is nothing worse than spending days or weeks undertaking detailed statistical analysis and preparing tables and figures for a report, only to discover that there are errors in your data set, meaning that you have to go back and do everything all over again.

TIP

Allow adequate time in your project to clean the data properly. This means

- Check for values that are outside the range of permitted values.
- Look at the distributions of variables and check for extreme values. Some extreme values may be genuine. Others may be a result of 'fat finger' syndrome (like typing an extra zero and ending up with 100 rather than 10 as a data point).
- Understand how to use 'missing values' in SPSS. These help you to identify gaps in the data and how to handle them (for example, the difference between 'I don't know', Not Applicable, or missing measurement).

If you find an unusual observation, check it with your supervisor or research colleagues. They may want to inspect your data to see that your observations are correct. Don't try and hide an unusual observation (or worse still, ignore it, or leave it out of the data set without telling anyone). Always be frank and open about letting others inspect your data, *especially* if you or they think there may be something wrong. We all make mistakes. It is no great shame if there are some errors in the data that we missed and that someone else helpfully spots for us. Be thick-skinned about this. The real embarrassment comes if we do lots of analysis and the errors in the data only come to light when we make a presentation of our results.

1.7.2 Never Present Endless Detailed Tables Containing Raw Data

It is your job as a scientist to summarize data in a coherent form (in tables, graphs, and figures), tell an interesting story about the relationships between the variables you have measured, and interpret the results intelligently for your reader, using appropriate statistical analyses.

Of course, you need to keep accurate records of observations, and make sure that your data set (spreadsheet) is stored securely and that you have backup copies of everything. Bulking up a report with tables of raw data is bad practice, however. No one will read them.

Chapter 15 provides lots of examples about how to summarize data to make the presentation of results interesting. It also shows how to present results according to the type of audience you are talking to. If I am presenting new results about the impact of school food on attainment to scientific colleagues, I will include lots of information about the methods that I used to identify my samples, make observations, and analyze the data, as well as details about the findings themselves. My scientific colleagues will need enough information to be confident that my data are unbiased, that I have used the right analytical approaches, and that the results are statistically significant. This is the same basic approach that I will take when I am writing a paper for submission to a peer-reviewed journal. In contrast, if I am presenting results on the same topic to a group of teachers, I will use lots of graphs and charts to summarize the results in a way that tells a good story. The underlying data will be the same, of course. But the teachers are likely to be bored by too much detail about methods – they probably just want to know the headline about whether better school food has a positive impact on attainment, and how big that impact is likely to be.

1.7.3 Significant Digits and Rounding

It always surprises me, when teaching undergraduate and postgraduate students, that they often don't know how to round numbers properly. So when asked to present a result to two decimal places, for example, either they provide a string of numbers after the decimal place (far more than two) in the mistaken hope that somehow that is 'better' or 'more accurate', statistically speaking. Alternatively, it becomes evident that the concept of 'rounding' is not familiar to them, and their answers vary like leaves blowing in the wind.

The underlying principle is that when undertaking calculations, it is useful to retain as many digits as possible during the course of the calculation. This is what happens when you use your calculator, Excel, or SPSS [11]. This will produce the most mathematically precise result. However, when the final value is presented, it should contain no more significant digits than the numbers from which it is derived.

For example, calculate the average height of a group of five students, each of whom had been measured to the nearest centimetre (Table 1.1).

The average (the arithmetic mean) of these five values is 164.4 cm. However, presenting the result to the nearest millimetre (tenth of a centimetre) would be misleading, as it would imply that your starting observations had a similar level of precision. You should, instead, round the value for the result to the number of significant digits with which you started. In this case, round 164.4 cm (four significant digits) to 164 cm (three significant digits, to the nearest whole centimetre). This is the value that you should report for your result, as it reflects the level of precision of your original observations.[12]

TABLE 1.1 Height of Five Students (cm)

163
152
176
166
165

---

[12] On the other hand, keep all the significant digits when doing your calculations. We will see how this works in later chapters.

TABLE 1.2   Rules for Rounding

Rule	Original Value	Rounded Value
If the final digit is less than 5, round to the value of the preceding digit	164.4	164
If the final digit is greater than 5, round to the value which is one higher than the preceding digit	164.6	165
If the final digit is equal to 5, and the preceding digit is odd, round up to the next **even** number	163.5	164
If the final digit is equal to 5, and the preceding digit is even, round down to the preceding number	164.5	164

The standard conventions for rounding are as shown in Table 1.2.

These conventions may differ from those which you have been taught, but they are the conventions followed by all calculators and all computers when undertaking computations.

Some people have been taught always to round up if the last digit is equal to 5, but the calculations in Table 1.3 illustrate the error which is introduced if that rule is followed.

Although this error seems small, it can be substantial if we are dealing with small numbers. For example, if the original values had been 3.5, 4.5, 5.5, and 6.5, and we were rounding to whole numbers, the average would be equal to 5 for the original values and correctly rounded values (4, 4, 6, 6), but the average for the incorrectly rounded values would be 5.5 – an error of 10%!

Curiously, Excel and some statistical packages (e.g. Minitab) display numbers which are *always rounded up* when the last digit is 5. However, underlying calculations are based on the correct rules for rounding shown in Table 1.2. To ensure that your calculations are correct, always follow these rules.

Finally, be careful when reporting values from Excel or Minitab – even though the calculations will be right, the final displayed value may not accord with the rules above.

TIP

Use common sense to report final values according to the correct rules of rounding – don't just report what the computer tells you. This principle – using your common sense to interpret computer output – will come up again and again throughout this book.

TABLE 1.3   Impact of Rounding Styles on Mean Value

Original Value	Correctly Rounded to Nearest Even Digit	Incorrectly Rounded (Always Upward)
163.5	164	164
164.5	164	165
165.5	166	166
166.5	166	167
Average = 165	Average = 165	Average = 165.5 (rounded = 166)

1.8 READING

The concepts which underlie research design and statistics set out in this book may be very different from any that you have had to think about. Persistence will bring rewards, however, even if the topics seem difficult at first.

Very often, one author's treatment of a topic will seem totally incomprehensible, while another's will seem crystal clear. Below, therefore, is a list of books to which you might like to refer – try at least two on the same topic if you are having difficulty grasping a particular idea. Don't worry about the publication dates – the approaches to basic statistics have not changed for the last few decades. The volumes cited use examples from medicine rather than nutrition and dietetics, but the statistical principles remain the same.

The books marked with an '*' are particularly highly recommended. Note that a number of these

TABLE 1.4   Impact of Screening for Breast Cancer on 5-year Mortality in 62 000 Women

		Cause of Death			
		Breast Cancer		All Other Causes	
	n	n	Rate/1 000	n	Rate/1 000
Screening group					
Examined	20 200	23	1.1	428	21
Refused	10 800	16	1.5	409	38
Total	31 000	39	1.3	837	27
Control group	31 000	63	2.0	879	28

texts are now available as e-books, usually at a substantially reduced price compared with the hard copy.

ᴵ   Armitage P, Berry G, Mathews JNS. *Statistical Methods in Medical Research*, 4th edition. Blackwell Science. Oxford. 2001. Very thorough and wide ranging, with excellent explanations of the mathematics behind the statistics. Highly recommended.

*   Bland M. *An Introduction to Medical Statistics*. 4th edition. Oxford University Press. 2015. Good, basic introduction, wide ranging, with lots of useful examples including SPSS. Might be a bit difficult for beginners, as he tends to jump straight in without too much underlying explanation.

ᴵᴵ   Bowling Ann. *Research Methods in Health*. 4th edition. Open University Press. Buckingham. 2014. This text provides an excellent overview of issues in both quantitative and qualitative research. Together with Ann Bowling's other text ('Measuring Health', 4th edition, McGraw Hill Education, 2017), it provides a practical and straightforward guide to research design for the health sciences.

Campbell MJ, Machin D, Walters SJ. *Medical Statistics: A Textbook for the Health Sciences (Medical Statistics)*. 4th edition. Wiley-Blackwell. Chichester. 2007. A comprehensive text, the book has lots of 'common sense' tips and useful comments sprinkled liberally throughout.

*   Campbell MJ. *Statistics at Square One*. 11th edition. BMJ Books. 2009. Useful little 'cookbook', good for quick reference to remind you of the underlying statistical formulae, but not very good about explaining the principles underlying the tests or why they work as they do.

Campbell MJ. *Statistics at Square Two*. 2nd edition. BMJ Books. 2006. This is a useful follow-on to Statistics at Square One. It explores more complex statistical analyses involving multiple variables and complex study designs.

Freedman D, Pisani R, Purves R. *Statistics*. 4th edition. Norton. London. 2014. Basic and very readable text. May at times seem long-winded, but lots of detailed examples and useful exercises (with answers).

Glantz SA. *Primer of Biostatistics*. 7th edition. McGraw-Hill. London. 2012. First rate text, very clear descriptions of tests with medical examples and problems for solving.

Corder GW, Foreman DI. *Nonparametric Statistics: A Step by Step Approach*. 2nd edition. Wiley. 2014. Very good at explaining the fundamentals of nonparametric statistics.

*   Juster, Norton. *The Phantom Tollbooth*. Harper Collins. New York. 2008. Illustrations by Jules Feiffer. A wonderful allegory of scientific thinking concerning two kidnapped Princesses: Rhyme and Reason. The illustrations by Jules Feiffer perfectly complement Milo's struggle to make sense of the world. The ideal fantasy for when you're fed up with statistics.

Mead R, Curnow RN and Hasted A (editor). *Statistical Methods in Agriculture and Experimental Biology*. 3rd edition. Chapman and Hall CRC Press. London. 2002. The authors worked in the Applied Statistics Department of the Food Research Institute at Reading, so the examples are geared towards food science.

Moser CA and Kalton G. *Survey Methods in Social Investigation*. 2nd edition. Heinemann Educational. London. 1985. Detailed and practical advice on survey techniques and design. Nonmathematical. A classic.

* Norman GR and Streiner DL. *Biostatistics: the Bare Essentials*. 4th edition. People's Medical Publishing House. USA. 2014. Clear, funny, and irreverent. Goes into the lower reaches of the upper echelons of statistics (i.e. covers the basics plus some of the more advanced stuff).

* Riegelman R. *Studying a Study and Testing a Test: How to Read the Medical Evidence*. 5th edition. Lippincott Williams and Wilkins. 2004. Good for interpreting the medical literature.

1.9 EXERCISES

Answers to these exercises can be found in Part 4, at the end of the chapters.

1.9.1   Rounding and significant digits

a. Round the following numbers to two decimal places. Use the rules plus common sense.

12.2345
144.5673
73.665
13.6652
99.4545

b. Round the same numbers to three significant digits.

1.9.2   Interpreting data: does screening save lives?

62 000 women in a health insurance scheme were randomly allocated to either a screening programme for breast cancer, or no screening. After 5 years, the following results were observed (Table 1.4):
a. Does screening save lives? Which numbers tell you so?
b. Among the women in the screening group, the death rate from all other causes in the 'Refused' group was almost twice that in the 'Examined' group. Did screening cut the death rate in half? Explain briefly.
c. Was the study blind?

1.9.3   Hypothesis and null hypothesis

In a study designed to assess whether undernutrition is a cause of short stature in poor inner-city children:
a. State the hypothesis (H_1)
b. State the null hypothesis (H_0)
c. Consider:
   i. confounding factors
   ii. sources of systematic bias
c. Consider ways to minimize the effects of confounding and systematic bias

REFERENCES

1. Popper Karl R. *Conjectures and Refutations. The Growth of Scientific Knowledge.* 5th edition. Routledge. London. 2002.

2. Fisher RA. *Design of Experiments*. 7th edition. Oliver and Boyd. London. 1960.

3. Juster Norton. *The Phantom Tollbooth*. Random House. New York. 2000.

4. Bradford Hill A. The environment and disease: association or causation? *Proc R Soc Med.* 1965 May; 58(5): 295–300.

5. Bradford Hill A. *A Short Textbook of Medical Statistics*. 11th edition. Hodder and Stoughton. London. 1985.

6. Fedak KM, Bernal A, Capshaw ZA, Gross S. Applying the Bradford Hill criteria in the 21st century: how data integration has changed causal inference in molecular epidemiology. *Emerg Themes Epidemiol.* 2015; 12: 14. doi: https://doi.org/10.1186/s12982-015-0037-4 https://www.ncbi.nlm.nih.gov/pmc/articles/PMC4589117/

7. Shein-Chung Chow, Jen-Pei Liu. *Design and Analysis of Clinical Trials: Concepts and Methodologies*. 3rd edition. Wiley.London. ISBN: 978-0-470-88765-3. 892. January 2014

8. Medical Research Council. *Developing and Evaluating Complex Interventions: New Guidance.* Medical Research Council. London. 2008. https://mrc.ukri.org/documents/pdf/developing-and-evaluating-complex-interventions/

9. Rothman K. *Epidemiology: An Introduction.* 2nd edition. Oxford University Press. 2012.

10. Margetts B and Nelson M. *Design Concepts in Nutritional Epidemiology.* 2nd edition. Oxford University Press. 1997.

11. IBM SPSS Statistics. Version 24. © Copyright IBM Corporation and others, 1989, 2016.

CHAPTER 2

Populations and Samples

After studying this chapter you should be able to:

- Describe a population and a sample
- Know how to draw representative samples from populations
- Name and use the basic measures of central tendency and variation which are useful when describing populations and samples
- Understand some basic arithmetic symbols and equations that will be used throughout the book

2.1 DEFINING POPULATIONS AND SAMPLES

Very few studies are carried out on entire populations, for two reasons. First, we rarely have the time or the resources[1] to measure everyone. An exception to this is the national census, where the whole purpose is to find out about every person in the population. It is worth noting that this is such a time consuming and expensive operation, that it is carried out in most countries only once every 10 years. Second, most of what we need to know about the population can be found out by studying representative samples drawn from the population. Not only does this save a huge amount of time and effort when carrying out scientific research, it also enables us to undertake far more studies with the resources available. In Chapter 12, we will look at how to calculate how large a sample needs to be in order to achieve a specific research aim.

---

[1]Most of the time when we use the word 'resources' we are talking about money to pay for things – research staff, computers, printing, telephone, equipment, etc. It may also include an infrastructure (like a University Department) where some of these things could be obtained, or the time that is available to carry out a project in terms of expertise, supervision, project funding, etc.

Statistics in Nutrition and Dietetics, First Edition. Michael Nelson.
© 2020 John Wiley & Sons Ltd. Published 2020 by John Wiley & Sons Ltd.
Companion website: www.wiley.com/go/nelson/statistics

2.1.1 Population

Population: *A large collection of individual items*

In everyday terms, a *population* is usually thought of as the people who live in a particular country or region. In statistical terms, however, a population is any large collection of individual items. These could be people, or rats, or leaves, or colonies of bacteria, or birth certificates, or electoral wards, or schools, or GP surgeries, or local authorities, or cities and towns, or practically anything else you could think of. There is no lower or upper limit to the number of elements in a population, although we generally tend to think of them as 'large'.

Some populations can be defined by selected characteristics, and so again do not fit in with the everyday notion of what we think of as a population. For example, we could talk about the population of elderly men living in warden-assisted accommodation, or all non-insulin dependent diabetics over the age of 65 living in the United Kingdom. In research terms, it is necessary to define closely the population to which your work relates. Generalizations made on the basis of the research (properly carried out) will then unambiguously relate to the defined population. This also helps to prevent *over*-generalizations, in which the results are extended to groups in the population to which they do not properly relate.[2]

In your reading, you will find texts that distinguish between finite and infinite populations. Much of the theory on which the statistical tests are based assume that populations are infinite, but clearly that does not hold true for the populations you are likely to be dealing with in research. For the purposes of this textbook, therefore, the distinction between finite and infinite populations will not make any material difference to the calculations which you will undertake.

[2]Newspapers have a terrible habit of over-generalizing the results of scientific studies. 'New cure for diabetes' might turn out to be a study carried out using cells isolated from mouse pancreas, bearing little or no relation to a cure for diabetes in humans.

Inevitably, there is ambiguity about how small a group can be and still constitute a population. Would you regard all pregnant women using health services in a given catchment area as a population? It could be, and any results based on a sample drawn from that population would be generalizable to that population. Would you regard all pregnant women attending a particular doctor's surgery as a population? Probably not: this would be more properly regarded as a subgroup of all pregnant women, or pregnant women living in that GP's catchment, but not a population. Indeed, if your intention was to draw research conclusions relating only to the women attending that particular surgery, this would be akin to a case study. When such doubts arise, you should consult with statisticians and other researchers to make sure you have defined your population correctly, and that it is sufficiently large to justify any generalizations that you want to draw.

2.1.2 Samples and Sampling Frames

Sample: *A selection of items from a population*

In its simplest terms, a *sample* is a subset of a population, selected with no restrictions as to size or representativeness. In practice, of course, the usual aim is to select a sample that *is* representative of the population from which it is drawn. By representative, we mean that the sample contains items with characteristics that are in the same proportion (or vary in the same way) as in the population as a whole. Because a sample is only a subset of the population, these characteristics are unlikely to be *exactly* in proportion to the characteristics in the population. But we shall see in later chapters that we can check to see if our sample is representative of the population or not.

If a sample *is* representative, we will be able to make statements about the population based on what we have observed in the sample, using the types of logic discussed in Chapter 1. There are several sampling techniques to improve the likelihood that samples are representative of the population, and these are described below.

Sometimes, clever sampling can be used to identify groups which are not representative of the population as a whole but which contain people with special characteristics. This can save large amounts of time and effort. Causes of breast and uterine cancer have been studied in nuns, for example, to exclude (in the main) components of risk that relate to pregnancy, childbirth, or breast-feeding. Seventh Day Adventists choose not to drink alcohol or eat meat, fish, or poultry (they are lacto-ovo-vegetarian); they provide groups for assessing disease risk in comparison with other groups in the general population who are not vegetarian and who do drink alcohol. This overcomes the problem of finding adequate numbers of nondrinkers in the general population (many of whom avoid alcohol for medical or cultural reasons), or people who avoid meat, fish, and poultry (but may have reasons for doing so which are associated with other aspects of a healthy lifestyle).

Sampling frame: *A list or form of identification of the elements of a population*

In order to select a sample from a population, we need to have a way of listing or ordering all the items in the population. A *sampling frame* is a list of all the elements of a population. From it, we can draw representative samples of the population. It should be a complete list of the elements of the population, without blanks, and accessible.

Typical sampling frames are lists of patients in doctors' surgeries; school registers; telephone directories (although the increased use of mobile phones has made telephone directories less useful than in the past); electoral registers; and postal codes. Some sampling frames are numbered from 1 to N, where N is the total number of elements of the population. It is then possible to draw up a list of random numbers between 1 and N, and to choose the sample by selecting the items with the corresponding numbers in the sampling frame.

Other sampling frames might consist simply of an unnumbered list, or a set of index cards each of which relates to one element of the population.

Choosing a sample from this type of sampling frame is best done using *systematic sampling*. The principle of systematic sampling is described in more detail below.

Every sampling frame has its flaws. Lists of patients in doctors' surgeries will include only those people in the population who are registered with a doctor. Patients who have either moved or died but not had their name removed from the list may be inadvertently included.[3] School registers will apply only to children of school age and may not include every child living in a given area, as some may be attending school elsewhere (or not attending school at all). Telephone directories include only people who have telephones. Electoral registers contain only adults who are registered to vote. Postal codes identify offices and institutions as well as private residences. Most lists of postal codes allow nonresidential codes to be excluded, but equally, some residences may not be occupied. Census data is perhaps the most obvious and complete sampling frame of the population, but it is held strictly confidential and is not, therefore, accessible for most research purposes. It also becomes progressively more and more out of date as the years pass and members of the population change their status or move house, and does not reflect changes in household composition due to births and deaths, children leaving home for college or work, etc.

An important part of any sampling procedure, therefore, is to ensure that the sampling frame includes all (or as many as possible) of the people or items that you want to include. In some instances, it may be necessary to construct your own sampling frame by conducting a mini-census. For research using animals, it is assumed that the animals of a particular species or strain are part of a well-defined population which share common physiological and genetic characteristics. (Reports of animal experiments in the scientific literature always specify both the species and the strain of animals used, and often the source of the animals

---

[3]Often referred to as 'ghosts'.

as well.) It is then assumed that any group of animals of a given sex and age will be physiologically representative of the population from which those animals were drawn.

2.1.3 Inclusion and Exclusion Criteria

One of the most important keys to success in research is the careful selection of both populations and samples. In order to generate unambiguous conclusions, it may be appropriate to exclude certain people from a population, or to select a sample on the basis of subjects who satisfy a set of inclusion criteria. The underlying concept is referred to as *eligibility*.

In the study on diet and peripheral artery disease (PAD) described in Chapter 1, age and gender were important factors to take into account in the creation of a strong study design which allowed the hypothesis to be tested when two groups were being compared. If the study were to be carried out, who would be included in the population, and who would be selected for the sample?

The population might be defined using a single *inclusion criterion*, such as 'all subjects who were referred to the Vascular Clinic in Hospital X, South London'. This would include most patients living in that locale who were referred to the hospital because they had problems with peripheral circulation. If the clinic was a regional centre for treatment, however, the population defined by attendance at the Vascular Clinic would then include patients referred from other hospitals in the southeast of England. If the purpose of the study was to investigate the influence of anti-oxidant vitamins on PAD, this is potentially a good population from which to select a sample. The assumption would be that those attending the clinic were physiologically and socially representative of the surrounding population. Generalizability would be good. Findings from the study in this clinic should be widely generalizable to patients with PAD elsewhere in the country *unless* there were something special about living in the southeast of England. What if the impact of lifestyle on disease appearance or progression (e.g. smoking,

diet, access to public transport) varied regionally? These factors would need to be measured and taken into account in order to be confident about the generalization one wanted to make.

For the purposes of the study, the population may include subjects with PAD whose age, lifestyle, or medical complications influence the disease appearance, severity, or development. We should select our sample to limit the influence of these factors so that they do not undermine our ability to test our hypothesis. Who, then, should be included in the sample and who should be excluded?

Vascular disease takes a great many different forms. Suppose we decide that only one form (PAD) is of interest. So the first *exclusion criterion* is anyone who does not have a clear diagnosis of PAD. Secondly, patients may have characteristics or complications which will interfere with our ability to test the hypothesis. For example, medical complications may be more common in older patients. So it may make sense to restrict the sample to subjects under 75 years of age in order to get a clearer picture of the influence of the vitamins on the disease process. Thirdly, PAD is more common in people with diabetes for reasons related to insulin production, metabolism, and vascular integrity. So it makes sense to exclude subjects with diabetes so the influence of these factors does not obscure the effect of the vitamins on PAD, or at least to separate in the analysis those with diabetes from those without diabetes (but this will have an impact on the total number of observations needed for the study). Finally, we may want to *include* only those patients who have been referred to the clinic for the first time, in order for our hypothesis testing not to be confounded by treatments which may have been given in the past.

Every study needs to have populations and samples which are clearly defined by their source, and by a list of inclusion and exclusion criteria. This will enable other researchers to carry out similar studies in order to test the hypothesis independently. As we said in Chapter 1, being able to recreate an experiment and test the hypothesis a second or third time is important for science to progress.

2.1.4 Sampling Techniques

Simple Random Sampling

In *simple random sampling*, every sample of a given size n has an equal chance of selection. This is slightly different from saying that each element of the population has an equal chance of selection. We will see in Chapter 4 why this distinction is important.

Every sample, however, is not necessarily representative of the population. Just by chance, a sample could be drawn that contained 75% men and 25% women, even though there were equal numbers of men and women in the population. Common sense and experience tell us that large samples are more likely to be representative of the population than small samples. Again, the reason for this will become apparent when we look at probability distributions in Chapter 4.

The principle of simple random sampling is straightforward. A list is prepared of all of the items in the population. Each item is given a unique identifier or label, say a number from 1 to N, where N (the upper case letter) is the number of items in the population. This constitutes the sampling frame. A list of n random numbers is generated, where n (the lower case letter) is the number of items which are to be included in the sample.[4] Each of the random numbers should appear only once in the list, so that no one in the population is selected twice.[5]

There are many techniques for generating random numbers. The traditional image is of a rotating drum containing N ping-pong balls. The ping-pong balls are numbered from 1 to N. The drum is rotated to mix the balls thoroughly, and a ball is removed. The process is repeated n times (where n is the number of items we want to include in our sample). The list of randomly generated numbers is made up from the numbers on the selected ping-pong balls. The balls are removed from the drum as each element of the sample is identified (so the sampling is 'without replacement'). Unfortunately, this technique is not very practical if you have thousands of items in the sampling frame, or if you don't happen to live near a bingo hall where you can get access to lots of ping-pong balls with the right numbers on the them and a huge rotating drum that can contain them all.

Fortunately, statistical software packages (SPSS or Excel, for example) can be used to generate lists of n random numbers with values between 1 and N (you need to specify both n and N in the command).[6] Or you can use lists of pre printed random numbers, and select the first n numbers from the list.[7] If the sampling frame consists of a set of index cards with people's names on, you could alphabetize the list and choose every ith card, where i was your sampling interval. Alternatively, you could shuffle the cards as thoroughly as you could, and then select the first n cards. Whichever technique you use, the principle is to draw a truly random sample from the population.

EPSEM and Non-EPSEM Simple Random Sampling

In order to keep life from being dull and boring, there are, in fact, two forms of simple random sampling. The first is called **EPSEM** sampling (Equal

---

[4]In statistics, it is important to distinguish between upper case and lower case letters, as they are often used to describe different things. The same will be true when we get round to using Greek letters.

[5]This is known as sampling 'without replacement', that is, once an item is notionally removed from the population for inclusion in the sample, it cannot be selected a second time. Sampling 'with replacement' would allow a subject (or more usually, an observation or measurement from a particular subject) to be put back into the sampling frame and eligible to be selected on subsequent occasions. Almost all sampling for research purposes is 'without replacement'.

[6]Make sure that the list of random numbers generated does not have repeats. Excel, by default, produces lists of numbers 'with replacement'. If a number appears more than once in the list as you are selecting the elements to include in your sample, simply ignore the repeated number and go on to the next (non-repeated) number in order for your sample to be representative of the population.

[7]Given the widespread availability of software to generate random number lists, pre-printed lists of random numbers are now rarely used. Again, if you are using pre-printed lists of random numbers, remember to ignore the repeats.

Probability **SE**lection **M**ethod). In EPSEM sampling, every item in the population has an equal chance of being selected. Its primary attribute is that the sample is *unbiased*: in theory, for a given measurement, the sample average should be close to the population average, and the variation in the measurement of interest from one subject to the next should also, on average, be similar in both the sample and the population.[8]

In practice, however, EPSEM sampling may not produce a sample that yields an answer that is representative of what is happening in the population. The alternative is **non-EPSEM** sampling or **PPS** sampling (**P**robability **P**roportional to **S**ize). 'What was the matter with EPSEM sampling?' you ask. There is nothing the matter with EPSEM sampling provided that you *want* every item in the population to have an equal chance of being selected. If every element in the sampling frame represents an individual, then EPSEM sampling is fine. But let us take an example in which EPSEM sampling would not be appropriate. Suppose the Regional Health Authority wants to know the average distance from a person's home to their nearest health centre. Let the *population* (the items in the sampling frame) consist of towns and villages. Assume that there are five times as many villages as there are towns within the Region. If every town and village has an equal chance of being selected, the final sample will (in theory) contain five times as many villages as towns. If we ask 50 adults in each town or village how far it is to their nearest health centre, it is clear that the result will be heavily biased towards people who live in villages. To obtain an answer that better reflects the average travelling time for everyone who lives within the Region, we need to have a sample in which the chance of selecting a town or village is proportional to the number of people who live there.

Thus, sampling would be proportional to size. The final sample would contain towns and villages in proportion to the number of people living in them, as towns (with bigger populations) would have a greater chance of being selected than villages. The application of this technique to sampling should be carried out with the support of a statistician.

An alternative strategy is to use stratified sampling (see below) and then to weight the results.

Systematic Sampling

A variation on simple random sampling is **systematic sampling**. In systematic sampling, we select every ith item in the sampling frame. How do we define the interval, i? Suppose that the sampling frame consists of a set of 10 000 cards with people's name on (one name per card), ordered alphabetically by surname, and that we want a sample of 500 people. It would be virtually impossible to shuffle 10 000 cards thoroughly and then take the first 500. Equally, it would be very tedious having to count through the cards to find those corresponding to a list of n random numbers (assuming we had numbered the cards from 1 to 10 000). Instead, we could divide N (10 000, the total number of elements in the sampling frame, i.e. in the population) by n (500, the desired sample size). We calculate $i = 10\,000/500 = 20$, which means we select every 20th card in the set. The value for $i = N/n$ is known as the *sampling interval*.

There is an issue with this approach. If we always start with the first element in the population, then we are ignoring the other 19 elements in the first interval of 20 elements. It would not be right always to start with the first card, because most of the people in the sampling frame would then never have a chance of being selected. So we need to make a decision about where to start, based on random selection. We choose a random number between 1 and 20 (using SPSS or Excel to generate a random number between 1 and 20, or using random number tables) to find out which card in the first 20 should be selected. Thereafter, we would work our way systematically through the cards, taking every 20th

---

[8]It is very rare for the sample and population averages to be exactly the same, or for the variation in measurements between observations in the sample to be exactly the same as the variation between observations in the population. We will explore this idea later in this chapter, and again in Chapters 4 and 5.

card until our sample of 500 had been selected. Thus, if our random number generator told us to start with card number 7, we would then choose card numbers 27, 47, 67, and so on, until we got to the end of our sampling frame.

Systematic sampling is well suited to those circumstances in which an enumerated list of items in the population is not readily available, but where we do have a physical collection of items to choose from. It would be appropriate, for example, to use systematic sampling in a doctor's surgery in which patients' notes are kept on filing shelves. If we know the total number of patients' notes (N) and the size of the sample we wish to select (n), we can find $i = N/n$ and select every ith set of notes. It wouldn't matter how the files were ordered – by number or alphabetically – provided all of the patients' files were on the shelves at the time the sample was being selected (i.e. we would do the sampling outside surgery hours, so that the patients who were more likely to be seeing their doctor and whose notes were temporarily not on the shelves wouldn't be excluded). Systematic sampling can also be used with geographic sampling, in which we take every ith house in a street.

There are, of course, some problems with systematic sampling. If every ith house is on a corner and we are carrying out a survey on noise pollution, we may not get a very representative picture because people living in a corner house may experience more cars shifting gear as they approach the corner. Any periodicity in the sampling frame will be a problem if the periodicity is equal to i. Otherwise, systematic sampling should provide a representative sample.

Another type of systematic sampling is alphabetic sampling (taking all of the people from the list of names in the doctor's surgery whose last name begins with 'A', for example). It is not a good sampling technique, however. Certain letters may relate to particular subgroups within the population, or include a large number of people with the same surname who are genetically related. Alphabetic sampling may thus fail to produce a sample which is representative of the population from which the sample was drawn. The letter 'O', for example, will

be associated with many Irish names (O'Brien, O'Malley, etc.); the letter 'M' with Scottish names (McTavish, MacBride, etc.); and the letters 'J' and 'W' with Welsh names (Jones and Williams). The same applies to first names, which are often culturally or social class related (Darren and Tracy versus Benjamin and Samantha). It is best not to use alphabetic sampling. The exception, of course, would be a study in which you were trying to relate particular names to a particular outcome.

Stratified Sampling

By its very nature, simple random sampling can give rise to samples which are *not* representative of the populations from which they are drawn, especially if the samples are small.[9] Suppose, for example, that we want to estimate serum vitamin C levels in the population. We could draw a simple random sample from the population, measure serum vitamin C and calculate the average. We know, however, that smoking reduces circulating levels of vitamin C. Just by chance, we could end up with a simple random sample in which half of the subjects were smokers, even if the true proportion of smokers in the population was, say, 20%. If this happened, our calculated average would be an underestimate of the true average vitamin C level in the population.

To overcome this problem, we would use stratified sampling. First, we would identify smokers and nonsmokers in the sampling frame. This would normally be done by administering a simple screening questionnaire. Then, within each stratum[10] (smokers and nonsmokers), we would use simple random sampling to select the required number of individuals for the study. If we had the resources to study

---

[9] I keep talking about 'small' and 'large' samples. There are no strict definitions. But a 'small' sample might be one of 30 or fewer items, whereas a 'large' sample might be 100 or more. The issue of how big a sample needs to be for a study to achieve its research aims is discussed in detail in Chapter 12 on Power and sample size.

[10] *Stratum* is the singular form of *strata*, just as *datum* is the singular form of *data*. So we say 'strata are' and (just to remind you) we say 'the data are' not 'the data is'.

100 subjects, we could select 20 smokers and 80 non-smokers (i.e. make the final sample reflect the proportion of smokers and nonsmokers in the population). Alternatively, we could select 50 smokers and 50 nonsmokers. That would help to ensure that we had equally good data on vitamin C levels in smokers and nonsmokers. To find the average for the population, we would calculate a weighted mean (see Section 2.3) when we produced our results.

There are three particular merits to stratification:

1. It can help to reduce the likelihood of drawing a sample which is not representative of the population.

2. It allows us to *over* sample particular strata in the population which contain proportionately few people or elements. This can help us to improve the reliability of the estimates of the variable we are interested in every stratum in the population.

3. It allows us to calculate *weighted* and *unweighted* estimates of average values within our samples. The techniques for weighting observations and calculating the relevant averages within each stratum and for the sample as a whole are discussed in Section 2.3.

In theory, of course, it is only worth stratifying a sample if variable A is associated with the one in which we are interested (variable B). In the previous example, variable A was 'smoking' and variable B was 'serum vitamin C level'. We know that smoking has a deleterious effect on levels of vitamin C in serum, so stratification is appropriate. If the different strata in the population do not differ with regard to the variable of primary interest, then do not stratify – it is a waste of time and effort.

Here is another example. Suppose we were interested in the relationship between iron status in pregnancy and level of antenatal care. It would be worth stratifying the population according to the number of previous pregnancies because that might have an influence on iron status independent of the level of antenatal care. It would not be worth stratifying the population according to eye colour, however, because there is no relationship (that I know of) between iron status and eye colour.

For small samples, it is best to use stratified sampling. In the smoking and vitamin C example, this would help us to ensure that we obtain equally reliable estimates of serum vitamin C in our two strata. The final result would then be weighted to reflect the proportion of smokers and nonsmokers in the population. Where larger numbers of subjects are being recruited and the estimates of the variable are likely to be reliable in every stratum, simple random sampling, or stratified sampling with the number of subjects proportional to the numbers in the population would be appropriate, and calculation of a weighted average would not be required. If we had resources to study 1000 subjects, for example, and our sample contained roughly 200 smokers and 800 nonsmokers, the 200 observations of serum vitamin C in the smokers would be sufficient to give us a reliable estimate.

Staged or Cluster Sample

Sometimes it may be very difficult to arrange for physical access to a truly random sample which covers a wide geographical area. For instance, if the aim was to conduct a national survey of school children, we could in theory generate a list of the names of all school children in the country and draw a simple random sample. There are two problems with this approach. First, compiling the list of all school children would take a lot of effort. Second, the resultant sample would be widely scattered geographically. If the study involved seeing each child individually, field workers would have to travel long distances between subjects.

It would make much more sense logistically (and perfectly good sense statistically) to concentrate our efforts on relatively few schools. We could achieve this by sampling first at the level of parliamentary constituencies, then towns and villages within the selected constituencies, then schools within the selected towns and villages. In theory, if each of the selections is a truly random and representative selection (of constituencies, towns, villages, and schools), then the final sample of children chosen from registers of the selected schools should be representative of children across the country as a whole. The selection at each stage would use PPS sampling so that we did not overrepresent small constituencies or towns. The final sample would be highly *clustered* geographically (hence the term 'cluster sample'). Once the sample had been selected, we might check the geographical distribution to make sure that the sample reflected the distribution of pupils across the country as a whole and did not miss out particular regions or types of area.

It is important to note that at each stage we would be generating a sample that was representative of the population. We might also consider some stratification:

- by region at the level of constituency
- by size at the level of town
- by type of school (primary, secondary, state, private) at the level of school
- by gender, ethnic group, and social class at the level of children.

This would help to ensure better representativeness of our final sample. If we oversampled particular strata at any of the sampling stages (for example, we might want to ensure that we had enough observations to give reliable estimates of nutrient intake amongst nursery school children living in poor inner city areas) then our final calculation of results would need to use appropriate weighting. As you can see, the sampling for major national surveys can be a complicated business! The statistical analysis of clustered samples is more complex than the analysis comparing two groups, for example, as it needs to take into account possible similarities of characteristics within a cluster. A statistician's help will definitely be required.

Quota Sampling

You are walking down the street, minding your own business, when your path is blocked by someone who manages to make themselves appear as wide as the pavement. They are armed with a clipboard and pen. Or you are sitting in the peace and quiet of your own home one evening when the doorbell rings, and before you know it you have spent an hour talking with a complete stranger about personal deodorant, dog food, eating out, your favourite breakfast cereal, and whether or not you support a single European currency. Who are these people? They are the Market Survey Brigade, finding out on behalf of their sponsors the answers to innumerable questions about your personal views and lifestyle. You are in the province of the Opinion Polls.

You may have noticed that sometimes before they launch into their seemingly endless list of questions, they ask a series of deeply personal questions concerning your age, gender, where you live, whether or not you work locally, the type of work you do, etc. The purpose of these questions is to help them fill *quotas*. These people do not have a sampling frame from which they can select a truly representative sample. Instead, they have to rely on their introductory questions in order to obtain a balance of age, gender, and other criteria which will help them to obtain a sample which is likely to be representative of the population or from which weighted averages can be calculated. The need for these questions arises because the timing and location of their work will influence the sample composition. If I were to stand in my local high street at 10:00 o'clock in the morning and stop people at random (truly at random), I would obtain a sample which was predominantly female (mothers who had just dropped their children off at school), or elderly (people who are retired), or people whose business allowed them to be out on the street at that hour, or people on their way to the doctor or dentist. I would not see school teachers, or factory workers, or very many men. In order to generate a sample which is more likely to be representative, these introductory questions are necessary to limit the numbers in the sample in each category.

At the simplest level, quota sampling might be based on age and gender. Attached to the clipboard might be a little grid that looks like this:

Sex	Age (years)	
	25–44	45–64
Male	||||||||||	||||||||||
Female	||||||||||	||||||||||

Each of the 10 marks in the boxes indicates a person. When the field worker has asked their introductory questions, they will put a preliminary tick against one of the marks to indicate that an interview has been started with a person in that category. When the interview has been completed successfully, they will confirm the preliminary tick by changing it to a cross. When responses have been collected from ten people in one category, any other people in that category will be rejected at the screening stage. When all of the interviews have been completed and the questionnaires returned to the office, the final results will be weighted to reflect the balance of gender and age in the population.

Where the interviewers position themselves, the time of day, and the streets chosen for door knocking will all influence sample composition. These factors will normally be decided by the sampling team in the office running the study. It is easy to see that if I do all of my interviewing on the pavement outside Harrod's Department Store in London I will get a very different social class mix than if I do my interviewing outside the local Social Security Office. If Social Class is a factor which I want to take into account, then I will have to choose a number of different sites for my interviewing, or add additional categories to my quota sampling scheme which include social class (based on occupation, say).

A Final Word About Sampling

The aim of sampling is to enable the characteristics of a population to be inferred from sample data. Appropriate care must therefore be taken during the sampling procedure to ensure that this is possible.

Some people have the misguided notion that if they simply increase the sample size, they will overcome any problems about representativeness. If the sample does not include representative subgroups of all segments of the population, however, no amount of increase in sample size will compensate. For example, if we were to carry out a study to assess the relationship between exercise and risk of heart disease, and we selected our sample from hospital patients who have recently been admitted with a heart attack (a convenient and motivated sample, it must be acknowledged), we would clearly be missing from our sample all those people who may have some form of heart disease but who were not admitted to hospital (e.g. people seen in out-patient clinics, or people with angina seen by their GP). Any generalizations that we made about exercise and heart disease would relate only to that group of people whose heart disease led to hospitalization. This problem is known as *selection bias*. No amount of increase in sample size will compensate to generate a more representative sample. We are consequently in danger of misinterpreting our findings if we try and generalize them to the whole population. Put simply, selection bias leads to misinterpretation (Box 2.1).

Similarly, if a particular subgroup within a study systematically fails to complete the study (e.g. subjects who are employed find that they cannot take the time to come into College to complete a series of physical fitness tests), then a problem of bias may arise retrospectively, even though the initial sample seemed representative. It is the final *achieved* sample which is important in relation to generalizability.

Lastly, it is important that the sampling frame is complete and includes all the members of the population that we wish to sample. Telephone directories used to be a popular sampling frame, but with the rise of mobile phones, listings of land lines omit substantial portions of the population, and their

---

BOX 2.1

The danger of selection bias

Selection bias ⇒ Misinterpretation

completeness is age-related (households with older residents are more likely to have a land line). Postcode sampling was mentioned in relation to cluster sampling, providing a robust geographically complete listing of households, but it is important to exclude nonresidential postcodes (i.e. businesses) from the sampling frame. GP lists are also a good source of sampling frames for a given community, but there are often 'ghosts' – people who have died or moved away but who remain on the lists. Take care when compiling the sampling frame to make sure that it reflects the population that you wish to study.

2.2 MEASURES OF CENTRAL TENDENCY

In Chapter 1 we observed that data are what we collect, and results are what we report. We need to start thinking about useful ways to summarize our data based on our sample observations.[11]

There is an inherent recognition that whenever we make a series of observations, the measurements will vary in some way around a central value. In a given sample, the observations will vary from one measurement to the next. If our aim is to get the best estimate of someone's usual blood pressure, for example, our sample might be repeat measurements of blood pressure in the same individual. Or we might want to compare growth in two groups of

children taking part in a dietary supplementation trial (treatment versus control group). Assuming that we had matched the children in the two groups for age and sex, we could take a single measurement of height and weight in each child at the beginning and end of the study, and compare the average change in height and weight between the two matched groups.

We often ask (innocently) 'What is the average?' But the word *average* can actually imply a number of different expressions. These are the so-called 'measures of central tendency' that indicate the centre of the distribution of values. Admittedly, 'measures of central tendency' is a rather clunky, inelegant expression. However, it does convey two useful concepts. First, it implies that there is more than one way to summarize where the middle of the distribution of values might be (hence 'measures' in plural). Second, the measures are approximations of the centre of the distribution of values (hence 'tendency'). Our aim is to use the observations in the sample to get a good estimate of what is going on in the population. This section describes how we can determine these various measures of central tendency. In Section 2.4, we will look at ways of summarizing how the observations vary around the centre of the distribution (based on the measure of central tendency that we think is appropriate for our data)

2.2.1 The Mean

The most commonly used measure of central tendency is the *mean*. There are in fact a number of different ways to calculate the mean. The one which is used most often is the *arithmetic mean*. When people talk about 'calculating the mean', it is the arithmetic mean that they are usually referring to. When other types of mean are being referred to, the word 'mean' must be prefaced by an adjective (e.g. *geometric, harmonic,* and so on – see below) to indicate how the mean was calculated. The main emphasis throughout this textbook will be on the *arithmetic mean*.

Say we have a series of values which represent the daily dietary fibre intakes in a group of seven

[11]At this stage in the proceedings, I want to include a warning. When preparing reports, DO NOT include endless tables of data, either in the main body of the text or in an appendix. I know that you may feel you have worked hard to collect your data, and you want to share the effort and the pain. But only you will love your data to this extent. Of course, it is vital that you collect your data based on careful observation, using appropriate measuring instruments (whether in the field or in the laboratory). However, it is typically only when a query arises over the results that someone may want to inspect your data to make sure that your conclusions are justified. In that case, you must be prepared to share your data in its entirety, and not try to hide or exclude any observations that you think are questionable. We will come back to this issue of outlying data points in later chapters.

women, estimated using a seven-day weighed food diary. Here are our seven values:

Dietary fibre intake (g/d):
9   14   13   12   17   18   15

What is the mean daily intake of dietary fibre in this group of women? Higher mathematics are not needed to undertake this calculation,[12] but I will spell it out for the sake of clarity:

$$\text{Arithmetic mean} = \frac{9 + 14 + 13 + 12 + 17 + 18 + 15}{7}$$
$$= \frac{98}{7} = 14$$

EQUATION 2.1   The expression to calculate the arithmetic mean of dietary fibre intake (g/d) in seven women, written out in full

We would conclude that the mean intake of dietary fibre in this group of women is 14 g/d. Three of the women have value for intake above the mean, three have values below the mean; and for one woman, her intake and the mean value are the same. So it looks like our mean value is a good indication of the middle of the distribution, which is what we were after.

The mean is something which comes up a great deal in statistical 'conversation'. It is useful, therefore, to have a way of summarizing both its calculation and expression. Let us look again at the dietary fibre example.

Variables

We have been talking so far about 'observations' and 'measurements', but I have also used the more conventional terminology 'variable'. Put simply, a *variable* is something we want to measure in our sample (e.g. height, blood pressure, dietary fibre intake, blood alcohol level). The nature of a variable is that

it *varies* from one observation to the next (hence 'variable', 'not fixed', or 'not the same' – different from a 'constant').

We also need a shorthand to describe variables, for three reasons. First, we don't want to have to keep writing out the variable name in full (for example, 'dietary fibre intake (g/d)') when we undertake statistical calculations. Second, we want to be able to distinguish between different sets of observations (different variables) within the same sample. The conventional shorthand is to use a letter toward the end of the alphabet and to put it in italics. For example, we might use the letter 'x' to refer to 'dietary fibre intake (g/d)'. If I had other sets of measurements (say energy intake or protein intake), I might use the letters 'y' and 'z'.[13] Third, we need to have a mathematical way of both summarizing and generalizing what we are doing. Using these kinds of labels for our variables makes that process much easier, as we shall see.

For the present example, let us use the letter 'x' (in italics) to denote the measure of our variable 'dietary fibre intake (g/d)'.

Back to the Calculation of the Mean

The first thing we need is a way of referring to each of our seven observations so we can distinguish between the first, second, third, and so on up to the seventh observation. This can be done by using our chosen letter to describe our variable, x, with a subscript numeral. The first observation, 9 g/d, could be referred to as x_1, the next observation, 14 g/d, as x_2, and so on up to the last observation, 15 g/d, which could be referred to as x_7. There is also an expression for the arithmetic mean itself, $\bar{x}$, which is spoken in English as 'x-bar'.

---

[12]Yes, I know, you learned this in Year 2 of primary school (or Second Grade in Elementary school, depending on where you live). I am starting very slowly here. But please bear with me. Things will get more challenging quite quickly, I promise.

[13]You can see that, very quickly, I am going to run out of letters at the end of the alphabet. In practice, any letter or combination of letters will do, provided it is clearly defined. So, I might use the upper case letter A to denote age (years), or DF to denote dietary fibre intake (g/d). You will also note that I am dropping the single quotes around my variables. The italic case makes it clear that I am talking about variables, provided I have defined them clearly in my report or paper.

We can now rewrite the expression for the mean as follows:

$$\bar{x} = \frac{9 + 14 + 13 + 12 + 17 + 18 + 15}{7} = \frac{98}{7} = 14$$

EQUATION 2.2   The expression to calculate the arithmetic mean ($\bar{x}$, or 'x-bar') of dietary fibre intake (g/d) based on observations in seven women, written out in full

But we could also express this more generally for any series of seven numbers. It would be written as:

$$\bar{x} = \frac{x_1 + x_2 + x_3 + x_4 + x_5 + x_6 + x_7}{7}$$

EQUATION 2.3   The expression to calculate the arithmetic mean ($\bar{x}$, or 'x-bar') of any seven observations, written out in full

Usefully, we can take the generalization of our expression still further. We have seen that we can refer to each of the observations as x_1, x_2, x_3 up to x_7. More generally, we could use the expression x_i (see footnote[14]), where i can take a value between 1 and 7. But if we had more than seven observations, we might want to refer generally to the total number of observations in our sample using the letter n (we have used this before to denote the number of observations in our sample). In this particular set of observations on dietary fibre intake, $n = 7$. But if we say there are n observations in our sample (not just seven observations), we could refer to the last observation as x_n. Thus, we could re-write our expression for the mean of a sample of size n using all our new terms, $\bar{x}, x_i$, and x_n:

$$\bar{x} = \frac{x_1 + x_2 + x_3 + \cdots + x_i + \cdots + x_n}{n}$$

EQUATION 2.4   The fully generalized expression for calculating the arithmetic mean based on n observations, written out in full

---

[14]We sometimes speak about the ith value of x, or x_i, which can stand for any value that the variable may take between the first value (where $i = 1$) and the last value (where $i = n$). 'ith' is spoken as if you were saying the word 'eye' with a 'th' at the end ('eyeth').

This is still rather cumbersome, however. It would be useful to have a single term for the numerator in this equation (the term above the line) that expressed the sum of all the values of x from x_1 to x_n. We use the term Σ (the upper case Greek letter 'sigma') to denote the phrase in English 'the sum of'. We can then say that the sum of all of the observed values for variable x from the first (x_1) to the last (x_n) is equal to:

$$\sum_{i=1}^{n} x_i$$

Sometimes the expression is written with the numbers to the side rather than above and below the letter Σ, like this: $\sum_{i=1}^{n} x_i$. The two expressions mean the same thing.

The expression 'the sum of the values of x from the first observation x_1 (where $i = 1$) to the last observation x_n (where $i = n$)' is fully set out in Equation 2.5:

$$\sum_{i=1}^{n} x_i = x_1 + x_2 + x_3 + \cdots + x_i + \cdots + x_n$$

EQUATION 2.5   The expression for denoting the sum of n observations

Now we have a *real* shorthand for denoting the arithmetic mean:

$$\bar{x} = \frac{\sum_{i=1}^{n} x_i}{n}$$

EQUATION 2.6   The shorthand expression for denoting the arithmetic mean

Equation 2.6 is equivalent to saying in English 'the arithmetic mean is equal to the sum of all the values of x from x_1 to x_n, divided by the number of observations n'. The numerator is usually simplified still further to Σx (spoken in English as 'the sum of x'), without the '$i = 1$' and 'n' as part of the expression. This is what I call the 'lazy' notation (there is less to write each time). So our final, fully simplified 'lazy' expression for the arithmetic mean becomes:

$$\bar{x} = \frac{\sum x}{n}$$

EQUATION 2.7   The 'lazy' shorthand expression for denoting the arithmetic mean

The expression in spoken English is still the same: 'the arithmetic mean (x-bar) is equal to the sum of x (the sum of our sample observations) divided by the number of observations in the sample'.

Strictly speaking, the term $\bar{x}$ is used to designate the arithmetic mean of a *sample*. A different term, μ (the lower case Greek letter 'mu') will be used to refer to the arithmetic mean of the population. As we shall see, the sample mean and the population mean are not necessarily the same. But more of this later.

We will be using the expressions $\sum x$ ('the sum of x') and $\bar{x}$ ('x-bar' or 'the sample mean') over and over again. If you do not understand them at this point, you should read the section 'Back to the Calculation of the Mean' again until this shorthand is entirely clear. Each time you see the symbols, do not quiver and quake – simply say out loud what they mean in English until it becomes second nature. It is a bit like learning a foreign language. Initially, the words on paper in the new language don't make sense, but after a while you look at them and their meaning becomes instantly recognizable.

2.2.2 The Median

The mean, of course, can be calculated for any set of values. But is it always the best 'measure of central tendency'? It certainly falls near the centre of the distribution when the values are distributed more or less symmetrically either side of the mean (as in our example above). But what happens if there are extreme values (either very high or very low values) in relation to most of the observations? The extreme values will tend to pull the arithmetic mean away from the centre, and it will no longer be the best indicator of the centre of the distribution.

To illustrate, suppose that we include in our observations above the dietary fibre intakes of two vegetarians whose intakes were 24 g/d and 31 g/d. The mean dietary fibre intake for all nine subjects is now equal to 17 g/d (rather than 14 g/d for the original seven subjects). The plot in Figure 2.1 shows the distribution of the values for dietary fibre on the horizontal scale.

Whereas before, the mean provided a good indication of the middle of the distribution, now, five values fall below the mean, and only three above. It looks a bit lopsided. Is there a better measure of central tendency that would provide a value more indicative of the middle of the distribution?

The answer is 'yes'. The value is called the *median*. The median is, by definition, the value which lies at the centre of the distribution of all of the observations, such that half of the observations are less than the median and half are greater than the median. Using our present example, the value of the median is equal to 15. Four values lie below the median, and four values lie above, and the median itself is the central value, 15 (Figure 2.2).

The median thus provides a better representation of the middle of the distribution for values which are not symmetrically distributed around the mean. As we have seen, the mean is unduly influenced by very large (or very small) observations, whereas the median is a much more stable measure of the centre of the distribution, uninfluenced by extreme values. It is worth noting that before we

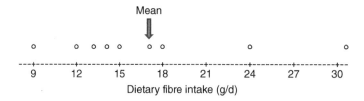

FIGURE 2.1   Distribution of observations of dietary fibre intake (g/d) showing mean.

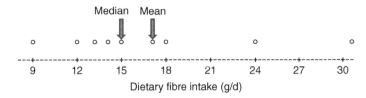

FIGURE 2.2   Distribution of observations of dietary fibre intake (g/d) showing mean and median

added the more extreme values of the vegetarians to our observations, the mean ($\bar{x} = 14$) and the median (14) were the same.

Where the mean and the median are similar, it is better to use the mean as the measure of central tendency; the mean is easier to manipulate mathematically, and provides a number of statistical advantages. (In Chapter 3, we will look at formal ways of identifying those times when we should calculate a mean, and those times when we should determine the median.)

There is no shorthand expression for the term 'median' (like $\bar{x}$ for the mean) – it is always written out in full. Nor is there a quick way of finding the value. It is always necessary to sort the values from smallest to largest (or largest to smallest, it doesn't matter), and find the value or values in the middle (the 'mid-most' value or values). Most of the time, of course, we will be using Excel or SPSS or other statistical package to determine the value. Alternatively, if you have relatively few values to sort and you don't have a computer handy, you can carry out a 'tally' (see Exercise 2.8.3 at the end of this chapter).

So, how is the median determined? It depends on whether there is an odd or even number of observations in the sample. We can use notation like the one that we developed for the mean to indicate which value in a series of observations is equal to the median.

Rank the observations (put them in order from smallest to largest). Call the smallest observation x_1 and the largest observation x_n. If there is an odd number of observations in the data, then the median value will be equal to x_i, where $i = (n+1)/2$ and n, as usual, is the number of observations in the sample.

If I have nine observations, for example, then $i = (n+1)/2 = (9+1)/2 = 10/2 = 5$, so the median will be the fifth observation, x_5. Four of the observations will be above the median, four below the

median, and the median will itself be the central value. Or we can say:

$$\text{Median}_{\text{Odd number of observations in sample}} = x_{\left[(n+1)/2\right]}$$

EQUATION 2.8   An expression for the median (x_i) for distributions with an odd number of observations, where $i = (n+1)/2$

This is not a very elegant expression, mathematically speaking. It does, however, provide a succinct summary of what the median represents. In practice, no one uses it other than to illustrate how the median is determined.

If there is an even number of observations, no specific value in the set of observations will lie exactly halfway. It is necessary, therefore, to follow the convention that says that the median is half-way between the two mid-most values, that is, the arithmetic mean of $x_{[n/2]}$ and $x_{[(n+2)/2]}$. So the expression for the median where there is an even number of observations in the set of values is:

$$\text{Median}_{\text{even number of observations in sample}} = \frac{x_{\left[n/2\right]} + x_{\left[(n+2)/2\right]}}{2}$$

EQUATION 2.9   An expression for the median for distributions with an even number of observations, where the two midmost values are represented by x_i, such that $i = n/2$ (for the lower of the two mid-most values) and $i = (n+2)/2$ (for the higher of the two mid-most values).

So if there are 10 observations, the median is equal to the average of the fifth value ($x_{(10/2)} = x_5$) and the sixth value ($x_{(10+2)/2} = x_6$). In practice, no one bothers to use these mathematical expressions for the median, as they are really rather

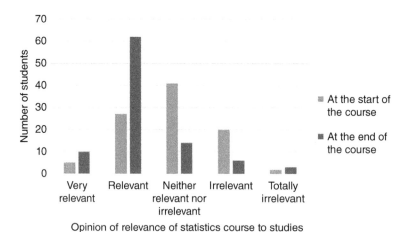

FIGURE 2.3   Illustration of mode: opinions of health science students regarding relevance of statistics course to their studies.

cumbersome; everyone just gets on with the calculations, or uses the computer.

To summarize:

1. The median provides a good representation of the middle of the distribution when there are a few values which are very much larger or very much smaller than the rest of the observations (i.e. the distribution of values is asymmetrical).

2. The median is less easy to manipulate statistically than the mean. You can add and subtract means (for example when calculating a weighted mean), but you cannot add and subtract medians in the same way.

3. The median takes into account only the *position* of values in a distribution, and ignores the relative *sizes* of the values. You are thus throwing away potentially useful information. We will come back to this issue about throwing information away in Chapter 7.

2.2.3 The mode

The *mode* is the value in a distribution for which there is the largest number of observations. In practice, it might be useful to know if there was a particular observation that kept occurring. For example, if you were

measuring opinions, you might find that for some questions every respondent gave the same answer. This could mean that the question was failing to discriminate a range of responses, or that virtually everyone really thought the same thing. So it could tell you about what people think; equally, it could alert you to possible problems with your measuring instrument.

At the start of each academic year, I ask the health science students[15] in my statistics class how relevant they feel the course will be to their studies. At the end of the course, I ask the same question. Figure 2.3 shows distribution of the opinions of health science students regarding the relevance of a statistics course to their studies at the start and end of the academic year.

A few students were very keen at the outset – it could be that they should have been taking a course in statistics, not health sciences. This very keen group has been joined by a few more by the end of the course who saw the application of statistics to their studies as 'Very relevant'. Most of the students were neutral at the start ('Neither relevant nor irrelevant'). As the course progressed and their understanding of statistics and its application improved, many of them changed their opinion about the

---

[15]These include trainee medics, nurses, physiotherapists, nutritionists, and dietitians.

relevance to their studies, and saw it as 'Relevant'. A handful didn't really see the point ('Irrelevant'), although these numbered fewer by the end of the course. Lastly, a few thought the course was a waste of time at the start, and continued to do so at its end. Whenever these students showed up for lectures, they sat at the back making rude comments, writing notes to each other, and throwing the occasional spit ball (no, not really – but they did make a racket from time to time when the material was especially difficult and they struggled to follow the lecture).

At the beginning of the course, the mode (the group with the largest number of observations) was the group that was initially neutral ('Neither relevant nor irrelevant'). By the end of the course, the mode was the group who thought the course was 'Relevant'. I usually interpreted this shift as a vote of confidence in the value of course.

The real problem with the mode is that it is not a very stable measure of central tendency. A few more observations in one category of response, or a few less in another, can cause a dramatic shift in the mode. Nor does it behave well mathematically. Like the median, it cannot be easily manipulated.

2.2.4 The Geometric Mean

The *geometric mean* (GM) is used for data which follow an exponential curve or logarithmic distribution. It is extremely useful for finding the mid-point of a series of observations that follow power or logarithmic functions. This is the case, for example, in serological studies in which the concentration of a titre decreases in a multiple relative to the dilution factor, for example, 2, 4, 8, etc. for successive two-fold dilutions; or for values showing population growth over time.

The geometric mean is the antilog of the mean of the logarithms of the observed values:

$$\text{Geometric Mean} = \text{antilog} \frac{\sum_{i=1}^{n} \log x_i}{n}$$

EQUATION 2.10 Formula for calculating the geometric mean

Again, this is not so scary if you say out loud what it asks you to do in English: 'take the log of each observation in the sample, from the first observation ($\log x_1$) through all of the subsequent observations ($\log x_i$) until you get to the last observation ($\log x_n$); add them all together ($\sum_{i=1}^{n} \log x_i$); divide by n; and find the antilog (the value x, such that, when you take $\log(x)$, you get the log that you calculated)'.[16] All of these operations can be done easily using a scientific calculator or a statistical spreadsheet like Excel or software like SPSS.

Negative or zero values are not suitable for this calculation, as they have no logarithm. You can get around this issue by adding a fixed amount (a 'constant') to every observation to make all of the values positive. Then calculate the logarithmic mean using the formula above. Finally subtract the constant from the antilog you calculate to find the geometric mean.

TIP: showing multiplication in a formula

In the expression shown in footnote 16 for computing the geometric means, the times symbol '×' may become confusing if the variable of interest is x. There are alternate ways of expressing multiplication in an equation. First, you can use a dot like this · in the middle of the line. The expression would then look like this: $\sqrt[n]{x_1 \cdot x_2 \cdot x_3 \cdot \ldots \cdot x_n}$. In Excel and SPSS, you need to use an asterisk * to indicate multiplication, so the expression becomes $\sqrt[n]{x_1 * x_2 * x_3 * \cdots * x_n}$.

---

[16]Another way of calculating the geometric mean is to take the nth root of the sample observations all multiplied together, where n is the number of observations in the sample: $\sqrt[n]{x_1 \times x_2 \times x_3 \times \cdots \times x_n}$. This can create exceptionally large values if you have lots of observations. Equation 2.10 is a much neater way of undertaking the same calculation using logarithms.

Finally, for simplicity of expression in statistics books like this or when writing an equation, you can omit the multiplication symbol altogether provided you don't need it for clarity of the expression. The geometric mean could then be written as:

Geometric Mean $= \sqrt[n]{x_1 x_2 x_3 \ldots x_n}$. This is the neatest and simplest way to indicate that you simply want to multiply values together. This is the convention that we will use throughout this book, except when a times sign is useful to clarify how an expression works or we need one to write syntax in SPSS or a formula in Excel.

2.3 WEIGHTING AND WEIGHTED AVERAGES

In the example concerning smokers and non-smokers in Section 2.1.4, above, one way to draw the stratified samples was to make the final proportion of smokers and nonsmokers in the sample equal to the proportions of these groups in the population (20 and 80, respectively). Thus, when the average serum vitamin C level was calculated for the entire sample, we could say that the sample estimates reflected the likely impact of smoking on serum vitamin C in the population as a whole. One danger of this approach is that the smaller stratum, containing only 20 smokers, may not yield as reliable a result as the larger stratum, containing 80 observations; we noted earlier that common sense tells us that large samples are likely to provide better estimates of what is occurring in the population than small samples.[17] If this is so, then it would be better to have equally good estimates from every stratum in the sample (i.e. 50 smokers and 50 nonsmokers). But if we selected equal numbers of subjects from each stratum, the final sample would no longer be representative of the population. We need a tech-

nique that will help us find the answer about what is going on in the population. The technique we will apply is called *weighting*.

Table 2.1 shows the values for the average serum vitamin C levels in a sample of 50 smokers and 50 nonsmokers. The table also shows the *unweighted* and *weighted* means based on the findings from a stratified sample in which there are equal numbers of smokers and nonsmokers.

The *unweighted* average can be found by calculating the sum of the observations in the whole sample and dividing by the number of observations in the sample (100), that is, $\bar{x} = \Sigma x / n$. The values in the table give us the average for each stratum. The sum of the values for each stratum (smokers and nonsmokers) can be found by multiplying the average for the stratum by the number of observations in that stratum. If we rearrange the expression for the mean, we see that the sum of the observations is equal to the mean times the number of observations, that is $\Sigma x = \bar{x} \times n$. For smokers, this is equal to $25 \text{mg/l} \times 50 = 1250 \text{mg/l}$; for the nonsmokers, it is $35 \text{ mg/l} \times 50 = 1750 \text{mg/l}$. Add them together to find the sum of all of the observations for the sample ($1250 \text{g/l} + 1750 \text{ mg/l} = 3000 \text{mg/l}$) and divide by the total number of observations in the sample (100 subjects). This yields an *unweighted* average of $3000 \text{mg/l} \div 100$ subjects $= 30 \text{mg/l}$. This value is the average for the *sample* (50 smokers and 50 nonsmokers), but it does not reflect the relative proportions of smokers and nonsmokers in the population (20% and 80%).

To find the best estimate of serum vitamin C levels in the population, based on our sample observations, we need to calculate a *weighted* average that reflects the relative proportions of smokers (20%) and nonsmokers (80%) in the population. To do this, we multiply the mean for each stratum not by the number of observations in the sample, but by the percentage of each stratum present in the population. We multiply the mean value for smokers by the percentage of smokers in the population: $25 \text{mg/l} \times 20 = 500 \text{mg/l}$. For the nonsmokers, the value is $35 \text{mg/l} \times 80 = 2800 \text{mg/l}$. This then allows us to find the weighted sum of the

---

[17]We explore this notion mathematically in Chapter 5.

TABLE 2.1 Numbers of Subjects Recruited and Serum Vitamin C Levels, According to Whether Subject Smokes or Not. Calculation of weighted and unweighted estimates of average serum vitamin C levels.

	Smokers	Nonsmokers	Sum of Observations Divided by Number of Observations
Percentage in population	20%	80%	
Number of subjects in sample	50	50	
Average serum vitamin C (mg/l)	25	35	
Calculation of unweighted average	25 × 50 = 1250	35 × 50 = 1750	(1250 + 1750)/100 = 30
Calculation of weighted average	25 × 20 = 500	35 × 80 = 2800	(500 + 2800)/100 = 33

observations that reflects the relative proportions of smokers and nonsmokers in the population (500 mg/l + 2800 mg/l = 3300 mg/l), but based on our sample observations. We then divide this total by the weighted number of observations (20% × 100 + 80% × 100 = 20 + 80 = 100). This yields the *weighted* average: the weighted sum of the observations (3300 mg/l) divided by the weighted number of observations (100), i.e. 3300 mg/l÷100 = 33 mg/l. Our unweighted estimate of the average serum vitamin C levels (30 mg/l) would be an underestimate of our best estimate of the true level in the population (33 mg/l).

If we sample using stratification and selecting equal numbers of observations in each stratum, we help to ensure that the estimates of serum vitamin C levels in each stratum have similar levels of precision. The weighted average gives us a better estimate of the average value for serum vitamin C in the population as a whole. Weighted averages not only give us better estimates of what is going on in the population; they also provide a better basis for comparing average serum vitamin C values between groups or populations with different proportions of smokers and nonsmokers.

It is best to use SPSS to calculate weighted means for large samples or when there are lots of strata or values that you want to use as weights (e.g. the number of children in classes in schools, or the number of community dietitians in a local authority). There are a few tricks you need to learn to make sure that the outcome is correct. We will

work through these tricks in some of the examples in later chapters.

2.4 MEASURES OF VARIATION: RANGE, QUANTILES, AND THE STANDARD DEVIATION

Most measurements in biological material (foodstuffs, people, etc.) vary from one observation to the next. This is true whether we are talking about a single item of food (from which we take multiple samples for analysis); or repeat observations within a subject, or observations in different samples of the same foodstuff; or observations in different subjects drawn from the same population.

For example, two consecutive readings of blood pressure in the same subject are rarely the same, whether measured minutes or days apart. Similarly, within the same person, the intake of dietary energy and nutrients differs from day to day. It will also be true that average daily energy intakes measured over a week will differ from person to person, even if they are of the same age, gender, body size, and have similar levels of physical activity.

In the same way that it is useful to have a single value which helps us to know where the centre of a set of observations lies (measures of central tendency like the mean, median, or mode), it is equally useful to have measures that tells us about the spread of values around the measure of central tendency. This section looks at measures of spread which are in common use.

2.4.1 Range

The range, strictly speaking, is a single value. It is the difference between the highest value and the lowest value in a set of observations. Figure 2.4a–d show histograms of iron intakes in four groups of UK teenagers, boys and girls aged 11–14 and 15–18 years. The range is similar in the four distributions:

- Males 11–14 years: 54.4 mg/d
- Females 11–14 years: 50.0 mg/d
- Males 15–18 years: 62.7 mg/d
- Females 15–18 years: 65.0 mg/d

When we compare age groups, the range for the 11–14 year-olds is slightly larger for boys than girls; for the 15–18 year-olds, it is larger for the girls. Within gender, it is slightly larger for older boys compared with the younger boys, and much larger for the older girls. Given that older children are likely to have larger intakes, these values make some sense. But they do not tell us anything about where the levels of intake fall in the distribution of all possible intakes.

The *limits* of the range (the lowest and highest values, which is what most people describe when

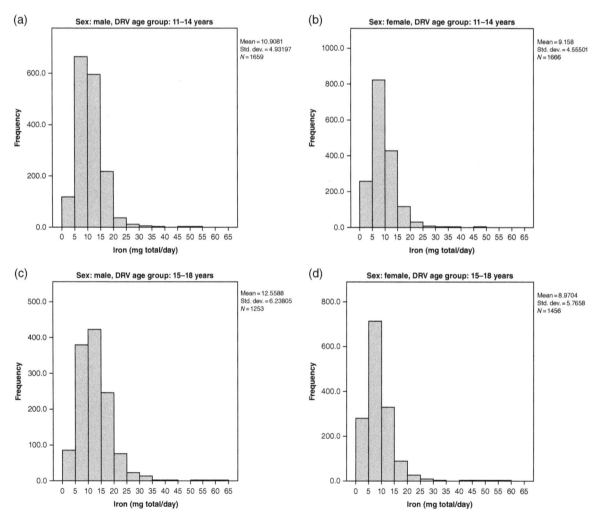

FIGURE 2.4   (a) Mean daily iron intake (mg/d), males 11–14 years. (b) Mean daily iron intake (mg/d), females 11–14 years. (c) Mean daily iron intake (mg/d), males 15–18 years. (d) Mean daily iron intake (mg/d), females 15–18 years.

TABLE 2.2 Tertiles, Quartiles, Range, and Limits of the Range for the Distribution of Iron Intakes Shown in Figures 2.4a–d

Age (years)	11–14		15–18	
Gender	Male	Female	Male	Female
Mean	10.9	9.2	12.6	9.0
Median	10.2	8.5	11.7	8.0
Range				
Range	54.4	50.0	62.7	65.0
Lower limit	0.1	0.0	0.0	0.0
Upper limit	54.5	50.0	62.7	65.0
Tertiles				
T1	8.4	6.8	9.5	6.4
T2	12.1	10.3	14.1	9.8
Quartiles				
Q1	7.7	6.0	8.4	5.6
Q2	10.2	8.5	11.7	8.0
Q3	13.4	11.4	16.0	11.0

they talk about the range) are more useful for interpreting the findings than the range itself. The range and the limits of the range are shown in Table 2.2. The lowest value is zero or close to zero. The highest value tells us the maximum reported intake. This is very helpful when looking at the spread of values around the mean or median.

The limits of the range may also raise important issues about the data and the way it was collected. Clearly, no one can survive if their daily intake of iron equals zero. The data from the diet diaries, however, suggest that some subjects may have recorded food intakes in which the computed iron content was less than 0.05 mg/d.[18] It leads one to question whether the subjects with these low values recorded consumption accurately, or if it was representative of their usual intake. The answer in both instances is likely to be 'no'.

What the range or the limits of the range do not tell us is how the *shape* of the graphs differ from

one another. We need something numerically more sensitive than the range or the limits of the range to describe this.

2.4.2 Quantiles

Most of us are familiar with the idea of 'percentiles'. Percentiles (or more correctly, *centiles*) are obtained by sorting a set of observations from smallest to largest, and then dividing it into 100 'chunks' or segments each of which contains an equal number of observations. If there were 1000 observations, for example, then each segment would contain 10 observations (10 below the first centile, 10 between the first and second centile, and so on). There are 99 centiles. If we know that a child's height is below the third centile, for example, we understand that they are very near the bottom of the distribution for height, and that 97% of children are taller. Centiles are helpful when dealing with large samples with hundreds or thousands of observations.[19]

Quantiles are used to divide distributions into any number of segments, from three to as many as you like.[20] These can also be used with large samples but are especially helpful for smaller samples. *Tertiles*, for example, divide a distribution into three equal segments. One third of observations fall below the first tertile; one third fall between the first and second tertile; and one third above the second tertile. *Quartiles* divide the distribution of values into four equal segments: 25% fall below the first quartile, 25% between the first and second quartile, and so on. *Quintiles* divide the distribution into five equal segments, and *deciles* into ten equal segments. Technically speaking, the number of quantiles is always one less than the number of segments. There are *two* tertiles, *three* quartiles, and so on.[21]

---

[18]When rounded to one decimal place, a value less than 0.05 mg/d will be rounded to 0.0 mg/d.

[19]If you have fewer than 100 observations in your sample, strictly speaking you cannot compute centiles.

[20]Of course, if you have only two segments, the value that divides the group into two equal sized chunks is the median.

[21]You will often find in the scientific literature authors who talk about observations 'in the first quintile of the distribution.' They really mean 'below the first quintile' or 'in the first fifth of the distribution.' Forgive them.

Table 2.2 shows the values for the tertiles and quartiles for Figure 2.4a–d. The tertiles are illustrated in Figure 2.5a–d.

We can see how quantiles provide useful information about the characteristics of the distribution not conveyed by the range or limits of the range. For example, when we compare quartiles for boys and girls aged 15–18 years, we see that the cutoff for the bottom quarter (Q1) is much lower for the girls (5.6 mg/d) than boys (8.4 mg/d). This means that 25% of girls have a reported iron intake of less than 5.6 mg/d, well below their likely requirement

(14 mg/d). Even if we allow for vagaries in the reporting of dietary consumption, this picture suggests that a substantial proportion of girls is likely to be iron deficient. And if we compare Q1 for girls by age, we see that it goes down with age (5.6 mg/d at age 15–18 compared with 6.0 mg/d at age 11–14) when we might expect it to go up. In contrast, the limits of the range suggested that intake was increasing with age amongst both boys and girls.

Thus, we can see that quantiles are more useful than the range when describing distributions. They give a sense of the way in which values are

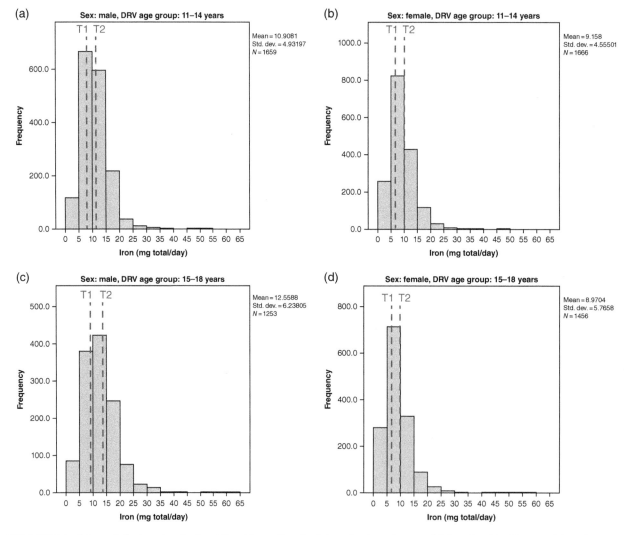

FIGURE 2.5   Mean daily iron intake (mg/d), with tertiles, for (a) males 11–14 years, (b) females 11–14 years, (c) males 15–18 years, and (d) females 15–18 years.

distributed and are less sensitive to the influence of extreme values. Probably the most commonly quoted quantiles are the first and third quartiles (Q1 and Q3), known together as the *inter-quartile range*. The inter-quartile range is often given together with the median to summarize the midpoint and the distribution of nonsymmetrical distributions of values. The second quartile (Q2) is, of course, the median (half of the values lie above Q2, and half below).

Quantile boundaries are determined in the same way as for the median, depending on the number of observations in the sample. Sometimes the quantile values will fall exactly on one of the observations (as was the case for the median when there was an odd number of observations in the sample), and sometimes between the two observations that are nearest to the value that divides the set of observations into equal groups (as was the case for the median when there was an even number of observations in the sample).

2.4.3 The Standard Deviation

The *standard deviation* provides a powerful way of summarizing how values are distributed around the mean. Essentially, it describes the *average* way in which the observations in a sample differ from the mean. The term 'deviation' simply means 'difference' [22] The standard deviation is one of the most fundamental and powerful concepts in the statistical repertoire.

TIP

The following section is extremely important to your understanding of the rest of this book!! If it doesn't make sense the first time, go back and read it again.

---

[22]Why statisticians feel the need to introduce jargon when plain English would do, I don't know. It's a bit like the misused jargon about quantiles – saying that 'subjects were in the bottom quintile' instead of saying 'subjects were in the bottom fifth' – it sounds more 'scientific' and frightens off the uninitiated. On the other hand, like some medical jargon, it makes it immediately apparent what you are talking about. 'Standard deviation' is one of those terms.

The standard deviation as a measure of variation works best for sets of values which follow a normal distribution (see Chapter 4). It can, however, be used with any set of values.[23] You will see it abbreviated as 'SD' or 'sd' or 'STD' or 'STDEV' depending on the article you might be reading or the software you are using. These all stand for the same thing.

Let us begin by applying common sense to the problem of finding a single value that describes how observations are distributed around the mean. The simplest approach, you might think, is to take the difference between each observation and the mean, and then find the average of the differences. Let us do that for the seven observations on dietary fibre intake cited in Section 2.2.1 and given in Table 2.3.[24]

In Section 2.2.1, we showed that the mean of the observations, $\bar{x}$, was equal to 14. The general expression for the difference between an observation and the mean is $x_i - x$. Out loud in English we would say, 'Take the difference between each observation and the mean', where x_i can stand for any observation in our sample.

If we are to calculate the average way in which the observations vary around the mean (the 'average deviation'), we need to find the difference for each of our observations in turn (x_1, x_2, x_3, x_4, etc.). If we have seven observations, we take the difference seven times. It is very important to take the difference in the same direction every time. The results are shown in Table 2.3

To find the average of the differences of each observation from the mean, we would do what we do to find any arithmetic average. We add our values

---

[23]We will discover in Chapter 4 that if a set of values does not follow the 'normal' distribution (also known as the Gaussian distribution or bell-shaped curve), we can apply transformations like log, square root, or an exponential function (raise to the power of 10 or *e*) and then test to see if the resultant distribution is normal (see Chapter 6). If a set of values does not follow the normal distribution and we cannot find an appropriate transformation, it is often (but not always) better to use median and quantiles to describe the distribution.

[24]I am using a very small data set in order to illustrate how the standard deviation is calculated. For large sets of observations, of course, we use statistical software.

TABLE 2.3   Dietary Fibre Intakes (g/d) in Seven Subjects, and the Differences Between Each Observation and the Mean

Original Observation x_i	Difference from the Mean $x_i - 14$
9	−5
14	0
13	−1
12	−2
17	3
18	4
15	1
$\sum x = 98$	$\sum(x - \bar{x}) = 0$

together (in this case, the differences between each observation and the mean) and divide by n, the number of observations. Using our new shorthand from Section 2.2.1, we could write this as $\sum_{i=1}^{n}(x_i - \bar{x})/n$. To use an even shorter shorthand, we can write the expression without the superscripts and subscripts: $\sum(x - \bar{x})/n$. I will refer to this simplified version of the expression as our 'lazy' notation.

When we add together our seven differences, we find that the total is equal to zero: $(-5) + 0 + (-1) + (-2) + 3 + 4 + 1 = 0$. In fact, it is not hard to prove that the sum of the differences of *any* set of values around the mean is equal to zero.[25] So, if we are to find an average of the deviations around the mean, we need to find another way to calculate it.

If we think about the problem, we are actually more interested in the *amount* of variation than the direction (whether it is positive or negative). So, we could just ignore the sign and look at the *size* of the

---

[25] $\sum(x - \bar{x}) = \sum x - \sum \bar{x} = \sum x - n\bar{x} =$

$\sum x - n\dfrac{\sum x}{n} = \sum x - \sum x = 0$

I will, from time to time, put in a footnote 'for the nerds.' Accept that it is ok to be nerdy, if you are that way inclined. If you are not nerdy, or you are having an unnerdy day, feel free to skip these asides.

difference. The mathematical expression that allows us to ignore the sign is called the *absolute value* or *modulus*. In its written form, it uses two parallel lines that tell you to ignore the sign. To give a quick example, the absolute value of 4 equals 4, that is, $|4| = 4$, and the absolute value of −4 equals 4, that is, $|-4| = 4$. So, for our expression of the differences between each observation and the mean, we could write $|x_i - \bar{x}|$, and the sum of the differences would be given by the expression $\sum_{i=1}^{n}(|x_i - \bar{x}|)$, or $\sum(|x - \bar{x}|)$ (using our 'lazy' notation). This expands to: $5 + 0 + 1 + 2 + 3 + 4 + 1 = 16$. If we divide this by 7, we get an average deviation of $16/7 = 2.286$.

This is all well and good. We have an average measure of the amount of deviation around the mean. If we look at the values for the differences in Table 2.3, we see that 2.286 is a good reflection of the amount of variation (between 0 and 5, ignoring the signs of the differences). The trouble with the modulus, however, is that it does not behave very nicely mathematically. We need to find a better way to get rid of the sign.

Statisticians' favourite trick for getting rid of the sign is to square each value. For example, $2^2 = 2 \times 2 = 4$, and $(-2)^2 = -2 \times -2 = 4$. So, let's add another column to Table 2.3 and include our new expression $(x_i - \bar{x})^2$, for each value. This is shown in Table 2.4.

If we take the average of the squared differences, we get $56/7 = 8$. This, of course, is very much larger than the previous value calculated for the average deviation (2.286) because we have taken the average of the *square* of the differences. It would make sense, therefore, (yes, of course it would) to take the *square root* of the answer we just found, that is:

$$\sqrt{\frac{\sum(x - \bar{x})^2}{n}} = \sqrt{\frac{56}{7}} = \sqrt{8} = 2.828$$

EQUATION 2.11   Calculation of the square root of the arithmetic mean for the observations given in column 3 of Table 2.4

The expression $\sum(x - \bar{x})^2$ comes up so frequently in statistics that it has its own name: 'the sum of

TABLE 2.4   Dietary Fibre Intakes (g/d) in Seven Subjects, the Differences Between Each Observation and the Mean (14), and the Square of Each Difference

Original Observation x_i	Difference from the Mean $x_i - 14$	Squared Difference $(x_i - 14)^2$
9	−5	25
14	0	0
13	−1	1
12	−2	4
17	3	9
18	4	16
15	1	1
$\sum x = 98$	$\sum(x - \bar{x}) = 0$	$\sum(x - \bar{x})^2 = 56$

EQUATION 2.12   Formula for calculating the standard deviation[26] or to be lazy about it:

$$SD = \sqrt{\frac{\sum(x - \bar{x})^2}{n}}$$

EQUATION 2.13   'Lazy' notation for calculating the standard deviation

The standard deviation is a fantastically useful and stable measure of the way in which a set of observations varies around its mean value. While you may still feel that the expression for the standard deviation looks horrendous, you now know what it means, and can put the meaning into plain English: 'For a set of n observations, take the difference between each observation (x_i) and the mean of all the sample observations ($\bar{x}$), square each difference, add the squares of the differences together ($\sum$), divide by n, and take the square root'.

TIP

If you are struggling to understand the equation for the standard deviation and how it is derived, do not despair. You may not 'get it' on first reading. If not, or thinking about it makes your head hurt, go away, have a cup of tea, and come back to it tomorrow. A good night's sleep will give your brain a chance to work out what is going on. Talk it through with someone who says that it does make sense.

If you did get it on first reading, hurrah! Well done!

squares'. This is shorthand for: 'the sum of the squares of the differences between each observation and the mean'. It is going to come up over and over again in this book. If its meaning is not clear, you need to look at this section again until you are familiar with the expression and its meaning.

Let's get back to the standard deviation. Like the average deviation, this seems to be a good measure of the average differences between each observation and the mean. Note that in this case, the standard deviation (2.828), based on the squares of the differences, is slightly larger than the average deviation (2.286), based on the absolute values of the differences. By squaring the differences, then finding the average of the squared differences and taking the square root, we give slightly more weight to the larger values.

Our expression for the standard deviation now looks like this:

$$SD = \sqrt{\frac{\sum_{i=1}^{n}(x_i - \bar{x})^2}{n}}$$

There is one final point to make about why it is helpful to take the square root of the average of the squares of the differences. When we squared the observations, we also squared the units. Thus, g/d became $(g/d)^2$ or g^2/d^2. This is a difficult unit to

---

[26]This is our first attempt at defining the standard deviation. There is actually a little more to it when we start to think about the differences between samples and populations.

interpret. It would be more helpful if our measure of spread had the same *units* as the original observations (as was the case for range and average deviation). Hence, since we squared the units at the start of this operation, it makes sense to take the square root when calculating a measure of the average amount of deviation. If we take the square root of (g/d)^2, that is $\sqrt{\left(g/d\right)^2}$, we get back to g/d, which is the unit we started with. Now our measure of deviation is on the same scale and has the same units as our sample observations.

2.5 THE RELATIONSHIP BETWEEN SAMPLES AND POPULATIONS

Life, of course, is always more complicated than you might like.

OH HELP. THIS SECTION IS *ALSO* EXTREMELY IMPORTANT TO YOUR UNDERSTANDING OF THE REST OF THIS BOOK!!

We need to refine our ideas about how observations in a sample relate to the population from which that sample was drawn. Of course, it is important that our sample is representative of the population and that we have valid measurements of the variables of interest. But our ultimate goal, when you stop to think about it, is to have the best possible understanding of what is going on in the population based on our sample observations. This is the cornerstone for the interpretation of statistical analysis.

2.5.1 Relating the Sample to the Population

At the start of this chapter, we said that one of the most important aims of sampling was to obtain a sample that was representative of the population. The reason for this goes back to the idea that we rarely have the need or the resources to measure every item in a population (except in a census).

Really what we want is to make observations in a sample that we can relate to the population as a whole using deductive logic. Only if a sample is representative of the population can our deductions be valid.

In a sense, what we are saying is that we are not really interested in the sample at all (apart from the fact that it is representative of the population and that the measurements that we make in our sample are relevant to our hypothesis and valid). We are really only interested in what the sample can tell us about what is going on in the population. What does this imply in terms of the calculation of the mean and the standard deviation?

First of all, if our sample is representative of the population, we can argue that the sample mean is likely to be close to the true population mean. It is unlikely, however, that the two mean values (for sample and population) will be exactly the same. We have already noted that large samples are more likely to have a mean value closer to the population mean than small samples. Equally important, we can assume that each time we draw a representative sample of a given size from the population, it will have a different mean value simply because we will have selected a different set of elements to measure. We will come back to this important concept in Chapters 4 and 5.

We have been referring to the mean value using the term $\bar{x}$ ('x-bar'). Strictly speaking, this is the term we use to denote the arithmetic mean of the *sample*. There is a different statistical term for the arithmetic mean of the *population*. It is given by the lower case Greek letter 'mu' (μ). It is defined in exactly the same way as $\bar{x}$, that is $\mu = \sum x/n$. The difference now is that n is the number of observations in the entire population. We can say that $\bar{x}$ (based on the sample observations) is our *best estimate* of μ (the true population mean based on the measurement of variable x in every element of the population).

Similarly, we can argue that if our sample is representative of the population, then the standard deviation, our measure of the spread of observations around the *sample* mean, is probably a good estimate of the way in which the observations vary around the *population* mean. Again, large samples will give us a better estimate of the standard deviation of the population than small samples. Whatever the sample size, however, it is unlikely that the standard deviation based on the sample observations will be exactly equal to the true population standard deviation.

Just as we now have two symbols that allow us to distinguish between what is happening in the sample (the sample mean, $\bar{x}$) and what is happening in the population (the population mean, μ), so the standard deviation is also going to need two symbols. We need one which denotes the *best estimate* of the true population standard deviation based on our sample observations, and one which denotes the true standard deviation based on measurements of every member of the population.

If we rewrite our expression for the measure of variation of values around the population mean μ instead of the sample mean $\bar{x}$, it would look like this: $\sqrt{\Sigma(x-\mu)^2/n}$. The value for n now refers to all the measurements of variable x in the entire population. You know this because we are using μ in the equation for standard deviation rather than $\bar{x}$. When we use $\bar{x}$ in the equation, you know that n refers to the number of observations in the sample.[27]

This new expression (written using our 'lazy' notation) is the equation for the true standard deviation in the population. It is represented by the lower case Greek letter 'sigma' (σ). So we can say:

$$\sigma = \sqrt{\frac{\Sigma(x-\mu)^2}{n}}$$

EQUATION 2.14   Formula for calculating σ, the standard deviation of the population

Of course, we are not usually in a position to measure every element in the population. We need to find an expression for the standard deviation based on our sample observations that will give us a good approximation of σ in the same way that we use $\bar{x}$ to approximate μ. The *best estimate* of the population standard deviation based on sample observations is given by the expression $\sqrt{\Sigma(x-\bar{x})^2/(n-1)}$, where n is the number of observations in the sample. Note that we are dividing by $n-1$ rather than dividing by n. We use the letter s to denote this expression, that is:

$$s = \sqrt{\frac{\Sigma(x-\bar{x})^2}{n-1}}$$

EQUATION 2.15   Formula for calculating s, the *best estimate* of the standard deviation of the population based on the sample observations

As we noted previously, the use of $\bar{x}$ in the equation tells you that we are dealing with sample observations (Box 2.2).

Just to note, the standard deviation of the sample is the one that we calculated when we first thought about how to compute a value of spread, given by the expression $\sqrt{\Sigma(x-\bar{x})^2/n}$ (Equation 2.13). In order to develop the concept, we divided by n to indicate that it was the average of our n differences between x and $\bar{x}$. However, this expression is of so little interest, statistically speaking, that there isn't even a special symbol for it like s or σ.

BOX 2.2

The definition of **s**
   Important!!

- **s** is the **best estimate** of the population standard deviation σ based on the sample observations.
- **s** is **NOT** the standard deviation of the sample.
- Dividing the sum of squares by $n-1$ yields a better estimate of σ than if we divide by n.
- **ALWAYS** use $n-1$ when calculating the standard deviation.

---

[27]Careful reading of any equation will help you to know if it relates to the sample or the population.

The reason why we use $n-1$ is discussed in Chapter 5 (I know, you can't wait!). Accept for the moment that you achieve a better estimate of σ by dividing by $n-1$ in Equation 2.15 rather than by n. **ALWAYS** use $n-1$ when calculating the standard deviation. As you can see, as n gets larger, the difference between n and $n-1$ becomes less and less important in terms of the calculated value for the standard deviation. But using $n-1$ will always give you a better estimate of σ.

2.5.2 Calculating the Values for s and σ

The expressions for the standard deviation that we have developed in the previous section are very good for expressing the concept of variability. They are less good, however, for the purposes of calculation. Having to calculate the mean, and then take the difference between each observation and the mean, square it, and then add the values together, is really rather tedious.

A judicious rearrangement provides a much more 'friendly' formula that gives exactly the same result. For the nerds among you, the numerator simplifies as shown in the footnote below.[28] The essence of what we need to know is given in Equation 2.16:

$$\sum\left(x-\bar{x}\right)^{2} = \sum x^{2} - \frac{\left(\sum x\right)^{2}}{n}$$

EQUATION 2.16   'User-friendly' expression for the 'sum of squares', the numerator in the calculation of the standard deviation (s)

---

[28]Don't worry if this seems a little complex. I put it in for those who are interested in the justification for our new expression:

$$\sum\left(x-\bar{x}\right)^{2} = \sum\left(x^{2}-2x\bar{x}+\bar{x}^{2}\right) = \sum x^{2} - 2\bar{x}\sum x + \sum\bar{x}^{2}$$

$$= \sum x^{2} - 2\left(\frac{\sum x}{n}\right)\sum x + \sum\left(\frac{\sum x}{n}\right)^{2}$$

$$= \sum x^{2} - \frac{2\left(\sum x\right)^{2}}{n} + \frac{n\left(\sum x\right)^{2}}{n^{2}}$$

$$= \sum x^{2} - \frac{2\left(\sum x\right)^{2}}{n} + \frac{\left(\sum x\right)^{2}}{n} = \sum x^{2} - \frac{\left(\sum x\right)^{2}}{n}$$

BOX 2.3

The difference between 'the sum of x-squared' and 'the sum of x *all* squared'.

Understanding the user-friendly expression for the sum of squares

The first term in the user-friendly expression, $\sum x^{2}$, is known as the 'crude sum of squares'. In speaking, we refer to this as 'the sum of x-squared'.

The second term, $(\sum x)^{2}/n$, is the 'correction for the mean'. In speaking, we refer to $(\sum x)^{2}$ as 'the sum of x *all* squared'.

Note that $\sum x^{2}$ ('the sum of x-squared') is different from $(\sum x)^{2}$ ('the sum of x *all* squared').

Σx^{2} is not the same as $(\Sigma x)^{2}$

BOX 2.4

Calculating 'the sum of x-squared' and 'the sum of x *all* squared'.

The first term, $\sum x^{2}$, the sum of x-squared, is the sum of the squared values of x.

- Square each value of x
- Add the squared values together
- In speaking, refer to this as 'the sum of x-squared'

The second term, $(\sum x)^{2}$, the sum of x *all* squared, is the square of the sum of the values of x.

- Add the values of x together
- Square the sum of x
- In speaking, refer to this as 'the sum of x *all* squared'

Read this Box as many times as necessary until the distinction between these two terms is clear!

For clarification, I have described the elements to the right of the equal sign in Equation 2.16 in Box 2.3, and set out the calculations in Box 2.4. I am emphasizing this particular point because these terms will come up again and again in later chapters.

We can now rewrite the expression for the standard deviation as follows:

$$s = \sqrt{\frac{\sum x^2 - \left(\sum x\right)^2 / n}{n-1}}$$

EQUATION 2.17 'User-friendly' expression for the calculation of s, the best estimate of the population standard deviation based on observations in a sample

Equation 2.17 is the one used by computers and calculators to find s. It involves much less arithmetic (because you do not have to find the mean and then take the differences between each observation and the mean). It's easy to compute $\sum x^2$ and $(\sum x)^2$ as you go along, rather than having to wait until all the values have been collected and then compute the arithmetic mean and take the differences from each observation. I refer to the method shown in Equation 2.17 as the 'short' method for calculating s (even though it looks longer), and to the expression in Equation 2.15 as the 'long' method (even though it looks shorter).

Let's work through an example using the dietary fibre intake data to illustrate how the new formula works. We will compare the two methods of calculation in Eqs. 2.15 and 2.17.

First, I have added another column to our table of values for dietary fibre intake (Table 2.5) to show the square of each observation, and their sum.

Now we have all of the values that we need to show that our two formulae for calculating the standard deviation s are equivalent:

- Sum of x: $\sum x = 98$
- Sum of x squared: $\sum x^2 = 1428$
- Sum of x all squared: $(\sum x)^2 = 98^2 = 9604$
- Sum of squares: $\sum \left(x - \bar{x}\right)^2 = 56$

If we plug the appropriate values into each of our two expressions, we should come up with the same answer for the standard deviation. I am going to use $n-1$ rather than n as the divisor, as we now know that that is the right thing to do to find the value for s, our best estimate of σ.

Method 1 (the 'long' method):

$$s = \sqrt{\frac{\sum\left(x - \bar{x}\right)^2}{n-1}} = \sqrt{\frac{56}{7-1}} = \sqrt{\frac{56}{6}} = \sqrt{9.3333} = 3.06$$

Method 2 (the 'short' method):

$$s = \sqrt{\frac{\sum x^2 - \left(\sum x\right)^2 / n}{n-1}} = \sqrt{\frac{1428 - 98^2 / 7}{7-1}}$$

$$= \sqrt{\frac{1428 - 9604 / 7}{7-1}} = \sqrt{\frac{1428 - 1372}{7-1}}$$

$$= \sqrt{\frac{56}{6}} = \sqrt{9.3333} = 3.06$$

TABLE 2.5   Dietary Fibre Intakes (g/d) in Seven Subjects, the Differences Between Each Observation and the Mean (14), the Square of Each Difference, and the Square of the Original Observation

Original Observation x_i	Difference from the Mean $x_i - 14$	Squared Difference $(x_i - 14)^2$	Square of Original Observation x_i^2
9	−5	25	81
14	0	0	196
13	−1	1	169
12	−2	4	144
17	3	9	289
18	4	16	324
15	1	1	225
$\sum x = 98$	$\sum\left(x - \bar{x}\right) = 0$	$\sum\left(x - \bar{x}\right)^2 = 56$	$\sum x^2 = 1428$

The second method may appear to be longer, but in reality it is less work, quicker and more accurate to calculate. Note that the two methods coincide in the final two steps.

This value for the standard deviation is larger than both the average deviation (2.286) and the earlier calculation when we divided by n rather than by $n-1$ (2.828). In statistical terms, this is a 'good thing'. You will see in Chapter 12 that this will help you to avoid errors which lead to incorrect inferences about whether or not your hypothesis is true.

2.5.3 Variance

It is often convenient in statistical calculation to use the formula for the standard deviation *before* taking the square root. This term is known as the *variance*. It is equal to the average of the sum of squares of the differences of each observation from the mean.[29] It is defined for populations and samples using the same symbols as before. The population variance is σ^2:

$$\sigma^2 = \frac{\Sigma\left(x-\mu\right)^2}{n}$$

EQUATION 2.18   Formula for calculating σ^2, the variance of the population

The use of μ tells you that our equation relates to the population, so it is correct to divide by n to find σ^2.

The *best estimate* of the population variance, σ^2, is given by s^2:

$$s^2 = \frac{\Sigma\left(x-\overline{x}\right)^2}{n-1}$$

EQUATION 2.19   Formula for calculating s^2, the best estimate of the variance of the population, σ^2

The use of $\overline{x}$ in the equation tells you that the observations are from a sample, so it is correct to divide by $n-1$ to find s^2.

We shall see examples of the use of the variance when we start to carry out statistical tests like the t-test (Chapter 6) and analysis of variance (Chapter 11).

2.5.4 Coefficient of Variation

I want to define one more term relating to variation in observations around the mean. This is the *coefficient of variation*, or CV. It expresses the standard deviation as a percentage of the mean. If you know μ and σ, then:

$$CV = \frac{\sigma}{\mu}\times 100$$

EQUATION 2.20   Formula for calculating the coefficient of variation (CV) based on the population mean (μ) and standard deviation (σ)

If (as is more likely) you know only $\overline{x}$ and s, then:

$$CV = \frac{s}{\overline{x}}\times 100$$

EQUATION 2.21   Formula for calculating the best estimate of the population coefficient of variation (CV) based on the sample mean ($\overline{x}$) and the best estimate of the population standard deviation (s)[30]

Because you multiple by 100 to find the CV, the final value for CV is sometimes expressed as a percentage, %CV.

The CV provides a useful way of comparing the amount of variation in related variables that may have different scales or orders of magnitude. For example, if you wanted to know which was more variable in a group of women, the intake of iron

---

[29]You may find in some texts that the variance is referred to as 'the mean square,' and the standard deviation as 'root mean square.' There seem to be quite a number of definitions of 'mean square' and 'root mean square' depending on your discipline and which statistical test you are referring to. It will come up again when we look at SPSS output. For the moment, we will stick with the term 'variance.'

[30]Sadly, or annoyingly, there is only one symbol for CV. There are no separate symbols for the CV based on the sample observations and those based on the observations in the population. This kind of inconsistency in statistical terminology crops up regularly. This is why you need to read statistical analyses very carefully, so you know exactly what is being talked about.

($\bar{x} = 10.2\,\text{mg/d}$, $s = 3.4\,\text{mg/d}$) or the intake of calcium ($\bar{x} = 804\,\text{mg/d}$, $s = 340\,\text{mg/d}$), it would be difficult to know just by looking at the numbers which set of intakes was more variable. But if you calculate the CV for each variable, it becomes obvious.

$$CV_{\text{iron}} = \frac{s}{\bar{x}} \times 100 = \frac{3.4}{10.2} \times 100 = 0.333 \times 100 = 33.3\%$$

$$CV_{\text{calcium}} = \frac{s}{\bar{x}} \times 100 = \frac{340}{804} \times 100 = 0.423 \times 100 = 42.3\%$$

Searching for sources of unexpected variation in a data set with a high CV may lead to useful discoveries concerning unusual or extreme observations. High values for CV (over 50%, say) will also help you to discover when distributions of values are non-normal, and for which other measures of central tendency and spread (e.g. median and limits of the range) might be more appropriate.

2.6 BE PATIENT AND DON'T GIVE UP

For those readers who have never tried to learn statistics before, I know that this can be hard work. The use of symbols for numbers can be confusing, especially when the same symbol is used to represent different things. We have already seen, for example, in the equations for σ and s, that the letter n is used to denote two different things, either the number of items in the population (for the calculation of σ), or the number of observations in the sample (for the calculation of s).

Frequently, the clue to the meaning of a symbol can be obtained from the context in which you see it. In this example, you would know that n in the calculation of σ refers to the number of observations in the population because the equation includes the letter μ, the symbol for the population mean. In contrast, the formula for s includes $\bar{x}$, which refers to the sample mean, so you could reasonably (and rightly) assume that n referred to the number of observations in the sample.

As you become more familiar with statistical formulae, these clues will become easier to spot. In

addition, there is a Glossary at the end of this chapter to help you remember the concepts and formulae that have been introduced.

Finally, it is important to remember that statistical formulae are tools to help you understand your data. We will introduce rules about when and where to use the formulae to best effect. As we go on, however, you will discover that rules are not always hard and fast, and that you may have differing statistical interpretations about your data according to which analytical approach you choose. This can be a source of frustration for many students. In time, you will discover that there is usually a 'best' approach to analysis. But it can also be seen that statistics is sometimes as much an art as a science (although it is fair to say that the rules cannot be bent too far before they break and that your statistical interpretation becomes invalid).

If you are in doubt, consult a statistician for clarity. As you progress through the book, you will understand how better to formulate your questions for a statistician. More important, you will understand better the answers that a statistician gives you about which approaches to take in your analyses.

Above all, don't give up. As I said in the Introduction, sometimes the presentation of a statistical concept or test in one textbook will seem totally obscure, and in another crystal clear. So be prepared to re-read sections of this book until you understand the concepts being presented. Alternatively, have a read of other textbooks (I'm not proud). The important thing is to learn how best to interpret your data as objectively as you can, and how best to understand articles in the scientific literature.

2.7 GLOSSARY

This chapter has introduced many new terms, symbols, and concepts, more than any other chapter. These are summarized in the Glossary, below. You may not remember all of them straight away, but we will return to them again and again in the rest of the book, so it might be worth turning down the corner of this page, or bookmark it electronically, so that you can find it easily for future reference.

Summary of terms, definitions, and formulae relating to populations and samples

Term	Definition	Formula or key
Populations and samples		
Population	A large collection of individual items	
Sample	A selection of items from a population	
Sampling frame	A list or form of identification of the items in a population	
Simple random sampling	Every sample of a given size n has an equal chance of selection	
EPSEM	Equal Probability Selection Method: option within simple random sampling	
PPS	Probability Proportional to Size: option within simple random sampling	
Systematic sampling	Selecting every ith item in the sampling frame: an option within simple random sampling.	i = number of items in sampling frame divided by number of items to be sampled
Stratified sampling	The sampling frame is divided into strata using one or more variables that are **associated** with the variable of interest. Simple random sampling is used to select items within each stratum.	
Cluster sampling	Items are selected from the population in such a way as to create geographical clusters, but the final sample is representative of the population as a whole.	
Quota sampling	Items are selected from the population until a given number is obtained with a pre-defined set of characteristics.	
n	n denotes the number of items in a population or sample	
N	Some authors use the upper case letter N to denote the number of items in the population. Others do not! Some statistical formulae use N to refer to the number of observations in a sample rather than a population. Be prepared to think about what N (or n) refers to each time it is used.	
Measures of central tendency		
μ	The lower case Greek letter 'mu' (μ) denotes the population mean, where n is the number of observations in the population	$\mu = \dfrac{\sum x}{n}$
$\bar{x}$	The sample mean, spoken 'x bar', where n is the number of observations in the sample. Also referred to as the 'arithmetic mean' of the sample. $\bar{x}$ (the sample mean) is the **best estimate** of μ (the population mean).	$\bar{x} = \dfrac{\sum x}{n}$

(Continued)

Term	Definition	Formula or key
Weighted mean	Calculated to generate an estimate of the mean more representative of the population when the numbers of observations in each stratum (subgroup) in the sample do not correspond to the relative proportions of the subgroups in the population.	
Geometric mean	The geometric mean is used as a measure of central tendency for data which follow logarithmic or exponential distributions	
The median	The value in the centre of the distribution of observations sorted from smallest to largest, such that half of the observations are below the median, and half are above. Good for sample observations that are not symmetrically distributed.	
The mode	The value (or interval) in a set of observations which contains the largest number of observations.	
Measures of spread		
The range and the limits of the range	The range is a single value which shows the difference between the smallest and largest observations. The limits of the range describe the smallest and the largest values of the distribution.	
Quantiles Tertiles: T1, T2 Quartiles: Q1, Q2, Q3	Values which are boundaries between equal size segments of a distribution of observations sorted from smallest to largest. There are two 'tertiles' (which divide a distribution into three equal segments), three 'quartiles' (which yield four equal segments), four 'quintiles', nine 'deciles,' and 99 'centiles'.	
The inter-quartile range	The first and third quartiles, Q1 and Q3, often quoted together with the median (Q2), to summarize the spread (and mid-point) of sets of observations that are not symmetrically distributed	
Modulus	The absolute value of a number. The modulus is positive, regardless of the original sign of the number (+ or −)	$|x|$
Sum of squares	The sum of the squares of the difference between each observation and the mean. Can be computed for populations (if μ is known) or samples (if $\bar{x}$ is known).	$\sum(x-\mu)^2$ or $\sum(x-\bar{x})^2$
Crude sum of squares	Used in the 'short' formula for standard deviation	$\sum x^2$
Correction for the mean	Used in the 'short' formula for standard deviation	$\dfrac{(\sum x)^2}{n}$
$\sum$	The upper case Greek letter sigma ($\sum$). It means 'the sum of'	$\sum$
σ	The lower case Greek letter sigma (σ). It denotes the population standard deviation, where n is the number of observations in the population	$\sigma = \sqrt{\dfrac{\sum(x-\mu)^2}{n}}$

(Continued)

(Continued)

Term	Definition	Formula or key
s	The letter s denotes the **best estimate** of the population standard deviation (σ) based on n observations in a sample	$s = \sqrt{\dfrac{\Sigma(x-\bar{x})^2}{n-1}}$ or $s = \sqrt{\dfrac{\Sigma x^2 - (\Sigma x)^2 / n}{n-1}}$
σ^2	The population variance (the square of the population standard deviation).	$\sigma^2 = \dfrac{\Sigma(x-\mu)^2}{n}$
s^2	The **best estimate** of the population variance based on the sample observations	$s^2 = \dfrac{\Sigma(x-\bar{x})^2}{n-1}$
CV	The true coefficient of variation in the population: the population standard deviation, σ, as a percentage of the population mean, μ	$CV = \dfrac{\sigma}{\mu} \times 100$
CV	The best estimate of the coefficient of variation: the best estimate of the population standard deviation based on the sample observations (s) as a percentage of the sample mean ($\bar{x}$). Sometimes (but not often) denoted as CV_s. Most of the time, CV is based on sample observations.	$CV = \dfrac{s}{\bar{x}} \times 100$

2.8 EXERCISES

2.8.1 Weighted means

A town with a population of 100 000 has a social class distribution as shown in Table 2.6. A sample of 50 households is drawn from each social class, and income assessed. Calculate the unweighted and weighted means of income for the town. Explain why the two values differ.

2.8.2 Mean and standard deviation

The following values show the time (in seconds) taken to walk 10 m by 12 patients attending a stroke rehabilitation centre: 14 18 29 34 22 25 15 22 33 20 11 21

Calculate:
a) the arithmetic mean ($\bar{x}$)
b) the Standard Deviation (s)
  - the 'long way' (using the original formula for s, Equation 2.15)
  - the 'short way' (using the revised formula for s, Equation 2.17)

TABLE 2.6   Income (£/yr) by Social Class in a Town with Population = 100 000

Social Class	Number in Town	Number in Sample	Income (£/yr)
I	8 000	50	50 000
II	20 000	50	25 000
III	50 000	50	15 000
IV	15 000	50	10 000
V	7 000	50	8 000

2.8.3 Data tabulation

A visual representation of a data set is often helpful to readers to understand how observations are distributed. Typically, you might tabulate (or 'tally') data, and then plot a histogram. While it is likely that you will eventually undertake this kind of exercise on the computer, it is useful to try it manually to understand the principles. We can use the values from the previous problem to illustrate the technique.

Time (in seconds) taken to walk 10 m by 12 patients attending a stroke rehabilitation centre:

| 14 | 18 | 29 | 34 | 22 | 25 | 15 | 22 | 33 | 20 | 11 | 21 |

a) Scan the data to find the smallest and largest observations.
   Smallest = 11 Largest = 34
b) Identify an interval into which to classify the data so as to obtain a suitable number of bars for a histogram. Somewhere between 5 and 15 bars is useful, depending on how many observations you have originally and depending on how 'smooth' or 'bumpy' you want your histogram to be. Sometimes you will need to try out different numbers of bars to obtain the appearance that you think is most helpful to readers.

First, find the range: take the difference between the largest and smallest value:

$$\text{Range} = 34 - 11 = 23.$$

Common sense tells us that if we make each band (or 'bin') 'five seconds' wide, then we will capture all of the observations in our tally. There will be five 'bins' for the tally and five corresponding bars in the histogram:

| 10–14 | 15–19 | 20–24 | 25–29 | 30–34 |

There are two conventions operating here regarding the notation for bin sizes. First, note that the values for the limits of the bin indicate seconds to the nearest whole number. This convention is more helpful than saying 10–14.999 999,…,15–19.999 999… and so on, which is not only tedious but becomes illegible when presented on a graph. Second, the lower limit of each bin is indicated using a starting number that is easy to grasp. For this data set, 5 bins would technically have been covered by $23/5 = 4.6$, and the bands 11–15.5, 15.6–20.1, 20.2–24.7, etc. Obviously, these are much more difficult to take on board than the more simple labels 10–14, 15–19, etc. Go for simplicity that helps you to accomplish the purpose of your presentation. There is more on this in Chapter 15.

c) Work systematically through the data, starting with the first observation and finishing with the last observation. For each observation, put a clash against the bin in which the observation falls, and then put a line through the observation in your data set so that you know you have dealt with it and can go on to the next one. For example, your data set and tally would look like this after the first three observations (Table 2.7):

~~14~~ ~~18~~ ~~29~~ 34 22 25 15 22 33 20 11 21

This approach is also the best in case you get interrupted during the tally – you won't lose your place and have to start again.

When completed, the tally and data set would look like this (Table 2.8):

~~14~~ ~~18~~ ~~29~~ ~~34~~ ~~22~~ ~~25~~ ~~15~~ ~~22~~ ~~33~~ ~~20~~ ~~11~~ ~~21~~

Finally, you produce a very simple histogram (Figure 2.6).

TABLE 2.7 Starting the Tally

Bin	
10–14	I
15–19	I
20–24	
25–29	I
30–34	

TABLE 2.8   The Completed Tally

Bin		No. of Observations
10–14	||	2
15–19	||	2
20–24	||||	4
25–29	||	2
30–34	||	2

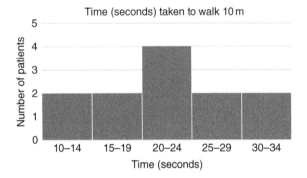

FIGURE 2.6   Histogram of time (in seconds) taken to walk 10 m by 12 patients attending a stroke rehabilitation centre.

This does not make for a very exciting histogram, but you get the idea.

Two points to emphasize: First, always work systematically through the data set, starting with the first observation and finishing with the last observation. This is far more efficient than using a 'hunt and peck' approach, in which you scan the entire data set for values that fall into the first bin, counting them up as you go along, then scanning it again for values that fall into the second bin, and so on. This latter approach creates two problems that are likely to lead to error. First, you may miss an observation on each scan of the data and miscount the number of observations that fall into a particular bin. Second, you are going to have to scan the entire data set five times, once for each bin. (If you had 10 bins, you would have to scan the data set 10 times.) This is hopelessly inefficient. And the more times you scan the data set in its entirety, the more chances there are that you make a mistake in your counting.

One last point. If you wanted to find the median, you know (don't you – yes, of course you do) that it lies somewhere in the middle interval. If you list the values from smallest to largest just for that interval (a lot less work than ordering the values for the whole data set), it is easy to find the median. In this case, the values are 21, 22, 22, and 25, so the median is equal to 22 (the mean of the two midmost values because the number of observations is even). Again, for a larger data set, this is something that you would normally use your computer for, but it is instructive to do this 'manually', as it were, to see the principle at work.

Now try this entire exercise on a larger data set. The data set on the next page (Table 2.9) is from a study of calcium intake in a group of Cambridge women 18–53 years of age.

1) Tabulate the data. Choose the number of bins that you think will make a good histogram. (**Hint** – try 14.) Define the intervals that will generate 14 bins (you'll need to know the minimum and maximum values in the data). Use sensible boundary values for your bins.
2) Plot a histogram.
3) Find the mean, standard deviation, median, first and third quartile, mode and any other statistics of interest to you using SPSS.

2.8.4   An exercise in Excel

The following exercise introduces commands ('syntax') in Excel to undertake calculations. Wherever possible, I use Excel rather than a calculator to undertake these kinds of calculations, even if I have only a few observations. First, you can see the values that you have entered (on a calculator, they disappear as you enter more values). Second, this example shows you how programmes like Excel and SPSS work in the background to give you computed results for things like standard deviation or mean or median. From time to time, it is helpful (and satisfying) to work manually through what a computer does so that you have a deeper understanding of the underlying calculations and statistics. Finally, this is an exercise in how to use Excel commands and menus to generate what you want.[31]

1) Download 'ch02exdata04' from the website and open it in Excel.
2) You are now going to use Excel to calculate the mean and the standard deviation the 'long' way (Equation 2.15) and the 'short' way (Equation 2.17) by computing the necessary values.

   a) Find $\sum x$. Look at cell B102. You use the Excel function '=sum(range)' or '=sum(value1, value2, value3, etc.)' to find the sum of a set of values. (You omit the quotation marks when you enter the formula in Excel.) I have entered '=sum(B2:B101)' to find $\sum x$, where 'B2:B101' shows the range of the values that I want to include.

   b) Find $\bar{x}$. In cell B103 I have entered the Excel function '=average(B2:B101)'. The Excel function to find the arithmetic mean is '=average(range)' or '=average(value1, value2, value3, etc.)'.

   c) For each value of x, find $x - \bar{x}$. In cell C2, I have entered the formula to find the difference between x_1 (the value in cell B2) and $\bar{x}$ (the value at the bottom of column B: '=B2-B$103'). I have completed the first couple of formulae for you in the spreadsheet.

   Click on the '+' character in the lower right-hand corner of cell C3 and drag the formula down the column for the rest of the observations. Alternatively, highlight cell C3, press Ctrl-C (to copy), highlight the remaining cells in the column for $x - \bar{x}$ (adjacent to the observations in column B), and paste the formula by

pressing Ctrl-P. The cell references in the formulae will update automatically.

   d) For each value of x, compute a value for x^2. In cell D2, enter the expression '=B2^2'.

TIP

Note that in the formula, there is a **$** in front of the row number. This holds constant the row number for that cell when I drag the cell formula down to copy it. So as I drag the formula down, the reference to the row number for x in Column B changes, but the reference to the value for $\bar{x}$ (in cell B103) does not change. You can put a **$** in front of a column reference as well to hold the column reference constant if you are dragging a formula to the right or left.

The carrot '^' means 'raise to the power of', and the '2' following it means 'find the square of the value'. (I have completed the first couple of formulae for you in the spreadsheet.) Click on the '+' character in the lower right-hand corner of cell D3 and drag the formula down the column for the rest of the observations. Or highlight cell D3, press Ctrl-C (to copy), highlight the remaining cells in the column for x^2 and paste the formula using Ctrl-P. The formula for $(x - \bar{x})^2$ is in cell E2: '=C2^2'. To copy the formula, click on the '+' sign in cell E2 and drag it down to row E101.

   e) You already know $\sum x$. Now find the formula $\sum(x - \bar{x})^2$ and $\sum x^2$: copy the formula in cell B102 to cells D102 and E102. Compute $(\sum x)^2$ in a cell somewhere near the cells where you have entered the totals for the columns. Refer to the example in (d), above, to generate the formula that will square the value of $\sum x$.

   f) You now have all the elements you need to calculate s based on your sample observations using Equation 2.15 and

---

[31]Ideally, you should take yourself off on an Excel course. Many IT departments in Colleges and Universities offer courses on the software that they support. Give up at least a day, and maybe some cash, and learn how to use Excel properly. It will pay dividends forever, even if you never use statistics again after this course.

Equation 2.17. I have put labels adjacent to the cells where you need to write your formulae.

For example, Equation 2.15 (the formula for s using the 'long' way) looks like this using Excel syntax: '=sqrt(E102/(100-1))'. Enter the formula (minus the quotation marks) in cell B111 and press Enter.

Work out how to use Excel syntax to calculate the formula for Equation 2.17 to compute s the 'short' way.

g) Check your answer using the Excel function '=STDEV.S(*range*)'. The '.S' finds the value for s based on the sample observations. All three values should be identical.

3) Use Excel to plot a histogram with 10 bars. Highlight the data from B2 to B101. Click on Insert, then the image of the histogram ('Insert Statistic Chart' should pop up), then on Histogram. Excel will paste the figure into your spreadsheet.

Tailor the histogram to make it look like the one you drew manually. First, find the values for the minimum and maximum values using Excel formulae (I have already inserted the headings on the left at the bottom of column A). An Excel formula always begins with an '=' sign. For example, the minimum value can be found using the Excel command '=min(range)'. For this example, 'range' is given by the expression 'B2:B101'. Again, omit the quotation signs when entering the formula. Second, right click on the *x*-axis in the histogram. Click on Format Axis. On the right-hand side you will see a panel that allows you to change the parameters for the figure. Play with these options to see what happens.

Does the histogram you created using Excel match the one you drew manually? If not, why not?[32]

4) Find the median. There are two ways to do this. You can order the values in the Excel spreadsheet from smallest to largest and find the average of the two mid-most values (there are 100 observations, an even number, so the median is between the two mid-most values). Or you can just use the 'MEDIAN' function in Excel without having to re-order the observations. If you haven't used the 'Sort' function in Excel before (on the right of the Home tab), play around with it to learn how to sort one column or two or more columns (especially important if you want to keep values in rows together).

Is the median bigger or smaller than the mean? What does that tell you about the distribution?

2.8.5 Sampling

Now that you have been introduced to some useful commands in Excel, we can you use your new skills to explore random and systematic sampling.

In the old days, before everyone had access to a computer, selecting a random sample from a population was a bit tedious. You would have gone to a book with pages and pages of tables of randomly generated numbers to find out which elements to select from your enumerated sampling frame. This would have allowed you to generate a truly random sample. If you were sampling 'without replacement' (that is, most of the time), it meant that if you came across the same number more than once in the list of random numbers, you ignored it after its first appearance and selected the next number in the list. Selecting a large sample became

---

[32]You will find that there are limits to the extent to which you can easily adjust the appearance of the x-axis in a histogram in Excel, i.e. without delving into the depths of the function you cannot specify the limits of the bins *and* their width *and* number. You will find that there is more flexibility in SPSS, although editing the figures is sometimes a little trickier than in Excel.

TABLE 2.9 Calcium Intake (mg/d) in 100 Cambridge Women 18–53

Subject Number	Calcium Intake (mg/d)	Subject Number	Calcium Intake (mg/d)	Subject Number	Calcium Intake (mg/d)	Subject Number	Calcium Intake (mg/d)
1	1318	26	679	51	795	76	887
2	674	27	764	52	1093	77	1313
3	1241	28	529	53	897	78	639
4	1073	29	1300	54	1101	79	661
5	703	30	1671	55	904	80	893
6	451	31	1193	56	373	81	874
7	361	32	683	57	596	82	794
8	600	33	697	58	757	83	773
9	1189	34	1025	59	701	84	1335
10	504	35	885	60	845	85	919
11	745	36	964	61	883	86	1045
12	743	37	519	62	798	87	874
13	783	38	1225	63	1688	88	1561
14	570	39	733	64	1127	89	1357
15	423	40	970	65	1253	90	1302
16	730	41	857	66	1283	91	715
17	430	42	977	67	946	92	1256
18	545	43	911	68	673	93	1087
19	861	44	798	69	897	94	871
20	391	45	1006	70	1640	95	411
21	650	46	1102	71	581	96	1177
22	546	47	929	72	1182	97	505
23	838	48	600	73	623	98	1186
24	757	49	635	74	1310	99	904
25	476	50	1002	75	933	100	749

problematic as you tried to avoid repeat numbers occurring in your list.

Nowadays (as they say), you use Excel, or your statistical software (like SPSS), or the internet, to generate a set of random numbers. If you have data from the population listed in a spreadsheet (like a set of postal addresses, or patient lists), Excel or SPSS can generate the random sample directly. This is better and faster than using the printed tables, of course, and less liable to error.

For systematic sampling, you need to take every jth subject in the sampling frame, where $j = N/n$, N is the number of items in the population (i.e. your sampling frame), and n is the number of subjects you want to select. If you want to select a sample of 20 subjects from a sampling frame of 3000 subjects, say, then you need to select every $3000/20 = 150$th subject. But where to begin? Again, you need to generate a random number between 1 and 150 **just once** at the start of the sampling process. This identifies the first element in the sampling frame to select. Thereafter, you choose every 150th element. When you get to the end of the sampling frame, you will have selected a sample of the desired size n.

The other tactic with the random number tables was to draw a physical line under the last number chosen. When you went back to the tables for more sampling, you didn't start at the beginning of the tables again (because the element of randomness would have been lost) but started from the number after the line you had drawn. In this way, you kept selecting new, truly random number sequences. Now, of course, each time you use the computer to generate a set of random numbers, they are truly random.

For the following exercises, use Excel to generate the random numbers that you need. Use the command '=randbetween(value1,value2)' to generate 10 random numbers in Excel.

a) Select a random sample of 10 values (without replacement) from the values in Table 2.9.
b) Select a sample of 10 subjects using systematic sampling. Use '=randbetween(1,10)' to identify the first subject for selection.
c) For samples drawn using the method described in (a) and (b), calculate the mean and standard deviation using your calculator.
d) Repeat (c) using the data in the Excel file *Ch02exdata04.xlsx*
e) Explore data in SPSS using *ch02e03.sav*. Generate your own syntax and output.

CHAPTER 3

Principles of Measurement

Learning Objectives

After studying this chapter, you should be able to:

- Distinguish between quantitative and qualitative data and research
- Describe and understand approaches to assessing reliability and validity in measurement and research
- Understand how to minimize threats to reliability and validity in measurement and research

3.1 INTRODUCTION

I need to confess at this point to being a dyed-in-the-wool quantitative scientist. For most of my research career, I have dealt with things that, in my view, could be 'measured': height, weight, food consumption, income, etc. Indeed, I started out as a rat biochemist, seeking to find ways of restimulating growth in animals that had been malnourished (in order to see if the same could be achieved in human children), measuring tissue growth, numbers of cells per gram of tissue, DNA and RNA content per cell, and other parameters. Latterly, I have strayed into areas where measurements are defined to a degree by convention: poverty, social class, what constitutes a good school lunch service, and the like. And in the last decade, I have come to appreciate the strengths of qualitative research, where words and their meanings and associations are of paramount importance in relation to researchers' understanding of a problem.

All of this is by way of a preamble to this chapter, and indeed to the rest of the book. The statistics and examples will focus unashamedly on quantitative measurement. Quantitative scientists like to think of their measurements as 'hard' data, as opposed to the so-called 'soft' data of qualitative research. Given that I am now a reformed character, with growing respect for qualitative research, I think this distinction between 'hard' and 'soft' data seems inappropriate. More to the point, the intricacies and subtleties of qualitative research are well described in numerous other texts [1, 2], and I direct you there rather than attempt to describe in detail their basis and techniques for analysis in this textbook. I will write a little something about qualitative research, just to provide you with some orientation as well as reassurance regarding qualitative studies.

Finally, it is fair to say this is a rather 'dry' chapter. There are no formulae, few figures, and not much to laugh at. On the other hand, many of the concepts being described are fundamental to a robust approach to scientific investigation and the successful interpretation of data. So, I ask you to take your time, and to persevere in your reading. The central ideas relate to types of research and measurement, how things can go wrong, what you need to do to avoid pitfalls, and how to start thinking about 'relevant' measures:

- are you measuring what you think you are measuring?
- are the measurements you are making the right ones for testing your hypothesis?
- are your measurements accurate?

We will come back to these ideas in Chapter 14. The exercises at the end of this chapter will help to clarify these issues, and I will try to insinuate a bit of levity.

3.2 TYPES OF RESEARCH

Quantitative research generally relies on numbers and objective measurements to test hypotheses. The nature of the relationships between variables, or differences between groups (be they human subjects, or groups of experimental animals, or biochemical samples), can be assessed using statistical tests. Quantitative research can be descriptive, but it is very often 'experimental' in character, testing the impact of an intervention on a particular 'outcome variable' of interest while attempting to control (keep constant) other relevant variables. This type of research has clearly defined explanatory (or 'independent') variables and response (or 'dependent') variables. Models for this type of research were outlined in Chapter 1. Qualitative research can also be used to explore the impact of interventions, but these are often not controlled in the same way as in quantitative studies. For example, a qualitative study might choose to explore how access to the internet has changed the ways in which people relate to each other, develop friendships, make food choices, and so on.

It has been argued that quantitative research does not always reflect reality. Often, selected variables are controlled in clinical or laboratory settings. For example, subjects may be fed a known quantity of a particular type of fat spread to a known schedule in order to observe its impact on circulating levels of cholesterol. Outside the clinical setting, not only may the quantity and frequency of consumption vary in a way that differs from the laboratory protocol, there will be other factors that affect cholesterol levels (e.g. fats other than the one being tested, physical activity, body weight) which vary from subject to subject in an uncontrolled way. This will affect the generalizability of findings based on the clinical experiment. It is the role of a good scientist to generalize honestly and sensibly, not to overstate the case, and not to let ego or the expectations of funding bodies influence conclusions.

Qualitative research, on the other hand, aims to establish the meanings of people's behaviour through language (verbal and nonverbal), and typically does not ascribe numbers to the observations. Sociological and demographic research often falls into this category. Qualitative research still tests hypotheses, but they are not usually evaluated by statistical testing or quantitative logic, but rather by the consistency of the evidence obtained and the nature of relationships that are elucidated.

In qualitative research, the bulk of data often consists of descriptive, subjective, verbatim responses. It is these that are analyzed and reported. Qualitative data are usually collected using questionnaires, structured or semi-structured interviews, guided discussion groups, and themed focus groups. Statistical interpretations are often not necessary or appropriate. Sophisticated software (NVivo, Nudist, MAXQDA, and many others) is used to contextualize and explore links between types of responses, and many software systems provide the opportunity to combine qualitative and quantitative analysis in a single framework. Numbers may be assigned to qualitative results as described in Section 3.3, creating opportunities to undertake statistical analyses of what are essentially qualitative data. But these are not necessarily a central feature of qualitative research. As is made clear below and in the exercises at the end of the chapter, not all numbers can be manipulated using quantitative or arithmetic approaches. The great strength of qualitative research ultimately lies in a researcher's ability to describe how qualitative data reveal relationships explored primarily through language.

Finally, it is important to mention that questionnaires are regularly used in both qualitative and quantitative research, and questionnaire design is critically important in both types of research. Helen Bowling has written two excellent textbooks on the basics of good question design and their testing and validation [3, 4].

3.3 TYPES OF MEASUREMENT

Both qualitative and quantitative research are likely to involve the collection of two classes of measurement, qualitative and quantitative. Qualitative data are essentially descriptive, be they of feelings, behaviours, views or opinions, or understanding of issues and concepts that inform and influence these. Quantitative data, in contrast, usually involve measurements of physical or directly observable phenomena. Quantitative data tend to be numerical. The results can usually be summarized using mathematical tools. The nature of the measurements, as categorized in Section 3.4, dictates the way in which data can be handled mathematically.

There is a degree of overlap between qualitative and quantitative data. In addition to notions concerning how respondents *feel* about things, and the appropriate analysis of language used to describe those feelings, views, or opinions, qualitative data often include simple descriptions of categorical data, such as gender, or nationality. A range of views or opinions ('Strongly agree', 'Agree', 'Neither agree nor disagree', 'Disagree', 'Strongly disagree') may be classified on a scale from 1 to 5. This can provide useful grouping of responses, and comparison of responses based on other variables (for example, to what extent is age a determinant of the way in which people respond). But there will be a limit to the way in which such data can be manipulated mathematically. There is no point in trying to compute 'average gender'; I can, of course, describe the relative proportions of males and females in a sample or population, and analyse results appropriately for each category. And while I might be tempted to compute an 'average opinion' based on the scores of the range of responses cited above, it is so lacking in information and detail about the way in which responses are distributed as to be unhelpful. Some numbers are labels (e.g. Zip Codes) and cannot be meaningfully manipulated mathematically (i.e. there is no point in computing an average Zip Code).

3.4 MEASUREMENT SCALES

Measurement scales describe the nature of the data collected. There are essentially four categories: nominal, ordinal, interval, and ratio. There are also two other ways we can describe data: continuous and discrete. Finally, when it comes to describing how data are distributed, we use the labels parametric and nonparametric. The meaning of each of these is described in this section.

3.4.1 Nominal Scales

Nominal scales provide a way of categorizing responses which are not necessarily ordered. If you ask your respondent to say what sex they are, the answers are likely to be male and female (unless you are specifically concerned with a study relating to gender and gender reassignment, in which case your range of responses might be broader). Or you might be interested in someone's city of birth, or the school they attend. There is no natural order to these responses, unless you assign one (e.g. you might subsequently choose to order city of birth by size of population, or latitude). But you will often see in data sets that numbers have been assigned to particular responses (e.g. Female = 2, Male = 1). This is not to imply that there is an inherent order to the responses. But many statistical packages (except those designed specifically for qualitative analysis) require numbers in the commands or in the data rather than words or text so that the syntax can be interpreted by the software. You can, of course, include text as part of a quantitative data set, but this may limit the types of analysis that you can undertake. For example, in SPSS, the full spectrum of the analysis of variance command (see Chapter 11) can only be captured if the groups being compared are labelled using numbers rather than text. If you want to compare responses between men and women, for example, it will be more efficient to use numbers (1 for male, 2 for female) rather than gender labels ('male' and 'female' or 'M' or 'F') to label groups.[1]

Mathematically speaking, nominal scales are the weakest, in the sense that I cannot manipulate any assigned numerical values mathematically – I cannot compute average gender, for example. That should not be taken to imply that nominal data are not as robust other types of data. They simply need to be handled in a different way.

---

[1] These considerations are important when you first design a study, as it may save time later if you don't have to tell the computer to assign values (i.e. having to tell the computer that 'Male' = 1 and 'Female' = 2). You may think it a little perverse if I now tell you that you can assign what are called *value labels* to your numbers, so that rather than having the number displayed to show results by category on your computer output, you can tell the computer to display the word 'Male' instead of a '1', and 'Female' instead of a '2'. Trust me, doing it this way round (entering data as numbers rather than text) is ultimately easier in terms of both programming and generating user-friendly (i.e. intelligible) output. And quicker.

3.4.2 Ordinal Scales

Ordinal scales are used to describe data that have an inherent order. I might choose to label portions of food from smallest to largest. The words 'first', 'second', and so on have meaning in relation to concepts such as tallest, hottest, biggest, etc. I might choose to order (or *rank*) observations using the numbers 1, 2, 3, etc. (up to n, where there are n observations in a set) in order to make clear how the observations stand in relation to one another.

A key characteristic of ordinal scales is that the differences between values do not indicate their relative size. If I were ordering food portion sizes from smallest to largest, for example, I would know that portion 2 is bigger than portion 1, but I could not say *how much* bigger. Equally, I wouldn't be able to say that portion number 4 in the sequence was twice as big as portion number 2. If I wanted to order children in a class according to their height, but I didn't have a measuring stick handy, I could get them to line up against a wall in height order, and assign the value '1' to the shortest child, '2' to the next shortest child, and so on up to 'n', where n was the number of children present in the class and the rank of 'n' referred to the tallest child. Equally, I could assign the value '1' to the tallest child, and 'n' to the shortest child.

For some of our statistical tests (especially the nonparametric ones), we *require* ordinal observations. We will look at this in detail in Chapter 7. The way in which I rank observations, from smallest to largest or largest to smallest, usually does not affect the statistical calculations, as we shall see later. You might choose to assign ranks according to the story you want to tell.

3.4.3 Interval Scales

Interval scales indicate two things. First, they indicate the relative order of observations (like ordinal scales). But unlike ordinal scales, they also indicate the true size of the interval between two values. Temperature in degrees Celsius, is an interval scale. The difference in temperature between 18 °C and 19 °C is the same as the difference in temperature between 24 °C and 25 °C. However, you cannot say that 20 °C is 'twice as hot' as 10 °C. This is because the origin (the starting point) of the Celsius scale is not zero. There is a 0 °C on the Celsius scale, of course, but this reflects the clever design of the scale. 0 °C is simply a marker for the temperature at which water freezes under standardized conditions. Similarly, 100 °C is simply the marker for the temperature at which water boils under standardized conditions. The degrees in between are allocated according to a standard amount of energy required to heat water from one degree to the next degree (again under standardized conditions). Of course, water can be made much colder than 0 °C by turning it into ice. Indeed, 'minus degrees' in Celsius can be used to describe all things which are colder than water at freezing point. Equally, I can have water much hotter than 100 °C (as steam, for example), and anything over 100 °C describes all things which are hotter than water at boiling point. So, while the interval between degrees Celsius is constant from one degree point to the next, the scale is a relative scale, telling us which things are hotter or colder than others; the size of the interval relates to a known, fixed quantity.

3.4.4 Ratio Scales

Ratio scales are, mathematically speaking, the strongest scales. They fulfil two conditions: they are interval scales (as defined above); and they have their origin at zero. Any interval scale which has its origin at zero is, in fact, a ratio scale.

Height is a good example. An adult who is 180 cm tall is 1 cm taller than someone who is 179 cm; and a child who is 90 cm tall is 1 cm taller than a child who is 89 cm. Crucially, the *ratio* of the heights is meaningful. The adult of 180 cm is, literally, twice as tall as the child of 90 cm.

All ratio scales are also interval scales, but interval scales are not ratio scales unless they have their origin at zero. We can illustrate the difference between the two types of scale using our previous example of temperature. Two temperature scales are in common usage: Celsius and Kelvin. The interval between degrees on the Celsius scale is the same as the interval between degrees on the Kelvin scale (i.e. they indicate the same difference in energy content between one degree and the next). As far as we know, nothing can be colder than 0 °K, or *absolute zero*. So, we can say that the Kelvin scale has its origin at zero. Something that is 600 °K is *twice as hot* as something that is 300 °K (i.e. contains twice the amount of energy).[2] Absolute zero on the Celsius scale is −273 °C. Using our example above of 600 °K and 300 °K, the corresponding values in degrees Celsius are 327 °C and 27 °C. Something that is 327 °C contains twice the energy of something that is 27 °C, but clearly the two values are not in the same ratio as the values on the Kelvin scale. The interval in degrees between the two temperatures is the same (300 °C) on both scales, meaning that the difference in energy content is the same whichever scale we use. But it is clear that one (Kelvin) provides us with a sensible ratio of relative energy content while the other (Celsius) does not.

3.4.5 Discrete Versus Continuous Scales

Discrete[3] scales can take only specific values. All nominal scales are discrete scales, as each observation can take only a designated value (be it text or a number) from a defined set. All ordinal scales are discrete, because the values for ranks will always be whole numbers. If your data have to do with counting the number of members in a group (children in a classroom, religious affiliation, etc.) your observations will also be in whole numbers, and so your data will be discrete.

Continuous scales can take any value within a valid range. If I am measuring weight, for example, the value might be anything from 500 g (for a very small newborn) to 200 kg (for a person who is grossly

---

[2]Bear in mind that I am not an astrophysicist, so what I am saying here about degrees Kelvin might be approved by Isaac Newton but not necessarily by Stephen Hawking.

[3]Make sure you get the spelling right on this. 'Discrete' means 'separate' or 'distinct'. 'Discreet,' on the other hand, means 'inconspicuous' or 'tactful'. These latter qualities clearly do not apply to data (whether text or numbers).

obese). Depending on the quality of the weighing scales I am using, I might be able to report weight to the nearest kg, or 100 g (one decimal place) or 10 g (two decimal places). If I am measuring children's height in a refugee camp, I might use a simple tape measure that allows me to record height with confidence only to the nearest cm. Alternatively, I might have available a more robust measuring device that allows me to report height to the nearest mm. Similarly, I might be able to weigh chemical reagents using an analytical scale in the laboratory, and report measurements accurately to 1/1000th of a gram. The value for weight can, in theory, take any value along a continuous scale; the number of significant digits or decimal places that I report depends on the quality of the measuring instrument that I am using. Ultimately, the sensitivity of a statistical test (for deciding if the difference in weight between two groups is statistically significant, for example) may depend in part on the precision of the measurements. More critically, a statistical test that is designed to accept continuous data may lead you to a false conclusion if you use discrete data, and vice versa.

Qualitative data are often thought of as discrete, but there are lots of examples where you might choose to have a continuous scale instead. Think of how one might collect information about general fitness using the question: 'How would you rate your fitness in relation to other people of your sex and age?' The answers might be discrete:

1. Much better than most people of my sex and age
2. A little better than most people of my sex and age
3. Similar to most people of my sex and age
4. A little less good than most people of my sex and age
5. Much less good than most people of my sex and age

Or I could also use a continuous scale to elicit the same kinds of response:

'Place an X on the line below to indicate where you would place *your* fitness in relation to other people of your sex and age'.

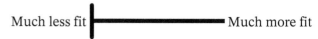
Much less fit ———————————— Much more fit

I might mark the middle of the horizontal line with a short vertical line or (more commonly) divide the horizontal line into 10 equal sections with 9 short vertical lines, just to help the respondents gauge better where they think their fitness falls. Adding lines on a continuous scale, however, tends to encourage respondents to choose only selected positions on the scale. Whichever scale you choose, try to collect the type of data that will best help you to test your hypothesis, and then use the appropriate statistical tests. Always consult with a statistician or experienced researcher before you make a decision.

3.4.6 Parametric Versus Nonparametric Distributions

The word 'parametric' is derived from the word 'parameter', a compound word derived from the Greek *'para-'*, meaning 'beside, subsidiary', and *metron*, meaning 'measure'. Sadly, this provides little insight into the meaning in statistics of 'parametric' and 'nonparametric'. I include it for its etymological interest.

More helpfully, the word 'parametric', when applied to distributions, can be taken to mean 'that which can be defined mathematically'. Probably the most famous parametric distribution is the so-called 'normal' distribution, also known as the Gaussian distribution (because Gauss was the first mathematician to describe its key characteristics[4]). It is also

---

[4] A normal distribution is defined as:

$$f\left(x,\mu,\sigma\right)=\frac{1}{\sigma\sqrt{2\pi}}\,e^{-\left(x-\mu\right)^{2}/2\sigma^{2}}$$

Don't worry, you won't be expected to remember or manipulate this, but you might give yourself a pat on the back if you recognized x, μ, and σ in the equation, our old friends: the sample observations (x_i), the population mean (lower case Greek letter *mu*), and the population standard deviation (lower case Greek letter *sigma*). π is *pi* (circumference of a circle divided by its radius), and e is the natural logarithm constant 2.718... etc., derived by the brilliant Swiss mathematician and physicist Leonard Euler (pronounced 'oiler'). (http://en.wikipedia.org/wiki/Contributions_of_Leonhard_Euler_to_mathematics)

known as the bell-shaped curve, simply because of its shape (Figure 3.1).

It is often referred to as the 'normal' curve because the distribution of many variables in the real world (height within age and sex groups, for example) roughly follow this distribution. The *x*-axis shows the value for each observation, and the *y*-axis shows how often each observation of a given size occurs in the distribution of values (the '*frequency*').

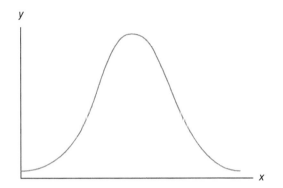

FIGURE 3.1   The Normal, Gaussian, or bell-shaped curve.

Values near the mean are likely to be observed more often than values a long way from the mean.

In addition to the normal distribution, there are other types of parametric distribution: the binomial, Poisson, logarithmic, exponential, equal probability ('uniform'), and so on. Each of these has a mathematical formula that describes them. We shall explore these in more detail in Chapter 4, as they are relevant to the statistical tests that we will encounter in Part 2.

Nonparametric distributions, by implication, have no underlying mathematical formula that describes them. This does not mean that they are not important in statistics. It does mean, however, that our approaches to statistical analysis must be specific to the type of distribution we are dealing with. Fruit consumption (g/d) as reported by male consumers aged 18 years and over in the National Diet and Nutrition Survey 2008–2011 [5] (i.e. excluding men who reported eating no fruit over the four-day survey) is a typical nonparametric distribution concerning food consumption (Figure 3.2).

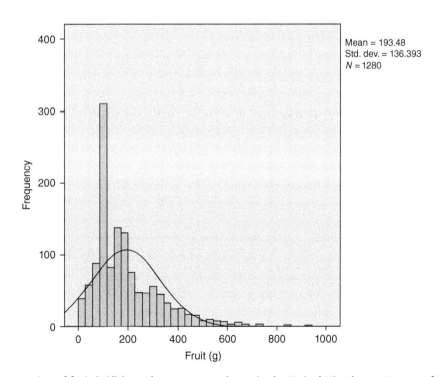

FIGURE 3.2   Consumption of fruit (g/d) in males 18 years and over in the United Kingdom, 2008–2011 [11].

The normal curve (based on the mean and standard deviation calculated from the 1280 observations from the survey) is superimposed so show how the observed distribution differs from what would be expected if the distribution were normal: there were far fewer subjects at the bottom end of the distribution than would be expected if the curve were normal (no one can have 'negative' fruit consumption, which is what the normal curve tells us to expect); there were more subjects than expected just to the left of the middle of the distribution (all the bars extend above the normal curve); and there were fewer subjects than expected in the upper half of consumption (the bars don't reach the line of the normal curve). Very helpfully, SPSS has statistical tests that you can apply to your data to find out if a set of observations can be analyzed using parametric tests, or if nonparametric tests would be more appropriate. We will explore these tests in Part 2.

3.5 RELIABILITY, VALIDITY, AND ERROR

Reliability and validity are important concepts in both quantitative and qualitative research. They can be defined as follows:

- Reliability: The extent to which you obtain the same answer using the same measuring instrument in a given set of circumstances. It is also referred to as repeatability or reproducibility or replicability. The measure of reliability is called *precision*.

- Validity: The extent to which a measurement is a true measure of what it purports to measure. The measure of validity is called *accuracy*.

We will return to the measures of precision and accuracy when we talk about measurement error. The meanings of all of these words – reliability, validity, precision, accuracy, and error – are very specific in statistics, and differ from the way in which these words are used in everyday speech.

The distinction between reliability and validity can be clarified using the images in Figure 3.3.

Let's start with the concept of 'validity' (Figure 3.3a). Assume that the 'truth' (Box 3.1) is represented by the black circle at the centre of the target.

If I have a measuring instrument that I know yields an accurate or true result for every measurement I take (say a set of scales that has been calibrated against standard weights, or a spectrophotometer calibrated for wavelength against standardized solutions), then if I use the scales or spectrophotometer according to instructions, I can expect to obtain a valid set of observations. Of course, I need to ensure that the measuring instruments are being used in a standardized way. My weighing scales should always be placed horizontally on a hard surface. If I am carrying out a survey in people's homes and I place the scales on a sloping floor or on a carpet, the scales are likely to yield an underestimate of the subject's true weight. Similarly, the spectrophotometer should be used in standardized conditions (not too hot, not too

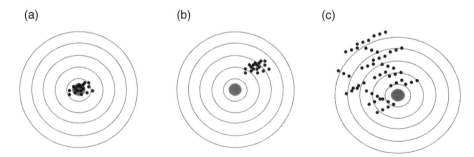

(a)   (b)   (c)

FIGURE 3.3   A graphical representation of the differences between observations that are valid, reliable, or neither. (a) Valid. (b) Reliable, but not valid. (c) Neither reliable nor valid.

BOX 3.1

'Truth'

I put 'truth' in quotation marks because we can never know the truth. This comes as a great disappointment to many students who come to a study of statistics (and science in general) hoping that it will reveal just that. We will explore this issue in Section 3.5.1 and in later chapters. Understanding how and why observations differ from the 'unknowable' truth is one of the primary objectives of statistical analysis.

BOX 3.2

Reliability is not the same as validity

Do not confuse reliability with validity!
Just because you can repeat a measurement and get the same answer, it doesn't mean that the observation is valid.

cold – the manufacturer will define the limits of what those conditions should be). If I use the spectrophotometer in nonstandardized conditions – working in a very hot or a very cold country, for example, where my spectrophotometer is not protected from the extremes of temperature – then the instrument may not yield accurate values.

Figure 3.3b represents observations that are reliable. Reliability concerns the extent to which the same measuring instrument yields the same result in the same circumstances. Suppose the scales mentioned above have not been calibrated correctly and give a result that is 0.5 kg heavier than the subject's true weight. If I weigh my subjects following the standardized procedures called for by the research protocol, I will obtain a set of results that may look as if they are valid (because they are highly repeatable), but in fact are all in error. If I repeated the measurements using the same set of scales on a second occasion, all I would be doing is replicating the error. I might mistakenly think that the results are valid (because I was able to replicate them); in fact, they are 'reliable' (repeatable) but not valid.

My favourite story to help distinguish reliability from validity concerns two thieves who have been brought to trial. They get together beforehand and agree their story. When the prosecutor says to the first thief, 'Where were you at 11:00 pm on the night of 19 December?' the accused says, 'I was in the Colchester Arms Hotel having a pint of lager with my mate here'. When the second thief takes the

stand and is asked the same question, he gives the same answer. Their evidence is 100% reliable. It lacks all validity, however, if in truth they were both in the High Street robbing a jewellery shop. It will be up to the prosecutor to calibrate their evidence against other objective measures (witnesses to the robbery, for example, or forensic evidence such as their fingerprints on the display cases in the jewellery shop window) (Box 3.2).

Reliability focuses on the performance (precision) of our measuring instrument. Validity, on the other hand, concerns the crucial relationship between the results that we observe and what we need to know in order to address our research question (i.e. the truth, or something close to it – the 'relevant' observation). This raises the whole question of: 'valid for what purpose?' We will come back to this when we consider project design and the concept of 'reference' measures later in this book.

Finally, Figure 3.3c shows results that are neither valid nor reliable. All I can say is that the measuring instrument used here was rubbish, and whoever is doing the research really needs to start again. Validation studies are often needed to ensure that a measuring instrument (a new food frequency questionnaire [FFQ], for example) is yielding results that are accurate.

I must issue an apology and a warning at this point. The rest of this chapter is 'super dry'. There are no laughs or amusing examples. No jokes or clever witticisms. I include the material because it is important that you recognize that measurements may not tell you what you think they tell you. Recognizing this basic fact is vital if you want to call yourself a scientist. More to the point, there is a vocabulary and an approach to understanding the way in which measurements may be misleading that are necessary to your ability to undertake robust research and use statistics well. So please take the time to read through these next sections and consider what they say. This will provide you with an understanding of the issues so that you can have an intelligent conversation with a statistician about how to address and measure error. You will be relieved to know that I will not go into the mathematical details of how to carry out the statistical tests discussed.

Again, if you have any doubts about whether a piece of research that you plan to undertake is likely to yield useful results, or even if you don't have doubts (maybe you should?), consult with tutors, lecturers, statisticians, fellow researchers, and others familiar with the territory you propose to explore. You could save yourself a lot of heartache (and possibly a lot of time and money) by thinking through the issues discussed in the rest of this section and understanding how you can undertake the best research that you can with the resources at your disposal. Above all, develop a healthy skepticism, keep an open mind,[5] and do your best to reach valid and generalizable conclusions that are supported by the evidence that you generate.

3.5.1 The Statistical Concept of 'Error'

Figure 3.3 raises issues about why measurements vary from the truth, and by how much. In statistics, the term *error* simply means 'variation from the truth'. This is very different from the meaning of the term in everyday language; the thesaurus in my computer comes up with 'mistake', 'fault', 'blunder', 'boo-boo', and so on. In statistics, the term 'error' does not imply that we have done anything wrong. Instead, it helps us to understand by how much our observations vary from the truth, or from what we were expecting, or from one measurement to the next when measurements are repeated. As we shall see in later chapters, these measurements of error

underpin the statistical tests which help us decide if, for example, two sets of observations really are different from one another, or if there is an association between one variable (e.g. eating school dinners) and another (e.g. educational attainment).

The underlying issue is that we can never determine the truth.[6] There are lots of reasons for this. First, no measuring instrument is perfect. Even if I use the same measuring instrument with the same subject in the same circumstances, I will come up with slightly different answers. For example, if I have a stadiometer for measuring height accurate to 1 mm, I should in theory be able to measure someone's height very accurately. But the height measurement will depend on how straight the subject is standing, the exact angle of their head, the time of day (we are taller in the morning than the evening), the angle at which I view the cursor on the stadiometer, and so on, all of which are likely to vary from one measurement to the next. In truth, I am likely to generate a range of observations that are not all identical.

Second, measurements often vary from one to the next because of minute to minute natural variation. If I take someone's blood pressure, it will vary from one reading to the next for a host of reasons – how relaxed or anxious the person is; when they last took exercise; whether they are sitting, standing, or lying down; their reaction to the person who is taking the blood pressure reading[7];

---

[5]But not so open that your brains fall out.

[6]Some people would argue otherwise. But they are comparing faith-based systems with those based on empirical observation. Also be aware that conspiracy theorists and others with a point to prove may cite selected 'scientific' evidence when in fact an objective overview of all the evidence available (a systematic review, for example) will tell a different story.

[7]There is plenty of evidence to show that if a person in a white laboratory coat takes a blood pressure measurement, it will on average be higher than if a person wearing everyday casual clothes takes the measurement. This is known, literally, as the 'white coat' syndrome. It relates to an element of anxiety that reflects a subject's concerns about what the professional in the white coat will think of them. It is a contributor to the 'subjective' and 'observer' effects that are part of the problem of bias, discussed in Section 3.6. As we shall see, the distinction between 'error' and 'bias' in not always clear-cut.

and so on. In order to get an 'accurate' reading (i.e. one close to the truth), especially for research purposes, we are likely to want more than one reading. As blood pressure readings often decrease as a subject gets used to the circumstances and procedures, the first reading may in fact be discarded, and the average of the next two or three readings used instead. Our aim in this instance would be to establish a person's 'usual' blood pressure, although as we shall see, the concept of 'usual' may itself be hard to define.

Third, there is natural variation that occurs from day to day, week to week, month to month and year to year. This would apply to blood pressure, but it is especially true of dietary measurements (food consumption and nutrient intake). Even if we had a perfect instrument for measuring diet (which we don't – I will come back to this issue in our discussion of *bias* in Section 3.6), people eat different foods on different days and in different seasons. Gradually, over time, there are changes in the foods that are available (only a handful of people in England in the 1950s ate yogurt or pizza – now they are commonplace). If I want to know what someone 'usually' eats, do I measure their diet for a few days, or a week, or a month, or one day a month for a year? If I want to generate the best representation of 'usual' consumption (which is what I need to know for each subject for the purposes of my research or clinical intervention), the time frame of what I mean by 'usual' may in part be defined by the research or intervention being undertaken.

Here are two other examples of what is meant by the 'truth'. If I am taking samples of blood or urine, the time of day at which I take a sample will have important implications for both reliability and validity. The level of glucose measured in blood taken while 'fasting' (before eating or drinking anything first thing in the day) will differ from levels measured in blood in the hour or two after a meal. Levels of cortisol typically decrease after an early morning peak, but they also vary with differing levels of stress and adrenal function. So, when I make comparisons between one group and another, or against a biochemical standard (for example, expected levels of blood glucose while fasting), it is vitally important that the measurements that I make are standardized (technique, measuring instrument, time of day, etc.) so that I can compare like with like.

Finally, on a more theoretical note, it is helpful to consider Heisenberg's uncertainty principle. This says that if we stop something to measure it, we change its characteristics.[8] In nutritional terms, if I ask someone to tell me about their diet, or to write down everything they eat and drink as they consume it, the fact that I have stopped their usual flow of food-based activity will in itself have an impact on what they report.

Using radio broadcasting as an analogy, you can think of error as noise in the signal. If there is a lot of hiss, you won't be able to hear the programme you are trying to listen to. Error equates to hiss; you are trying to get accurate results, but if there is too much error in your measurements, the accuracy of your results will be in doubt. The consequence of this is that you might fail to show a difference between two groups (when one exists), or fail to show the impact of a dietary intervention on a health-related outcome (when one exists). We will return to this problem in Chapter 12 when we look at *Power*.

---

[8]Heisenberg was referring to nuclear particles, but the principle applies to most of the natural world. In quantum physics, it turns out that I cannot know a particle's exact position and energy at the same time. The better I know the position, the more error (uncertainty) there is in the measurement of its energy, and vice versa. The more information I try and collect about someone's diet, the more I draw their attention to what they eat and drink, and potentially influence not only what they actually do but also what they choose to report. This uncertainty is different from the 'observer effect' (the 'white coat' syndrome mentioned in relation to blood pressure measurements), which also applies during a 24 hour recall, for example. In the world of nutrition and dietetics, making distinctions between uncertainty, bias and error can become very challenging. However we manage it, the main emphasis must be on how to make the best measurements we can to address our clinical needs or our research hypotheses, and to understand how the inaccuracies in our measurements may influence the interpretation of the results that we observe. See Section 3.6 for further discussion.

3.5.2 Random and Nonrandom Error

Random errors arise because of (i) natural sources of variation in the thing that we are trying to measure, and (ii) the performance of the measuring instrument itself. We can use our examples of blood pressure and food consumption to illustrate this.

Blood pressure varies from minute to minute, from day to day, and across different circumstances. So how and when should blood pressure be measured, and how many observations do I need to make? Similarly, because of variations in food consumption, how many days of dietary information do I need to collect to characterize a person's 'usual' intake? Is four days, a week, or one day per month for a year the best option? The answers to these questions will depend in part on the resources that are available, the willingness of the subject to provide more than one measurement, and the extent to which taking repeat measurements is feasible (is the subject willing to have multiple measurements made; is the subject physically available?).

Random error also includes the variations that occur in measuring instruments such as weighing scales, blood pressure meters, spectrophotometers, or dietary assessment tools. The better the quality of the measuring instrument, the lower the levels of random error associated with their performance. Random error would *not* include the elements of variation relating to 'white coat' syndrome, or because respondents choose to change their diet (or reporting of diet) based on their own internal prejudices about which foods they think of as healthy or unhealthy. (These relate to *bias* – see Section 3.6.)

Random error relates to the concept of *repeatability*: how much variation is there from one measurement to the next that I can attribute either to the natural variation in biological material (diet, blood pressure, circulating levels of metabolites, etc.) or to the level of precision in my measuring instrument? The more precise my measurement, the lower the amount of random error for a given set of measurements. I can carry out standardized tests with my measuring instrument (for example,

undertake repeat assessments of a standardized test solution to measure the variability in performance of a spectrophotometer). Or I can repeat my dietary measurements (collect seven 24 hour dietary recalls rather than four) to improve the precision of the estimate of dietary intake.

Nonrandom error relates to the concepts of validity and bias. In order to establish a measure of validity, I need to have a reference measure against which I can compare my observations. This is not as easy as it may sound. If I am measuring a subject's blood pressure on a given occasion using an automated cuff, how do I know that the cuff measurement (the digital readout on the screen of the machine) is accurate? If I compare the results obtained using an automated cuff with those from a sphygmomanometer (what we now think of as the old-fashioned manual method using an inflatable cuff, a hand-squeezed bulb, a column of mercury, a stethoscope, the doctor or technician's interpretation of the sounds, and their ability to read off the numbers on the mercury column at the moment the blood pressure sounds change), how do I know which one is more accurate? Is there another (perhaps more invasive) direct measure of blood pressure against which the automated cuff and the sphygmomanometer readings can be compared? In making comparisons between methods, I have already introduced an element of random error because I will need to measure blood pressure at slightly different time points (unless I can think of a way of collecting more than one measurement at the same point in time – which might be stressful for the subject, thereby pushing up their blood pressure – and introducing nonrandom error – but if all I want to know is whether the two methods give the same results; does that matter?). You can see how quickly the process of establishing validity can become very complicated.

The same issues apply in relation to dietary measurements. We talked above about the sources of random error in relation to dietary measurements. But the nonrandom error is much harder to identify, and potentially a much greater threat to our ability to conduct good research or clinical assessments. For example, it is now well-established that subjects who are overweight or obese or who score highly on dietary restraint[9] measurements are prone to under-report their consumption (i.e. miss out items from their records or recalls of diet). The conversation between a GP and her overweight patient that ends: 'But doctor, I hardly eat anything yet I seem to put on weight' is a good illustration.[10] All of us also have a little internal nutritionist that whispers 'Don't eat that, it's not healthy', or 'Eat more fruit and veg, it's good for you', and this has an impact not only on what we record or report but also what we choose to eat or recollect at the point at which diet is being measured. These are all examples of *bias*, a major problem in trying to obtain valid measurements. For a detailed analysis of the problem and how to address it in the sphere of nutrition and dietetics, see Nelson and Bingham [7] and Ocke and Foster [8].

3.5.3 Precision and Accuracy

Two further terms need clarifying. *Precision* is a measure of the replicability or repeatability of our findings. It provides an indication of the total amount of random error that arises from all sources (natural variation, plus the variability that arises from the use of a measuring instrument itself).

Precision, as we have said, is different from *accuracy. Accuracy* is a measure of how close to the truth our measurements are (taking into account both random and nonrandom errors). Having accepted that we can never know the exact truth, it is important to understand how far from the truth

our measurements are, and the impact that this has on the interpretation of our findings.

We have already seen how variability can be described using a measure such as the *standard deviation*. Other measures of variability can be used to determine how repeatable (precise) a measure is, and how valid (accurate). These measures were developed first in the fields of education and psychology, where the aim was to define constructs such as 'achievement' or a psychological state. These constructs do not necessarily have a 'right' answer, but being able to measure them in a repeatable way is essential if our aim is to test hypotheses. Building on the work in education and psychology, similar approaches can be used to determine precision and accuracy in other scientific disciplines such as nutrition and dietetics.

3.5.4 Measuring Reliability

There are four basic ways to determine reliability. All of them involve making comparisons – either through repetition of measurements or judicious comparisons of similar assessments to assess the same construct or concept. All the tests evaluate the two elements that are likely to affect the repeatability of a measurement: consistency (the replicability of the measuring instrument itself) and stability (replicability over time).

There is no perfect measure of repeatability. The results must therefore be interpreted using common sense. If the results from the tests tell us that our measurements are highly repeatable, then we need to go on to assess validity. If the tests tell us that the measurements are not repeatable (as in Figure 3.3c), then we know that we need to improve our measuring instrument.

Test-retest. This is the simplest method for measuring reliability. The measurement that we want to make is repeated at two points in time (say, hours, or days, or weeks apart, depending on the measurement in question and the purpose of the assessment of repeatability). The interval between the time points is critical. For example, if a subject was asked to complete an FFQ on two consecutive

---

[9]Dietary restraint is defined as a tendency to consciously restrict or control food intake, whereas dietary disinhibition is defined as a tendency to overeat in the presence of palatable foods or other disinhibiting stimuli, such as emotional stress (Source: Stunkard and Messick [6]).

[10]The laws of thermodynamics are pretty clear here. Energy is conserved. If someone increases in weight (i.e. stores energy), it is, in the main, because they consume more energy than they expend. Full stop. No other reason. If they are overweight it is not because they are 'big-boned', or have 'slow metabolism'.

days, they might remember their answers from one occasion to the next. This would potentially over-estimate the consistency of the questionnaire. Conversely, if the FFQ was administered four weeks apart, subjects' eating habits might have changed, leading to an underestimate of both consistency and stability. There is no right or wrong answer here, and good judgment needs to be applied. A week between FFQ measurements or repeat 4-day dietary records during a period of likely dietary stability (i.e. two weeks that do not include feast days or holidays or parties) is probably a sensible interval for testing overall reliability.

The measure of reliability for the test-retest assessment is usually referred to as the Coefficient of Stability. However, it may reflect elements of consistency as well as stability. The test result is expressed as a correlation[11] between the two sets of results. If subjects' answers were exactly the same on both occasions, the correlation coefficient would be equal to unity (that is, equal to 1.0). If the answers were very different on both occasions and there was poor repeatability, the coefficient would be close to zero. The correlation is likely to lie somewhere bet-ween zero and one. Measuring instruments that are precise have values closer to 1.0. If the responses are categorical (e.g. 'strongly agree', 'agree', 'undecided', 'disagree', or 'strongly disagree'), a different measure of agreement (such as *Cronbach's alpha*) should be used.

Parallel forms. This approach involves having two versions of the same measuring instrument. It is used more commonly in educational settings (e.g. two versions of an academic test that ask different questions but cover the same subject matter). But it can also be used where alternative sets of question are used to assess attitudes to food (understanding what people mean when they say a food is 'healthy' or 'unhealthy', for example, or assessing opinions about the impact of food processing on public health). If the two sets of answers agree closely, the instruments can be deemed to be reliable. If they

disagree, more interviews with respondents and testing of the questions with the target audience is needed to ascertain which set of questions provides answers that best reflect the construct or concept being investigated.

Parallel forms administered at the same point in time (or, more to the point, immediately after one another), can be used to estimate a Coefficient of Equivalence (consistency). A more complex varia-tion of this form of testing (effectively a combination of test-retest and parallel forms) is the administration of the parallel versions of the measuring instrument administered at two different points in time. This will yield a Coefficient of Equivalence and Stability.

Internal-Consistency Reliability. For long forms or questionnaires, it is possible to pose very similar questions at different points in the same form. Results from the two sets of similar questions can then be compared. This is a measure of Internal-Consistency Reliability, also known as the *split-half* method. There are specific statistical approaches to help understand this measure of replicability, depending on the type of questions being asked (coefficient of regression, Kuder–Richardson [for true and false questions], and Cronbach's Alpha method for categorical responses). All of them yield results between 0 and 1 (or 0.99, for some tests). A test result between 0.7 and 0.9 might be regarded as 'acceptable', but it depends on what is being measured and which sources of variability might be influencing the measurement.

Factors that decrease reliability. Anything that is likely to increase inconsistency in responses will decrease reliability. The main factors are:

a. *Response variation by the subject.* These may be due to physiological or psychological factors, such as motivation, effort or mood, or a change in responses (e.g. as a result of having attended a clinic for treatment for diabetes or overweight), or memory.

b. *Variations in test content or the test situation*, including lighting, distractions due to equipment or noise, room temperature, the setting itself, and interactions with other people.

---

[11]We will be looking at correlation coefficients in more detail in Chapter 10.

c. *Variations in administration*: variations in the physical environment, mentioned above, and variation in the technique or skill of different test administrators (the focus of inter-observer error assessment).

d. *Variations in the process of observation*: variation in the process of scoring responses as well as mistakes in recording, transferring answers or reading of scores.

For example, responses obtained in a neutral research setting may differ from those obtained in a domestic setting where background distractions may influence responses (e.g. a television is on in the room, children are demanding attention, partners are making uninvited comments on the responses). This can be a particular issue when conducting interviews over the telephone. Often, using a computer to gather information yields different results from a telephone conversation or a face-to-face interview.

3.5.5 Measuring Validity

Measures of validity (accuracy) require an understanding of how well the observations being collected reflect what is needed in order to test the research hypothesis in an unbiased way. There are three key measures of validity: content validity, criterion-related validity, and construct validity.

Content validity is demonstrated by showing how well the content of the test or of a measurement samples the subject matter about which conclusions are to be drawn. In education, for example, the aptitudes and skills required of a subject for successful test performance must be precisely the types of aptitudes and skills the educator wishes to develop and evaluate by specific test scores. In nutrition and dietetics, for example, respondents' aptitudes and skills may relate to their ability to describe what is meant by 'healthy' or 'unhealthy'. If the aim is to understand how respondents' views on 'healthy' and 'unhealthy' foods influence food choice and consumption, we must understand how respondents interpret these terms, and ascertain whether or not they have the background and vocabulary to describe them in relation to the research hypothesis.

Measures for establishing content-related evidence require *expert judges* to examine the test items and indicate whether the items measure agreed criteria, objectives, or content. The commonly used 'face validity' is a judgment that the items appear to be relevant, but more carefully collected evidence of content validity establishes the relationship more specifically and objectively.

Criterion-related validity addresses the question of the whether your measurements agree with those of a well-specified, predetermined criterion (a reference measure). Within the general definition of criterion-related validity there are two types of evidence:

a. *Concurrent evidence* of validity is demonstrated by comparing the results with one or more external variables (reference measures) considered to provide a direct measure of the characteristic or behaviour in question (e.g. a new method of assessing body fat may be correlated with established methods such as underwater weighing). Alternatively, the issue may be whether or not measurements of height or blood pressure collected in the field are valid. This will involve comparing measurements collected in the field using your study protocol and instruments with reference measurements obtained at the same point in time (for example, comparing measurements obtained using a portable field stadiometer and scales with those obtained using a fixed stadiometer and beam balance). Blood biochemistry assessed in the field using a finger-prick blood sample and portable assessment equipment (for blood glucose or haemoglobin, for example) must be compared with standardized laboratory procedures for these same measures. These comparisons are commonly based on correlations that relate the proposed field measurements to the validated reference measures. The Bland–Altman assessment of bias is also useful for seeing if results vary according to the size of the measurements (i.e. the method might be valid over only part of its range) [9].

b. *Predictive evidence* looks at the relationship between current measurements and what happens in the future (forecasts). It is often applied to measures of academic achievement, or predictions of response to therapy (psychological or dietetic).

Whether the reference data should be collected concurrently with the test data or at a later time depends on whether the test is recommended for assessment of present status or for prediction of future outcomes.

Construct validity is evaluated by investigating which qualities a test measures, that is, by determining the degree to which certain explanatory concepts or (unobservable) constructs account for performance on the test. Studies of construct validity are used to validate the model underlying the test. There are three steps:

a. *The inquiry*. From this model, what hypotheses may we make regarding the behaviour of subjects with high or low scores?
b. *Data collection*. Gather relevant data to test the hypotheses.
c. *Inference*. In light of the evidence, is the model adequate to explain the data collected?

If the model fails to account for the data, the test interpretation should be revised, the model reformulated, or the model rejected altogether. A good example is the predictive value of dietary restraint scores for determining success in weight loss or bias in dietary reporting. It provides some insight but does not wholly explain why some people are more successful at weight loss than others, or why some people are likely to misreport their consumption overall or for specific foods. How could the construct of dietary restraint be refined to improve its predictive value?

In summary, to investigate what a test measures, the simplest procedure is to correlate it with other, previously used tests measuring the same attribute (reference measures). A valid test should correlate highly with its closest (best matched) reference measure. Validity is clearly the single most important aspect of a measuring instrument and the findings that result from the data. If standardized tests and reference measures are used to assess validity, the evidence for the validity of the test measure (the one used in the actual project or study) will be strong. Correlations for criterion-related evidence should be 0.75 or higher. Correlations between 0.60 and 0.75 could be regarded as marginal; anything less than 0.60 suggests that validity is poor.

The previous two sections should really lead you to one conclusion: it is best to use measuring instruments that have already been shown to be reliable and valid. If there is uncertainty about the reliability and validity of an instrument (there is no published evidence, for example), then you can either choose a different measuring instrument with proven reliability and validity, or undertake the reliability and validity testing yourself. The latter is a potentially long and arduous process, and not to be undertaken lightly or without adequate time or resources.

3.6 BIAS AND GENERALIZABILITY

We now know that any measurements we collect need to be reliable and valid and free from bias. But there is more to come.

The central issue in any study is not simply whether the right measurements have been collected to test the hypothesis, but whether those measurements are relevant to the wider population from which our sample was drawn. Can we assume that what appeared to be true in our study sample is also true in the general population? Statistical analysis allows us to make that leap of faith (or not) in good conscience.

First, we need to recognize that there are two kinds of validity. 'Internal' validity helps us to be confident (i) that the observations that we have made are valid, in the sense that they are in accord with reference measures and reflect the (unknowable) truth, and (ii) the measurements are the right ones for testing our hypothesis. If both conditions are met, then we can answer the question: 'Is the difference between groups, or the association observed, or the outcome of the experimental intervention, valid in this specific instance?' Statistical analysis provides the tools to answer this question.

'External' validity, on the other hand, relates to the generalizability of the findings. Are the relationships we have observed in the sample likely to be the same in the population from which the sample was drawn? We need to answer the questions: 'To what populations, settings, treatment variables, and measurement variables can the observed findings be generalized?' and 'What relevance do the findings have beyond the limits of the experiment or results observed in our sample?' The answers to these questions will depend on the design and execution of the study, especially the sample selection and the relevance of the observations in the study to what happens in the real world.

Both internal and external validity can potentially be undermined by nonrandom error and extraneous variables (confounders). Nonrandom error often impacts on different subgroups in the sample in different ways. Suppose we are looking for an association between risk of cardiovascular disease and diet. We know that a subgroup of the sample with a higher risk of cardiovascular disease will be subjects who are overweight; but this same group is likely (on average) to under-report their food and drink consumption. Our ability to demonstrate associations between diet and disease risk (should they exist) will be undermined because of this mis-reporting. More important, generalizing the study findings to the population from which the sample was drawn will be inappropriate.

The following discussion is not exhaustive. It does, however, provide indicators of the care that needs to be taken both in designing a study and in the interpretation of study findings.

3.6.1 Protecting Validity

Internal validity can be undermined in three principal ways:

1. *Instrument bias.* We have talked about this before. Improperly calibrated weighing scales, for example, would be a source of nonrandom error that would have an impact on internal validity.

2. *Bias in selection and participation.* There are many sources of bias that can reduce the validity of a study, even if the study protocol is followed closely.

   a. *Sample representativeness.* Are the participants in your study (be they people, or rats, or schools) representative of the population from which the sample is drawn? If the aim of the study is to test the impact of a functional food on circulating levels of blood cholesterol, for example, subjects recruited using an ad in the local newspaper will constitute a very different group when compared with subjects selected randomly from a list of patients at the local family doctor's office.

   b. *Attrition (dropout rates).* How many subjects dropped out of the study? Are the subjects who dropped out different in character from those who stayed in the study? If you are comparing an intervention and a control group in an intervention study, is the attrition in both groups the same? If not, how do the groups differ at the end of the study, even if they were well-matched at the start?

   c. *Regression to the mean.* This is a phenomenon that occurs when subjects are selected by choosing those with extreme values (e.g. high blood pressure, high blood cholesterol levels). When they are measured a second time, the mean value for the group will in all likelihood be lower than when they were measured the first time. The observed change cannot be attributed exclusively to any intervention that may have taken place.

3. *Bias relating to study procedures and progress*

   a. *Learning effects and survey fatigue.* Subjects may need to be skilled in certain procedures in order to provide valid observations. The length of a recording process (e.g. the number of days over which diet is recorded; the length (number of separate food and drink categories) in an FFQ; the number of repeat 24-hour recalls) may also have an impact on the way in which subjects provide information. For example, when recording consumption of food and drink over seven days, reported intakes on days one, six, and seven are typically lower than on days two through five. This represents a combination of learning (some items may be missed or mis-reported on day one, until the field worker has a chance to check the records and point out some of the mistakes), survey fatigue (respondents get fed up recording their food and drink every day for seven days), and enthusiasm to do well in the recording process in the middle. Some studies have reported findings in which the information from Day 1 of the recording has been discarded, and it is regarded as a 'training' day (Day 0, rather than Day 1).

b. *Practice.* This is similar to learning effects but exists when subjects are asked to repeat a procedure (a test of knowledge, or a method of recording). Respondents are likely to improve their performance over time. This could lead to a misinterpretation of findings by suggesting that an intervention has caused the observed changes, when in fact the improvement is due to practice and not the intervention. In these circumstances, a control group or independent validation process can help to resolve the issue.

c. *Intervention effects.* If the study involves a dietary intervention, subjects may modify what they eat (i.e. deviate from normal habits or the study protocol) or modify what they recall about their consumption because of what they have read about possible associations between diet and outcome (whether or not they know the hypothesis being tested). This is a particular danger in case-control studies, where the cases may be seeking a dietary reason for their illness or disease or condition, whereas the controls are more likely to carry on with or report diet as normal. Controls may feel less engaged or committed in terms of study outcomes or treatment effects and drop out more often than cases.

Another issue is that it is difficult to 'blind' respondents in a food-based intervention study (except in a very limited range of circumstances, for example where the intervention is a smoothie with different ingredients [e.g. fatty acid content] but similar colour, taste and texture). Respondents may therefore know whether or not they are in an active treatment or placebo group, which may in turn affect either their dietary behaviour or reporting.

d. *Standardization and randomization of procedures.* Even when interviewers or clinicians have been thoroughly trained, differences in performance between observers may have an impact on the observations collected. For example, non-nutritionist interviewers may be less good than nutritionists at eliciting dietary information at interview [10]. Where there are two or more observers, randomization of observers to subjects is as important as randomization of subjects to treatment and control groups.

e. *Causality.* Where studies are trying to establish cause-and-effect between two variables, longitudinal studies provide better evidence than concurrent measurements, provided confounding variables are taken properly into account. Variables measured at the same point in time (increases in take up of school lunch and improvements in pupil attainment, for example) may show a positive association, but that doesn't necessarily mean the association is causative.

External validity (generalizability, or population external validity) is potentially affected by the three adverse influences on internal validity listed above, especially selection and participation biases. But there are other causes of poor external validity that can have an adverse impact on both the representativeness of the findings and their generalizability.

1. *Interaction effects.* The aim of most research is to generalize the observations or treatment to persons beyond the ones studied. Assessing the relationship between **diet and health** status or academic outcomes in a single class of Year 6 pupils from one school in London will clearly not be representative of all Year 6 pupils in all communities in England, as the intelligence, socio-economic status, and other characteristics of the pupils are likely to have an impact on the outcome of your study. Moreover, if one particular group of pupils in the class failed to complete all of the measurements (pupils with high levels of absenteeism, for example), this would also have an adverse impact on the generalizability. Random sampling of subjects from a variety of classes and schools (rather than taking the whole of one class from a single school) would help to improve generalizability. Staged or cluster sampling (randomly select schools, then classes within schools, then pupils within classes) would further improve generalizability (with the proviso that dropout rates were low, and similar across all schools).

2. *Confounding.* Confounding exists when the apparent association between an explanatory variable (dietary exposure, say) and an outcome variable (a health-related measure such as obesity or cardiovascular disease, for example) is actually explained by another variable that you may (or may not) have mea-

sured. Suppose you were testing the hypothesis that reducing high levels of short-chain fatty acid intake are associated with reduced serum low-density lipoproteins (LDL). You could look at this cross-sectionally (take a sample of men aged 45–54 at last birthday), or you could undertake an intervention study (change the nature of their fatty acid intake and see if their LDL changes).[12]

Let's say you choose to undertake a two-sample parallel intervention trial (see Chapter 1, Figure 1.3). You use your local family doctor's list of patients as a sampling frame, because you assume that the physiological reactions to changes in diet of the men in your local surgery would be representative of other men living in similar circumstances in your country. After sampling, the two groups of men are very similar for age, body mass index, socio-economic status and smoking. All of these variables are potential confounders. Each one of them is associated with both the exposure (the type of diet that your subjects consume) *and* the outcome measure – the serum LDL levels. A true confounder is always associated with both exposure and outcome. There may also be an interplay between confounders that makes their individual roles harder to identify (e.g. the relationship between socio-economic status, body mass index, and smoking).

You carry out your study over six months and demonstrate a statistically significant finding which shows that your treatment (reducing dietary short-chain fatty acid intake) has a beneficial impact on LDL levels compared with a placebo. Cooperation rates are similar in both groups, and at the end of the study the average age, BMI, socio-economic status, and smoking levels are still the same. But have you measured all of the potential confounders? What if, just by chance, a group of men in your treatment group decided to get fitter, and began training for a 10k charity run? Higher physical activity levels are associated with reduced serum LDL levels. If you didn't measure physical activity in your study, then the findings might

---

[12]Have a look at Chapter 1 for ideas on possible study designs.

overstate the association, not because you hadn't done the study properly, but because another factor (increased physical activity levels in the treatment group) explained at least part of the association observed between diet and LDL levels.

3. *Learning effects, practice, and fatigue.* The same issues that affect internal validity can also affect external validity. Pretesting, practice sessions, and survey fatigue may alter the way in which subjects in a study record information or respond to experimental treatments. As a result, what you observe in your study sample may be different from what is observed in un-pretested persons in the population from which the sample was drawn. For example, tests of cognitive function (CF) are designed such that different versions of the same test can be used to assess changes in CF over time. Performance in the second test, however, may benefit from having done the test previously, because the subject knows what to expect. Therefore it may not be valid to compare groups that have completed a particular type of test in previous research and groups that have not. Similarly, findings from groups who are regularly tested (e.g. taste panels) may not be generalizable to the population.

4. *Ecological external validity.* The word 'ecological' refers, in research terms, to the environment in which the observations are collected. We have already noted that the presence of an observer and experimental equipment may alter subjects' behaviour and outcomes. The *Hawthorne effect* refers to the tendency for people to act differently simply because they realize they are subjects in research. The *'John Henry'* effect refers to a situation when control groups discover their status and alter their behaviour to match that of the intervention groups (or, perversely, heighten their differences). Because the circumstances which occur in the research will not be replicated in the wider world, the impact of these effects will be to reduce the generalizability of the research findings in the population from which the sample was drawn.

5. *Multiple-treatment interference.* In Figure 1.5 (Randomized placebo-controlled cross-over trial), there is a 'washout period' in which the impact of any intervention in the first part of the study is allowed to dissipate before the alternate intervention (active treatment or placebo) is administered in the second part. But what if the active treatment results in a change which is not reversible (either within the timeframe of the study, or the effect is permanent)? Similarly, if a prior treatment (either within the scope of the research, or prior to the onset of the research) interacts with the active treatment within the research study, then the outcomes may be difficult to interpret. For example, in a dietary intervention study to improve outcomes for bowel cancer patients, the stage of the disease, surgery, and different types of chemotherapy or radiotherapy, are all likely to have an impact on appetite and hence compliance with the intervention, and hence study outcomes.

3.7 RELIABILITY AND VALIDITY IN QUALITATIVE RESEARCH

Reliability and validity are issues in qualitative research as much as in quantitative research. The issues may be more complex in qualitative research, however, for two reasons. First, the notion of 'replicate measures' of variables that are constructs or concepts is not straightforward because of the way in which such variables are derived. Establishing the characteristics of a variable such as 'prejudice' will reflect myriad aspects of population backgrounds. Replication of such measurements in the same individuals is much more complex than, say, taking repeat measure of height and weight because of the large number of potential influences on repeatability. Second, there may not be a simple reference measure against which to assess the validity of a new construct. Although the meanings of reliability and validity in qualitative studies have the same underlying sense as in quantitative research, their ascertainment differs, in part because of what constitutes 'data' in each approach.

3.7.1 Reliability in Qualitative Research

Reliability in qualitative research refers to the consistency of the researcher's interactive style, data recording, data analysis (textual and nontextual), and interpretation of participants' meanings within the data set. Reliability is immensely difficult to establish for qualitative researchers interested in a naturalistic event or unique phenomena. Failure to provide sufficient design specificity can create reliability threats to qualitative research.

External reliability in qualitative research is the extent to which independent researchers can observe the same phenomena in the same or similar situations. Detailed description is needed on five aspects of the design: researcher role, informant selection, social context, data collection and analysis strategies, and analytical constructs and premises.

Internal reliability in qualitative research design addresses whether, within a single study, different observers agree on the description or composition of events. Five strategies are used to reduce threats to internal reliability: low-inference descriptors (verbatim accounts of conversations and transcripts); two or more researchers (but three or more will increase the likelihood of problems relating to inter-observer error); participant researchers (aid from an informant); peer examination of results and publications; and mechanically recorded data using audio or video recording.

3.7.2 Validity in Qualitative Research

As is the case for reliability, the framework for establishing validity can be internal or external.

Internal validity. Some of the threats to internal validity in quantitative research are not considered threats in qualitative research.

History and maturation. For qualitative researchers, maturational stages can be regarded as varying according to cultural norms or historical periods. The researcher may be less concerned about what people are doing at some developmental stage than with how 'appropriate behaviour' is specified in a setting or an era and how individuals relate to these norms. In quantitative research, changes in the social or cultural framework in which measurements are collected may represent a form of confounding, especially where the aim is to understand how changes in dietary behaviours may impact on health or related outcomes. In these circumstances, a combination of qualitative and quantitative approaches may be beneficial to understanding.

Observer effects. Data obtained from informants and participants is valid even though it represents a particular view which may in part be influenced by the researcher. The influence of the observer is in itself a component of the data being collected. This issue is problematic only if the data are claimed to be representative beyond the context in which they have been collected, or where inter-observer error undermines consistent interpretation of the data.

Selection. When purposive sampling[13] is used, detailed description of the total possible sources of data is needed. The aim reflects the nature of the observations to be collected (maximize variation, minimize variation, select critical cases, etc.).

Experimental 'mortality' (attrition, or loss of subjects from a study) may be viewed as a normal event and becomes part of the data being reported. Attrition may be due to actual mortality (which might be a feature of the study itself), or more often loss of interest, or ill-health, or geographical (moving out of the study area). In both quantitative and qualitative research, attrition may lead to misinterpretation of the findings. If attrition is high, the remaining participants may no longer be representative of the population from which the subjects were drawn. Selective loss of participants, especially where losses are different in extent or character in groups being compared, can have a profound impact on the generalizability of the findings.

Alternative explanations need to be delineated (and are legitimized) through the search for bias or contamination during data collection and analysis.

---

[13]Purposive sampling, also known as judgmental, selective or subjective sampling, is a type of nonprobability sampling technique. http://dissertation.laerd.com/purposive-sampling.php

External validity Many qualitative studies use a form of case study design in which a single case, or even a group of cases, is not treated as a probability sample of the larger population. The aim in such studies is to characterize the nature of the phenomena being investigated and to understand its bearing on wider issues such as attitude, compliance, psychological state, or other subjective matters. Thus, threats to external validity for a qualitative study are those effects which limit its usefulness: *comparability* and *translatability*.

Comparability refers to the degree to which the research components are adequately described and defined for purposes of use in other situations. This typically involves demonstrating the extent to which measures are equivalent across a range of contexts [5]. *Translatability* refers to the degree to which the researcher uses theoretical frameworks and research strategies that are understood by other researchers [5]. (In some contexts, *translatability* refers to the ability to make translations between languages that are comparable, especially important in the context of multi-cultural research.)

3.8 CONCLUSION

This long, dry chapter has covered a lot of conceptual territory. The aim has been to provide a summary of ideas that you are invited to explore and to make the research process more robust. Of course, entire textbooks have been written that cover this material in much greater depth. Do not be shy of referring to these books for clarification and myriad examples, as they are likely to strengthen what you do and help you to make sure that the effort that you put into research bears fruit.

3.9 EXERCISES

3.9.1 Measurement Scales

For each of the following variables, name the type of measurement scale – Nominal (N), Ordinal (O), Interval (I), or Ratio (R) and state whether the

TABLE 3.1   Exercise on Measurement Scales

Variable	Nominal (N) Ordinal (O) Interval (I) Ratio (R)	Qualitative (Q) Quantitative and Discrete (D) Quantitative and Continuous (C)
Age at last birthday		
Exact age		
Sex (gender)		
Car registration number		
Height to nearest inch		
Exact height (cm)		
Weight at last birthday		
Race		
Place of birth		
Rank		
Iron intake (mg/d)		
Colour		
Postal codes		
IQ scores		

variables are Qualitative (Q), Quantitative and Discrete (D), or Quantitative and Continuous (C) (Table 3.1).

3.9.2 Exercise on Reliability, Validity and Error

Get together with six members of your class. Consider one measurement per group (e.g. height, fat intake, fasting serum glucose level). Decide how you would assess reliability and different aspects of validity. Identify sources of bias and error and think about how to measure these and how to minimize them.

REFERENCES

1. Creswell JW and Creswell JD. *Research Design: Qualitative, Quantitative, and Mixed Methods Approaches*. 5th edition (International Student Edition). SAGE Publications, Inc. London. 5 January 2018.

2. Moser C and Kalton G. *Survey Methods in Social Investigation*. Routledge. Abingdon. 2016.

3. Bowling A. *Research Methods in Health: Investigating Health and Health Services*. Open University Press. Maidenhead. 2014.

4. Bowling A and Ebrahim S. *Handbook of Health Research Methods: Investigation, Measurement and Analysis*. Open University Press. Maidenhead. 2005.

5. Goodwin WL and Goodwin LD. *Understanding Quantitative and Qualitative Research in Early Childhood Education*. Teachers' College Press. New York. 1996

6. Stunkard AJ, Messick S. *Eating inventory Manual*. San Antonio, TX: The Psychological Corporation. 1988.

7. Nelson M and Bingham SA. Assessment of food consumption and nutrient intake. In: Margetts BM and Nelson M. *Design Concepts in Nutritional Epidemiology*. 2nd edition. Oxford University Press. Oxford. 1997.

8. Ocke M and Foster E. Assessment of dietary habits. In: *Public Health Nutrition (The Nutrition Society Textbook)*. 2nd edition. Wiley-Blackwell. London. 2017.

9. Bland JM and Altman DG. Measuring agreement in method comparison studies. *Statistical Methods in Medical Research*. 1999; 8 (2): 135–160.

10. Nelson M, Dick K, Holmes B, Thomas R, Dowler E. *Low Income Diet Methods Study. Final Report for the Food Standards Agency*. King's College London. London. June 2003

11. Public Health England. National Diet and Nutrition Survey. 2008–2011. https://www.gov.uk/government/statistics/national-diet-and-nutrition-survey-headline-results-from-years-1-2-and-3-combined-of-the-rolling-programme-200809-201011.

CHAPTER 4

Probability and Types of Distribution

Learning Objectives

After studying this chapter you should be able to:

- Understand the meaning of 'probability'
- Identify a range of types of data distribution
- Know how to estimate the probability of events occurring
- Understand how sample size and probability distributions are related
- Understand how to transform the distribution of a variable

4.1 INTRODUCTION

We all talk about the chance of something happening:

- I am more likely to win an Olympic gold medal or be struck by lightning than I am to win the national lottery

- I am less likely to have a heart attack if I walk or cycle to work
- Cats named Oscar are more likely to have accidents than cats with other names[1]

We can assign probabilities to certain events happening. If I toss a fair coin, the probability of it landing face up is 50%.[2] If I throw a single dice (or 'die', to be linguistically correct about it), the probability of it showing four dots on the upper face is 1 in 6. There are more boys born (51%) than girls.[3]

---

[1]Coop pet insurance statistics, 2017. What I don't know is what happens to the cat's risk of having an accident if your cat is named Oscar and you change his name to Norman.
[2]For the nitpickers: Yes, I know, there is a slim chance that it could land on its edge rather than face up or face down, so the real probability is slightly smaller than 50%.
[3]There are lots of theories about why this is the case. Male mortality is higher than female mortality right from birth, which is why there are many more women alive in their 80s and 90s than men. At puberty, the number of boys and girls is roughly the same. Go figure. The 51%–49% statistic in England goes right back to the early nineteenth century when the data were first collected.

Statistics in Nutrition and Dietetics, First Edition. Michael Nelson.
© 2020 John Wiley & Sons Ltd. Published 2020 by John Wiley & Sons Ltd.
Companion website: www.wiley.com/go/nelson/statistics

Sometimes the questions can be more complex: What are the chances that a group of primary school children given free breakfast will do better at school than a similar group of children who do not receive a free breakfast?

For a given event (the toss of a coin, the throw of a die, the birth of a child), the probability of a *particular* outcome has to be between 0 and 1. If an event has a probability equal to zero, it never happens (the probability of the earth crashing into the sun in the next 15 minutes is zero). If an event has a probability equal to 1, it always happens (we all get older, never younger). We can also say that the *total* probability of all possible outcomes (heads or tails; one, two, three, four, five, or six in the throw of a die; being born a boy or a girl) will always equal one.[4]

The main aim of this chapter is to explore the different patterns of probability that occur in the world, and to understand why certain outcomes are likely to occur. This will then help us to know, from a statistical point of view, when an event is likely or unlikely. This in turn relates to the null hypothesis, and the principle of using statistics to decide whether to accept or reject the null hypothesis.

Just before we go on, we need to distinguish between the way we use words in everyday speech to indicate the chance of something happening, and their meanings in statistics. We use words like chance, probability, possibility, odds, likelihood, and risk to talk about how often we think something will (or will not) happen. In statistics, these all have specific meanings and mathematical definitions. Make sure that you are using the right term to express the concept that you want to convey (Box 4.1).

---

[4]Of course, we need to include the very small probabilities of a coin landing on its edge, or a die landing balanced on one corner, or the birth of a child who is hermaphrodite or intersex.

> **BOX 4.1**
>
> **Definitions in statistics of terms that express the chance of something happening**
>
> **Chance**: The possibility of something happening. It can range from 'never' to 'always' and is often expressed as a percentage.
>
> **Probability**: The extent to which an event is likely to occur, equal to the ratio of the occurrence of the cases of interest to the number of all possible cases. Values are between 0 and 1. In this book, *probability* is denoted by the upper-case letter P.
>
> **Odds (or odds ratio)**: This is the ratio of the probability of an event occurring over the probability of it not occurring ($P/(1-P)$). In case-control studies in epidemiology, it is used to express how often an event is likely to occur in cases compared with controls. Values can be above or below one and are always positive (asymptotically approaching zero).
>
> **Likelihood**: A way of expressing the probability of observing an event (or set of events) given the observations made. It is estimated using the observations themselves (answering the question: 'What is the underlying model that would give rise to these events occurring?') rather than estimating probabilities by making *a priori* assumptions about the way in which observations are distributed (the probability distributions that we will examine in this chapter).
>
> **Risk**: The term encompasses a range of concepts (absolute risk, attributable risk, relative risk). Like the odds ratio, it looks at the chances of events happening as a ratio of probabilities. Values can be above or below one and are always positive (asymptotically approaching zero).

4.2 TYPES OF PROBABILITY DISTRIBUTION

Probability distributions describe the distribution of outcomes commonly observed in the world generally (and, unsurprisingly, in nutrition and dietetics). We shall look at four:

- Uniform
- Binomial
- Poisson
- Normal or Gaussian (the bell-shaped curve)

There are many other probability distributions (harmonic, logarithmic, the august-sounding Pascal, the exotic Bernoulli, and a favourite of mine the Degenerate). There are also distributions for the statistical tests that we shall learn to use (*t*, chi-squared, and so on) that are derived from these. Understanding the nature of probability is key to our understanding of how to select and apply the statistical tests that will be introduced in later chapters in this book.

The first three probability distributions that we shall consider are for discrete variables that take positive integer values. The normal distribution (and many others) applies to continuous variables. As we shall see, the Binomial and Poisson distributions can approximate the normal distribution when the number of observations is very large.

One very important fact applies to all the distributions that we shall look at. The total probability of all possible outcomes for a given variable is equal to 1.0. The coin will come up heads or tails (0.5 + 0.5); the die will fall with one face upward $\left(\frac{1}{6}+\frac{1}{6}+\frac{1}{6}+\frac{1}{6}+\frac{1}{6}+\frac{1}{6}\right)$; all children born will be either male ($P = 0.51$) or female ($P = 0.49$); children taking an academic test will have a result somewhere between the lowest possible score (0) and the highest possible score (100).[5] Throughout this book,

---

[5]See the caveats in footnote 4.

BOX 4.2

The sum of probabilities for all observations of a given variable *x*

For variable *x*,

the total probability of all possible outcomes is given by the expression

$$P = 1.0$$

we will use the upper-case letter *P* to denote probability (Box 4.2).

4.2.1 Uniform Distribution

The uniform distribution describes situations in which there is an equal probability of each of the possible outcomes occurring. When you toss a coin, you would expect that, after many tosses, the coin would come up heads half the time and tails half the time. The probability is the same ('uniform') for both possible outcomes. Denoting probability using the letter *P*, the probability of tossing heads is $P_{\text{Heads}} = 0.5$; and the probability of tossing tails is $P_{\text{Tails}} = 0.5$. Most important, the total probability is $P_{\text{Heads}} + P_{\text{Tails}} = 0.5 + 0.5 = 1$. I have accounted for all the possible outcomes (heads or tails).

Here is another example. If I throw a die, there is an equal chance (on average) of seeing a one, two, three, four, five, or six on the upward face. For every throw of a die, the probability of the die falling with any one face upward (if the die is not crooked) is equal. Again, using *P* to denote probability, and the subscript number to indicate the number of dots on the upward face, I can say that $P_1 = P_2 = P_3 = P_4 = P_5 = P_6 = 0.16666666$. Again, you can see that the probabilities of each of the possible outcomes are identical: they are 'uniform'. When I add them all together, I see that $P_1 + P_2 + P_3 + P_4 + P_5 + P_6 = 1.0$. The total probability of the die landing with one face upward is equal to 1.0.

Figure 4.1 shows the uniform probability distribution for throws of a die with six faces. The *x*-axis shows

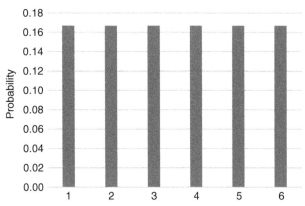

FIGURE 4.1 Probability distribution of the outcomes of throws of one die with six faces.

the possible outcomes (number 1 through 6); the y-axis shows the probability for each outcome occurring, equal to one-sixth ($P = 0.16666666$). Graphs of probability distributions follow this same format: the possible outcomes on the x-axis, and the probability of each outcome shown by the height of the line measured on the y-axis. This graph makes very clear the meaning of the term 'uniform': all the lines (the probability of each outcome) are of the same height.

4.2.2 Binomial Distribution

Some events can have only one of two outcomes (A or not A, diseased or not diseased, plus or minus, up or down, etc.). You can carry out a number of 'trials' to help you decide if what you have observed is likely or not likely. For example, if you toss a coin, it has an equal chance of coming up heads or tails. But if you toss a coin 20 times, you don't always get 10 heads and 10 tails. Sometimes you will get 9 heads and 11 tails, or 13 heads and 7 tails. You could, in theory, just by chance, get no heads and 20 tails. What is the chance of getting each of these results? If you can answer that question, then you can decide whether what you observed might have happened just by chance, or if you have observed something that deserves investigation. As we shall see later in this chapter, we can define what we mean by 'happened just by chance'.

Here is an example. You have been using a well-established programme to help obese adults lose weight. In previous years, around 60% of your subjects lose 4 kg or more in six months. In each group of 10 subjects, typically between four and eight subjects lose this amount of weight. Because your local health trust is short of money, however, you have been given additional responsibilities and you no longer have time to administer the programme yourself. You decide that the only way to continue the programme is to use community volunteers. How will you decide if your volunteers have been effective at administering the weight-loss programme? What if their success rate is 30% compared to your 60%? Would you continue using volunteers? They take time to train, and anyway, you want the obese adults in your health district to have an effective resource to help them lose weight. The binomial theorem can help you decide whether to continue to use the volunteers.

Assume the marker for the success of your intervention is an achieved weight loss of 4 kg in six months for each subject. Each obese subject can be regarded as a 'trial' (just like each toss of a coin) with one of two possible outcomes: 'success' (losing 4 kg or more in six months), or 'not success' (not achieving this level of weight loss). Say a typical group size for your weight loss programme is 10 obese subjects.

Let's think statistically. Each group of 10 obese adults can be regarded as a sample drawn from the population[6] of obese adults in your health district. Use the letter 'n' to denote the sample size; in this case, $n = 10$. We use the letter 'r' to denote the number of successes in each group. Most of the time, in your experience, somewhere between 4 and 8 subjects achieve success; the average is 6. In theory, of course, each time you draw a sample where

---

[6]Remember, a 'population' is one that you define. In this case, we are saying the population is 'all obese adults in your health district'. But not all obese adults will come forward to sign up for the weight loss programme. So maybe a better definition of the population is 'obese adults in your health district who choose to join a weight loss group'.

$n = 10$, you could have anywhere between 0 and 10 successes. What is the least number of successes to expect before you question whether the volunteers are effective at administering the programme?

The binomial distribution describes the probability that within a sample of size n there will be r observations with the characteristic which we are interested in. Although in theory r could take any value between 0 and n, common sense tells us that r in our sample is likely to reflect the characteristic in the population from which the sample was drawn. The proportion of the characteristic of interest in the population (in this case, 60% with successful weight loss, or 0.60) is denoted by the Greek letter π.[7]

Table 4.1 shows the probabilities of observing a given number of successes in any sample of 10 subjects drawn from a population in which $\pi = 0.6$.

The number of successes (between 0 and 10) is shown in the first column. The probability of observing that outcome, based on the binomial distribution, is shown in the second column. Look in the first column at the row headed '6'. The second column shows that the probability of observing 6 successes in a group of 10 subjects is $P = 0.2508$. Put another way, around one quarter of the time (0.2508, or 25.08% of all possible outcomes) you would expect 6 out of 10 subjects to be successful in losing weight. In other samples of 10 subjects, you might have only 4 successes ($P = 0.1115$ or 11.15%, i.e. just over one tenth of the time) or 5 successes ($P = 0.2007$ or 20.07%, i.e. around one-fifth of the time). Other times, you might achieve 7 or 8 successes ($P = 0.2150$ or $P = 0.1209$, respectively). These probabilities represent the proportion of samples (when $n = 10$) drawn from a population in which $\pi = 0.6$ that you would expect to see with a given value for r, allowing for random sampling variation.

The probabilities are shown graphically in Figure 4.2. As you can see, the greatest probabilities

---

[7]This use of π is different from the conventional use to indicate the value 3.1415926…, the ratio of the circumference to the diameter of a circle. As with the values for the population mean (μ) and the population standard deviation (σ), the Greek letter is used to denote what is happening in the population.

TABLE 4.1 Probabilities of 'Success' in Samples Where $n = 10$ and $\pi = 0.6$, Based on the Binomial Distribution

Number of Subjects Losing 4 kg or More in Six Months	Probability of Outcome for a Given r	Cumulative Probability of Outcome for a Given r
r	P	$P_{cumulative}$
0	0.0001	0.0001
1	0.0016	0.0017
2	0.0106	0.0123
3	0.0425	0.0548
4	0.1115	0.1662
5	0.2007	0.3669
6	0.2508	0.6177
7	0.2150	0.8327
8	0.1209	0.9536
9	0.0403	0.9940
10	0.0060	1.0000
Total	1.0000	

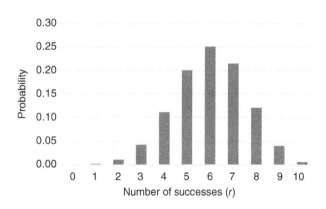

FIGURE 4.2 Probability distribution of the number of 'successes' (r) in samples where $n = 10$ and $\pi = 0.6$.

are for samples in which $r = 5$, 6, or 7, and least for samples where $r = 0$, 1, 2, 3, 9, or 10. This makes intuitive sense, given that $\pi = 0.6$. Note that the distribution is not symmetrical.

Now we have a tool that can help us decide if the volunteers are doing well enough to allow them to continue administering the weight loss programme. If they typically manage 4 or more successes, you might say that is good enough for them to carry on, because their results are within what you would expect to see if you yourself were administering the programme. But suppose they typically achieved only 3 successes or fewer ($P_{cumulative} = 0.0548$). Based on your own experience, this is a result that you would expect to see only around 5% of the time. If that was the best they could do, you might say 'that's not good enough', and choose to adopt a different approach to providing weight loss services. Now you have a statistical analysis of what you observed to make a rational judgement about what to do, instead of just saying 'I don't think 3 successes out of 10 is good enough'.

There are two more points to make before we leave this discussion of the binomial distribution. There is, of course, a formula for calculating the probability of finding r objects with the chosen characteristic in a sample of n observations drawn from a population in which π represents the proportion of objects with the chosen characteristic (Formula 4.1). (I just re-read the previous sentence and realize it contains quite a lot of information. You might want to read it again, just to make sure you follow what I am saying.)

$$\text{Probability of } r = \binom{n}{r} \pi^r \left(1 - \pi\right)^{n-r}$$

EQUATION 4.1   The binomial formula

I used this formula to calculate the probabilities in Table 4.1.[8]

The first expression to the right of the equals sign, $\binom{n}{r}$, is known as the binomial coefficient. It is spoken 'n choose r'. It means, 'Given a set of n observations, how many ways are there to choose r items from the set'. The binomial coefficients are given in Pascal's triangle.[9] Pascal was not the first to develop the coefficients, but he was the first to apply them to this calculation of

probabilities. I will not challenge your patience or mathematical aptitude by showing you exactly how he did this. Suffice to know that Appendix A1 shows you the *cumulative* probability P for all values of r in sample sizes from 1 to 20, for values of π (the proportion of objects with the chosen characteristic in the population) from 0.05 to 0.95, in 0.05 increments. The cumulative probabilities are generally more useful than the probabilities associated with a given value for r.

In the example above concerning the weight loss groups, we might want to ask, 'What is the probability of a volunteer achieving success with 3 *or fewer* subjects (rather than exactly three subjects) when the expectation was that they would achieve 6?' Look in Appendix A1.

_____

Pascal's Triangle for the first six rows looks like this:

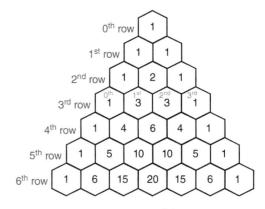

The values in each row relate to $\binom{n}{r}$ ('n choose r'), where n is the row number and r corresponds to the position of the binomial coefficient in the row. Look at the third row, for example. Let's say $n = 3$. How many ways can we choose r items out of 3? Say $r = 0$. There is only one way to choose zero items out of 3 (I don't choose any of them), hence the value for $\binom{3}{0}$ in the first cell in the row is equal to 1. There are three ways to choose one item out of three (I can choose the first item, or the second item, or the third item), hence the value for $\binom{3}{1} = 3$. There are three ways to choose two items out of three: the first and second, the second and third, and the first and third, so $\binom{3}{2} = 3$. And there is one way to choose three items of out of three: I choose them all, so $\binom{3}{3} = 1$.

You now begin to appreciate why I put this in a footnote. You can read more about Pascal's triangle and how it is created (there's a nice little graphic) on Wikipedia: https://en.wikipedia.org/wiki/Pascal%27s_triangle

_____

[8] I confess I did not work these out manually – I used Excel.
[9] I put this in a footnote because it is not essential for your understanding of the binomial distribution, but it is here for those of us who like this kind of thing.

Find the block of values where $n = 10$. Now find the row where $r = 3$, the average rate of success of your community volunteers. Read across to the column headed 0.6, the proportion of outcomes you are expecting in your sample if it is drawn from a population in which the success rate in achieving weight loss is 60% (that is, $p = 0.6$). The value for P, that is, the probability of the outcome observed in the volunteer groups, is $P = 0.0548$. This is equal to the sum of the first four rows in Table 4.1, and corresponds to the value in the binomial table (Appendix A1) for $n = 10$, $r = 3$, and $\pi = 0.60$.[10]

The other point to make is that you may not know the value for π (the true proportion of objects with the chosen characteristic in the population). If you don't know π, you can estimate it based on sample observations, and call it p.[11] Lower-case p denotes the proportion of objects with the chosen characteristic observed in a single sample (where $p = r/n$) or over several samples whose results are combined:

$$p = \frac{\sum r}{\sum n}, \text{ where } \sum r = r_1 + r_2 + r_3 + \cdots + r_i$$
$$\text{and } \sum n = n_1 + n_2 + n_3 + \cdots + n_i$$

EQUATION 4.2 Estimating p based on sample observations where the numeric subscript denotes the results from a specific sample (1, 2, 3, etc.) and i is the number of samples whose results are being combined[12]

Finally, for the sake of completeness, the *variance* of $r = np(1 - p)$, and (of course) the standard deviation is equal to the square root of the variance: $\left(SD = \sqrt{variance} = \sqrt{np(1 - p)}\right)$. These express the way in which we expect observations to vary around the mean. Note that these formulae for variance and standard deviation are different from the ones introduced in Chapter 2 which, as we shall see shortly, relate to the normal distribution.

4.2.3 Poisson Distribution

The Poisson distribution describes the occurrence of random events in time or space. Yes, it is named after a Frenchman named 'Fish'.

The Poisson distribution applies to things like radioactive emissions, or growth of bacterial colonies on agar plates. For example, if we are expecting 4 radioactive decays per second on average, what is the probability of obtaining 8 radioactive decays in one second? Or, perhaps more relevant to nutrition, if you typically had 3 referrals per month for Type 2 diabetes in adolescent children in your hospital clinic, what is the probability of getting 7 referrals in one month?

Let's consider the example of clinic referrals for adolescent Type 2 diabetes. We start by ascertaining the average number of referrals per month over the last year. The mean value is $\mu = 3$.[13] If the event (referrals) is truly random over time, sometimes we would see more than 3 referrals per month, and sometimes fewer. This is shown clearly in the Poisson distribution (Figure 4.3).[14] In this example, you can see that most months will have somewhere between 2 and 4 referrals; sometimes you might get only 1, sometimes 5.

---

[10]Of course, in the future, you are more likely to use Excel or other software to estimate P. I have taken you through the steps manually so that you understand the principles that underlie the calculation of P and that allow you to plug in the right values for n, r and p when requested.

[11]'Oh, help!' you might say, 'another p!'. One of the problems in statistics is that we quickly run out of unique letters to represent some of the basic concepts. So, the case of a letter (upper or lower case), and whether or not it is in *italics*, becomes important. Throughout the book, we will use upper-case P to denote *probability*, and lower-case p to represent *proportion*. Except when we don't – but then I'll let you know.

[12]Remembering, of course, that 'Σ' means 'the sum of'.

[13]Again, the Greek letter (the lower-case letter mu, μ) is used to denote the mean of the events (referrals per month) in the population, just as we used it to express the arithmetic mean. As with the example concerning the successes in the weight loss groups, sometimes our best estimate of the population mean can be obtained using sample data observed over the previous year or two.

[14]For the nerds. The probability of the occurrence of the observed value x, given the mean μ in the population, is given by the expression: $P(x; \mu) = e^{-\mu}\mu^x/x!$, where x is the number of events observed in a specific time period, μ is the average number of events in the time interval in the population, e is Euler's number 2.71 828 (the base for natural logarithms), and $x!$ is x-factorial ($1 \times 2 \times 3 \times \cdots x$). Sometimes the expression is given using the Greek letter lambda (λ) instead of μ for the population mean. This is not a ploy by statisticians to confuse you. It just seems to depend on which text you read.

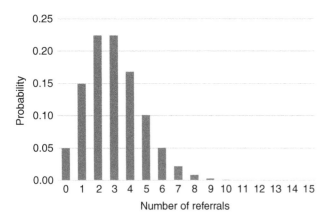

FIGURE 4.3   Probability distribution of referrals per month for Type 2 diabetes, $\mu = 3$.

But it would be unusual to see as many as 7 ($P = 0.0216$), and even more unlikely to see 8 or more (and the probabilities above 9 are all close to zero). Pause for a moment, think this through, and you will see that this accords with common sense.

Just for information, the variance of the Poisson distribution is equal to the mean for the population, μ, and the standard deviation, as before, is equal to the square root of the variance, $SD = \sqrt{\mu}$.

4.2.4 Normal (or Gaussian) Distribution: The Bell-Shaped Curve

The normal distribution is an exquisite jewel in the statistical landscape. It describes a myriad of common distributions, such as height of people of a given age and sex, day-to-day variations in energy intake, or nutrition knowledge scores in the workplace. It relates to continuous variables, but it can also be used to describe the distributions of some discrete variables, such as the scores on a test, provided the range of scores is great enough.[15] It is central to many

decisions about accepting or rejecting the null hypothesis. And it provides the under-pinning for a great number of statistical tests, some of which we shall learn about in the next few chapters.

The underlying principle is very simple. If a variable follows the normal distribution, the probability of observing a value which is close to the mean is greater than the probability of observing a value which is a long way from the mean. The exact probability of observing a value x which is a given distance away from the mean is given by a formula which relates the value itself (x) to the mean (μ) and the standard deviation (σ) of the population.[16] When plotted, values that follow a normal distribution have a characteristic bell shape, hence the other common name for the normal distribution, the Bell-shaped curve.[17] It is also called the Gaussian distribution because (surprise, surprise) it was described by Carl Friedrich Gauss [1], although other mathematicians in the eighteenth and nineteenth centuries also developed an understanding of how it was derived [2].

If a variable is normally distributed, you are more likely to see values of x close to the mean than values which are a long way from the mean. Think of this in relation to height in a group of children of the same sex and age. Most of the children will be similar in height and clustered toward the middle of the distribution. There will be some, however, that are shorter than most, and some that are taller than most. Figure 4.4a

---

[15]There is no fixed rule about what 'great enough' might be; after a time, you will get a feel for the times when you can use the normal distribution to approximate your data (whether continuous or discrete) and times when you cannot. We will look in Chapter 6 at the Kolmogorov–Smirnov test to help you decide if a distribution is normal or not. Go back to Section 3.4.5 in Chapter 3 to remind yourself of the differences between discrete and continuous variables.

[16]For the nerds: The probability density function for the normal distribution:

$$P(x) = \frac{1}{\sigma\sqrt{2\pi}} e^{-(x-\mu)^2/(2\sigma^2)}$$

What does this say in English? The probability of observing a given value of x in a normal distribution, $P(x)$, is equal to 1 divided by the standard deviation σ times the square root of 2 times π (this time we are talking about $\pi = 3.14159$), times e (where $e = 2.71828$) raised to the power of *minus* the square of the difference between the given value x and the population mean μ, divided by 2 times the variance σ^2. I promise you will never be asked to calculate this by hand. But if you put this page under your pillow and sleep on it, in the morning you will wake up feeling normal.

[17]There are, as we shall see, other bell-shaped curves, but the name is usually reserved for the normal distribution.

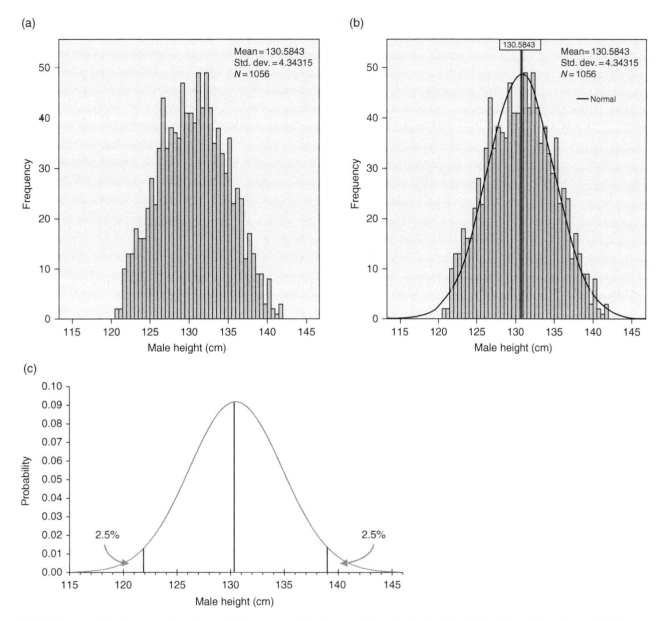

FIGURE 4.4   Distribution of height in 1056 boys aged 10–11 years living in England in 2015–2016: (a) Raw data (b) With normal curve (c) showing probability rather than frequency.

shows the height distribution of 1056 boys aged 10–11 years old in the National Child Measurement Programme in 2015–2016. This fits exactly with what we would expect to see with a normally distributed variable. In fact, we can superimpose the normal curve (Figure 4.4b), based on the normal formula given in footnote '16'. Some bars in the histogram fall a little bit

short of the curve, and some poke out above the curve. But generally speaking, it looks like a good fit.

The Area under the Normal Curve

Now things start to get really interesting and, from a statistical point of view, brilliantly helpful.

Suppose you have an 11-year-old boy in your clinic whose parents are worried he is very short for his age. When you measure his height, you find he is 120 cm tall. How can you decide if his growth is a cause for concern? You might go to the WHO growth charts [3] and plot height against age. If his height was below the third centile, say, you might want to investigate why he was not growing as fast as his peers. Alternatively, you might have data on growth in the local population, including the mean and standard deviation for children at this age. If his height was in the bottom 2.5% of the distribution, you might want to take some action. But what *is* the cut-off point for height that defines the bottom 2.5%? How can you work out if the child is in the bottom 2.5% of the growth distribution based on the local data?

You could, in the first instance, put all the measured values for height in the local population in order from smallest to largest, and find the value at which 2.5% of the children are shorter. Far more efficient, however, is to use normal theory to define the cut-off.

Think back to what we said earlier in the chapter about the total probability of all possible outcomes for a given variable being equal to 1.0. In the case of children, their height[18] measurement must fall somewhere in the distribution of height in the population for children of a given age, no matter how tall or short for age they may be. We looked at the histogram of the height data for boys in England aged 10–11 with the normal curve superimposed (based on the observed mean and standard deviation) (Figure 4.4b). The total area under the normal curve represents all the possible outcomes (height measurements) for boys in the population of 10–11 year-old boys living in England. We can say that the total probability of all possible outcomes (the total area under the curve) is equal to 1.0.[19]

The vertical line in Figure 4.4b is drawn at the mean. Because the normal distribution is symmetrical around the mean, the line separates the area under the curve into two equal halves. There is a 50% chance of a child's height being below the mean, and 50% chance of it being above the mean.

In Figure 4.4c I have dispensed with the histogram, and plotted the normal distribution with mean = 130.5843 cm and standard deviation = 4.343 15 cm. Instead of *frequency* on the y-axis, I have shown the *probability*[20] of each observation occurring using the normal probability density function given in footnote '16'.[21] In addition to the vertical line at the mean, I have added two more lines which define the areas under the curve in the two tails equivalent to 2.5% of the total. How did I know where to draw these lines?

Calculation of Areas under the Normal Curve

A key characteristic of the normal distribution is that the area under the curve is related to the distance from the mean in terms of the number of standard deviations. We can generalize this idea by introducing the concept of the *standard normal deviate*, defined by the letter u. This expresses the distance of a given observation x from the mean μ in terms of the number of standard deviations, σ:

$$u = \frac{x - \mu}{\sigma}$$

EQUATION 4.3   The standard normal deviate u based on μ and σ

---

[18]For children under the age of 2, we usually talk about length rather than height, but the same principle applies.
[19]This is equivalent to saying that the total probability of all the possible outcomes for the throws of a die represented in Figure 4.1 is also equal to 1.0.

[20]You will also see this axis labelled as *probability density* or *probability density function*.
[21]I have not done this manually for 1056 observations. Instead, I used Excel to compute the values using the formula in footnote 16. I put the height data in column A. In cell B1 I typed the command: '=NORM.DIST(A1,130.4843,4.34315,FALSE).' This returns the probability of occurrence of the observation in Column A, row 1, for a given mean and standard deviation, assuming the variable is normally distributed. I dragged the formula in B1 down Column B to get a probability for each observation in Column A. The term 'FALSE' makes the function return the probability of a given observation occurring. The word 'TRUE' would return the cumulative probability from the lowest to the highest value. We will come back to this concept shortly.

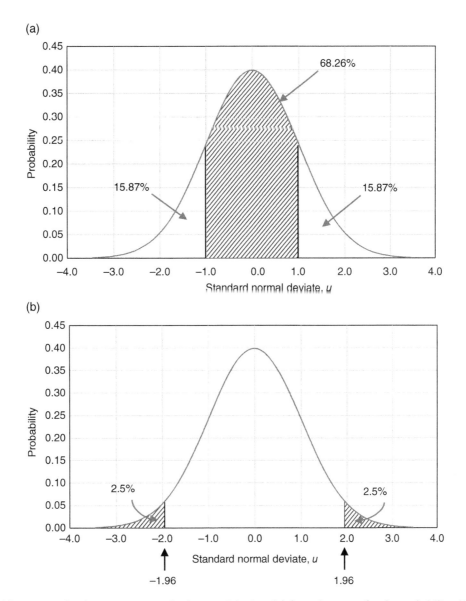

FIGURE 4.5   (a) Areas under the curve ±1 standard normal deviate (u) from the mean for the probability distribution of a normally distributed variable with mean (μ) and standard deviation (σ). (b) Areas under the curve more than ±1.96 standard normal deviates (u) away from the mean for the probability distribution of a normally distributed variable with mean (μ) and standard deviation (σ).

We can then talk about the areas in the tails of the normal distribution in relation to the values for u. For example, 68.26% of the area under the curve (that is, 68.26% of all possible outcomes for the variable x) lies between ±1.0 standard deviation (standard normal deviates) on either side of the mean. This means that 15.87% of the area under the

curve[22] lies 1.0 standard deviation or more above the mean. The remaining 15.87% of the area under the curve lies −1.0 standard deviation or more below the mean (the unshaded areas under the

---

[22] That is: $\dfrac{100 - 68.26\%}{2} = \dfrac{31.74\%}{2} = 15.87\%$

curve in Figure 4.5a). These relationships hold true for *every* normally distributed variable with mean μ and standard deviation σ.

In statistical terms, there are more useful areas under the curve to know about. For example, we may want to know if an observation is in the bottom 2.5% of all possible observations (that is, in the left-hand tail of the curve for a normally distributed variable). Or in the bottom 1%, or 0.1%. If we know x, μ and σ, we can compute u, and refer to the cut-off points for the values of u given in Table 4.2.

For example, Table 4.2 tells us that 5% of the area under the curve lies outside ±1.96 standard deviations (standard normal deviates [u]) on either side of the mean, and 95% of the area under the curve lies between these two values. If the total area outside these limits is 5%, because the normal distribution is symmetrical, then the area in each tail is equal to 2.5% of the total area under the curve. So, if an observation x has a corresponding value of $u \leq -1.96$, we know that the value for x lies in the bottom 2.5% of all possible observations. If x is less then μ, the value for u will be negative, meaning that we are looking at areas under the curve in the left-hand tail of the distribution. If x is greater than μ, the value for u will be positive, and we are looking at areas under the curve in the right-hand tail of the distribution. Similarly, 1.0% of the total area under the curve lies outside ±2.576 standard normal deviates either side of the mean, and each tail contains 0.5% of the area under the curve.

The areas under the curve for $u = \pm1.96$ are represented graphically in Figure 4.5b. For a population with mean of $\mu = 0$ and standard deviation $\sigma = 1$, the shaded tails are defined by the standard normal deviate equal to ±1.96, and the area under the curve in each tail is 2.5%.

Let's get back to the height data for boys that we have been examining. The cut-off point x for the bottom 2.5% of the area under the curve will be given by the formula:

$$x = \mu - 1.96\sigma = 130.5843\,\text{cm} - 1.96 \times 4.34315\,\text{cm}$$
$$= 122.07\,\text{cm}$$

We can expect 2.5% of boys this age in this population to be less than 122 cm tall. The boy in clinic who is 120 cm tall therefore has a height which is in the bottom 2.5% of the height distribution of boys this age in the population. We might want to find out what is contributing to his short stature.

This calculation determined where I put the lines in Figure 4.4c. For the left-hand tail with 2.5% of the area under the curve, the formula above yielded a value of 122.07 cm for the cut-off. For the right-hand tail with 2.5% of the area under the curve, the line for the cut-off is given by the formula:

$$x = \mu + 1.96\sigma = 130.5843\,\text{cm} + 1.96 \times 4.34315\,\text{cm}$$
$$= 139.10\,\text{cm}$$

Areas in the Tail of the Normal Distribution

Table 4.2 is a subset of a much larger table that allows you to know the area under the curve for any value of u (Appendix A2). There are many practical applications of these values. They allow you to derive useful information about a normally distributed variable for which you know only the mean and standard deviation. Let's see how the table works.

Appendix A2 shows values for the standard normal deviate u to one decimal place down the left-hand side. The second decimal place is given across the top of the table. The values in the body of the table are for $\frac{1}{2}P$, corresponding to the area under the curve in one tail of the normal distribution, as shown in the figure on page 341. Suppose I want to know

TABLE 4.2   Areas Under the Curve Based on the Standard Normal Deviate, u

u	Inside	Outside	
		In Both Tails	In One Tail
±1.96	95.0%	5.0%	2.5%
±2.576	99.0%	1.0%	0.5%
±3.291	99.9%	0.1%	0.05%

the area under the curve (the chances of observing a value at or above the value for u) for $u = 1.96$. I find the row headed 1.9 (for the first decimal place) and the column headed 0.06 (for the second decimal place). At the intersection of this row and column I find the valuc 0.0250. This gives the value for the shaded area under the curve (out of 1.0). If I multiply by 100, I find that the area under the curve when $u = 1.96$ equals 2.5% of the total area.

There are no values in the table for standard normal deviates less than zero. But the normal distribution is symmetrical around the mean. If my calculated value for u was negative, I would find the value for $\frac{1}{2}P$ based on the absolute value of u. Because the original value for u was negative, the tail of interest would be on the *left hand* side of the curve, and I would be looking at the probability of finding values of x *less than* the negative value for the standard normal deviate. This is exactly what was illustrated in Figure 4.5b.

Let's look at an example. In the 2007 survey of low-income households in Britain [4], the reported mean daily iron intake of women aged 19–34 was $\mu = 8.5\,\text{mg/d}$, with a standard deviation $\sigma = 3.4\,\text{mg/d}$.[23] The Reference Nutrient Intake (RNI)[24] for iron for this group of women is 14.8 mg/d; the Lower Reference Nutrient Intake (LRNI) is 8.0 mg/d [5].[25] You can now use the values of the areas under the normal curve in Appendix A2 to estimate the percentage of women who had intakes less than the RNI and the LRNI.

If mean iron intake is equal to $\mu = 8.5\,\text{mg/d}$, and $\sigma = 3.4\,\text{mg/d}$, we can calculate the value for u for intakes corresponding to 14.8 mg/d (our RNI cut-off point, equal to 'x' in our formula):

$$u = \frac{x - \mu}{\sigma} = \frac{14.8 - 8.5}{3.4} = 1.85$$

---

[23]Don't forget that standard deviations also have units, just like the mean.

[24]Reference Nutrient Intake: the level of intake sufficient for 97.5% of people in the population.

[25]Lower Reference Nutrient Intake: the level of intake sufficient for only 2.5% of the population.

Look up the value $u = 1.85$ in Appendix A2. Find the intersection of the row headed 1.8 (the first two digits of u), and the column headed 0.05 (the value of u in the second decimal place). The value in the table is 0.0322. This corresponds to the shaded area under the curve designated by $\frac{1}{2}P$. If we express 0.0322 as a percentage, we can say that 3.22% of women are likely to have an intake above 14.8 mg/d, that is, in the tail to the right of our cut-off point of 14.8 mg/d. If the total area under the curve is 1.0, a bit of simple maths tells us that the area to the left of the cut-off point (corresponding to women with intakes below 14.8 mg/d) is $1 - 0.0322 = 0.9678$. In percentage terms, this suggests that 96.78% of women in this age group have iron intakes below the Reference Nutrient Intake. This is a worrisome finding.

We can now find out what proportion of women have intakes below the LRNI. The mean and standard deviation are as before, but our cut-off (x) this time is the LRNI, 8.0 mg/d:

$$u = \frac{x - \mu}{\sigma} = \frac{8.0 - 8.5}{3.4} = -0.147$$

When we look in Appendix A2, we see that the values for u are all positive. How do we interpret a negative value like -0.147? First, we ignore the sign. Look up the value for 0.15 (our calculated value for u, 0.147, rounded to two decimal places). Find the intersection of the row headed 0.1 and the column headed 0.05. The corresponding value for the area under the curve is 0.4404. Second, we need to apply a little common sense. Remember that the normal Distribution is symmetrical. If the area under the curve for positive values of u lie to the *right* of the cut-off point (the shaded area under the curve), then the area under the curve for negative values of u will lie to the *left* of the cut-off point. If we express the value for the area under the curve as we did in the previous example, then we can say that 44.04% of women have daily iron intakes below 8.0 mg/d. This is of deep concern, as we would expect only 2.5% of women in this age group to have iron requirements less than 8.0 mg/d. Given the consequences of iron deficiency [6], this would appear to represent a major public health problem.

4.3 SAMPLING ERROR

The previous exercise demonstrated how it is possible to deduce facts about the population based on just two pieces of information, the mean μ and the standard deviation σ. We now want to carry out a similar exercise in which we deduce information about the mean of a *sample* in relation to the true population mean.

Think back to Chapter 2. Our aim in measuring observations in a sample is to make reasonable statements about what we think is happening in the population. We might simply want to be able to say something about the population mean based on the sample mean.

Every sample that is drawn from a population will, of course, have its own mean, $\bar{x}$. The value of $\bar{x}$ will almost always be different from the population mean, μ. Common sense tells us that, most of the time, the value of $\bar{x}$ will be close to μ.

Sometimes, just because of random sampling variation, the value of $\bar{x}$ will be a long way from μ. What does the shape of the distribution of the values for $\bar{x}$ look like? What factors influence the shape of the distribution? From the answers to these questions we will eventually be able to go on to make decisions about whether a particular sample observation is unusual. In turn, this might help us to make some decision about a particular group of subjects. For example, if we discovered that a group of elderly patients in hospital had a mean serum vitamin C concentration very different (lower) compared with the free-living population in the same age group, it might spur us to make an intervention to improve vitamin status in hospital patients. Exactly what we mean by 'very different' is the subject of the next chapter. For the moment, we just want to understand how the means of a set of samples drawn from one population are likely to be distributed.

Common sense tells us that the larger the sample size, the closer the value of $\bar{x}$ is likely to be to the population mean μ. Think about the distribution of the means of lots of different samples drawn from the same population. If all of the samples are large (say $n = 1000$), it is likely that the values for $\bar{x}$ will be tightly clustered around μ. If the samples are small (say $n = 10$), the values are likely to be much more widely distributed around μ. This is because there is a much greater chance that in small samples, the observations might all come from one end of the distribution of values in the population. For large samples, this is much less likely to happen. Thus, we can say that *as the sample size gets larger, the distribution of values of $\bar{x}$ is likely to get narrower.* Or more simply: *as n increases, $\bar{x}$ approaches μ.*

What other factor will influence the way in which the values for $\bar{x}$ are distributed? If the values of the original observations x are widely distributed, then it makes sense to think that the values for $\bar{x}$ would also be widely distributed. If the values for x were all tightly packed together around μ, then it makes sense to think that the values of $\bar{x}$ will also be tightly packed around μ. Our measure of the spread of the values of x is, of course, the standard deviation σ. Thus, *as the value for σ increases, the distribution of the values of $\bar{x}$ is likely to get wider.* Or to put it more simply: *as σ increases, the values for $\bar{x}$ diverge from μ.*

We can summarize the italicized statements at the ends of the last two paragraphs mathematically. We need to adopt a new term, the *standard error of the mean (or SEM or SE or se)*. The Standard Error of the Mean is the measure of the spread of values of $\bar{x}$ around μ. Most of the time, we use its abbreviated name, the Standard Error. We define SE as:

$$SE = \sqrt{\frac{\sigma^2}{n}}$$

EQUATION 4.4 Definition of the Standard Error of the Mean

Thus, we can say that the spread of values of $\bar{x}$ around μ is directly proportional to σ and inversely proportional to the square root of n. We can simplify this expression and say: $SE = \sigma / \sqrt{n}$

This is the most common way of expressing the standard error.

4.3.1 The Distribution of the Values of Sample Means $\bar{x}$

The idea that we consider next is one of the most profound in the whole of this book. Imagine drawing a sample of size n from a population. Refer to the sample mean as $\bar{x}_1$. Now draw another sample. This has a mean of $\bar{x}_2$. You can do this for as many samples as you like. Each sample that you draw is likely to have a mean value different from the previous samples. You can demonstrate that if you take the mean of all the possible samples of a given size n from the parent population, that the mean of the *sample means* will be equal to μ. This is the same μ that you determined when you calculated the mean of all the observations in the population, $\mu = \Sigma x/n$.

Now consider Box 4.3. **The information in Box 4.3 is extremely important!!**

The corollary is that the values for the areas under the curve in Appendix A2 apply to the standard error in exactly the same way as they apply to the standard deviation.

Let's follow this through. Earlier, we showed that the distance of a given observation x from the mean μ in terms of the number of standard deviations, σ, can be expressed as the standard normal deviate, u (Equation 4.3). We saw that for a variable that follows the normal distribution, 95% of observations of x would lie within ±1.96 standard normal deviates (u) either side of the mean.

The relationship described in Box 4.3 says that 95% of observations of $\bar{x}$ for a given sample size n lie within ±1.96 *standard errors* either side of the population mean μ. If that is true, then we can develop a new equation for the standard normal deviate (u) based on the relationship between $\bar{x}$, μ and standard error that parallels the relationship between x and μ and standard deviation. Our equation for u thus can be expressed as:

$$u = \frac{\bar{x} - \mu}{\sigma / \sqrt{n}} = \frac{\bar{x} - \mu}{\text{SE}}$$

EQUATION 4.5   The standard normal deviate (u) based on $\bar{x}$, μ, σ, and n

So, if you know μ, σ, and n, you can predict where the values for $\bar{x}$ are likely to lie 95% of the time.

We now have a tool that tells us what to expect when we observe a single sample with a mean of $\bar{x}$. If the value is near to the population mean (and by 'near', I mean within ±1.96 standard errors either side of the population mean), we can say that it is a 'likely' finding. If the sample mean is outside of this interval, we could reasonably refer to it as an 'unlikely' finding (something that we would expect to see less than 5% of the time). We will pursue this idea in the next chapter.

4.4 TRANSFORMATIONS

As we discussed in Chapter 3, there are two basic types of variable distributions: parametric and non-parametric. *Uniform, binomial, Poisson*, and *normal*

BOX 4.3

A key characteristic of the Standard Error

The standard error has the same relationship with μ as the standard deviation.

For a variable x which follows the normal distribution;

and for samples of a given size n each with a mean of $\bar{x}$;

95% of the values of $\bar{x}$ will be within ±1.96

standard errors either side of the population mean μ.

distributions are all examples of parametric distributions. Each one is characterized by a mathematical formula that relates the value of x to the probability of its occurrence. Nonparametric variables, by analogy, do *not* have a mathematically defined probability distribution.

Every statistical test relies on a model of the way in which data are distributed. It is vitally important to characterize data according to its type of distribution, and then undertake statistical analyses using those statistical tools that are appropriate.

The most powerful[26] statistical tests that we discuss in this text are based on the normal distribution. There are many circumstances, however, in which a variable does not follow the normal distribution. Some continuous distributions are skewed to the right or (more rarely) to the left, but are nonetheless parametric (i.e. have an underlying mathematical function that defines their distribution). Log-normal distributions, for example, are parametric but skewed to the right. Other distributions may lack symmetry altogether or be discrete.[27] Of course, if we use normal-based statistical tests to evaluate nonnormally distributed data, we risk misinterpreting our findings and coming to the wrong conclusion about whether to accept or reject the Null Hypothesis.

For continuous variables that are nonnormal in character, we can do one of two things. We can choose statistical tests that do not depend on a normal distribution for their application. But because these tests are weaker, in the sense that they use only some of the information available, we are more likely to accept the Null Hypothesis when, in fact, we should be rejecting it. The alternative is to *transform* the skewed data in such a way that the resulting distribution is close enough to normal to warrant the use of normal-based statistical tests. The latter is the preferred option, because it means we can use more powerful tests and improve our ability to demonstrate that our findings did not arise just by chance.

Intake of preformed vitamin A (retinol), for example, is often skewed to the right because it tends to be concentrated in relatively few sources of food that are eaten infrequently (like liver). When such foods are included in an individual's diet, their intake will be very much higher than the average. Figure 4.6a shows the distribution of retinol intake (µg/d from food only[28]) in 486 women aged 35–49 years living in low-income households in the United Kingdom in 2003–2005. The mean and the median are indicated, and the normal curve based on the mean and standard deviation superimposed.

The data are clearly nonnormal in character. First, the median is substantially less than the mean. If a variable is normally distributed, the mean and median are similar. In relation to the superimposed normal curve (based on the mean and standard deviation of the reported retinol intakes), there are many more observations poking above the curve below the mean, and fewer than we would expect to see above the mean. Compare this with the good fit that we saw in Figure 4.4b, where the number of observations for the different height measurements agreed well with the expected distribution based on the normal curve.

If there were some way of 'squeezing' the data into something resembling a normal distribution, we could use normal distribution-based statistics for our analyses. This 'squeezing' process would have to ensure two things:

1. that the relative position of the observations was preserved, and

---

[26]By 'powerful', I mean they help you to make valid decisions about accepting or rejecting the Null Hypothesis using the maximum amount of information available.

[27]Some variables may be discrete (e.g. the number of children in a class can take only whole number values) but have normal characteristics (e.g. show a distribution around the mean that is symmetrical and bell-shaped). It may therefore be appropriate to use normal-based statistical tests with this type of data. We will also discover that even for nonnormally distributed variables, the distribution of the values of the *sample means* may approximate a normal distribution. This means we can use the concept about where we would expect to find sample means in a wide variety of statistical settings. Consult your local statistician for advice!

[28]The data are for retinol intake from food only. If retinol supplements were included, the tail would be very long indeed.

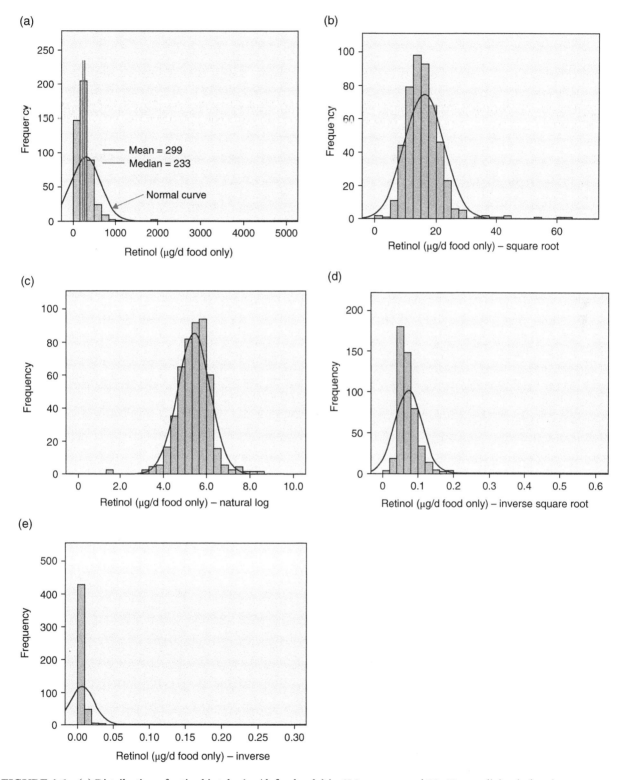

FIGURE 4.6 (a) Distribution of retinol intake (μg/d, food only) in 486 women aged 35–49 years living in low-income households in the United Kingdom in 2003–2005. (b–e) Distribution of retinol intake (μg/d, food only) in 486 women aged 35–49 years living in low-income households in the United Kingdom in 2003–2005, four transformations: (b) square root; (c) natural log; (d) inverse square root; (e) inverse.

2. that the change in proportional spacing between observations is the same for all observations.

These two requirements preserve the core characteristics of a *ratio* variable.

There are numerous mathematical techniques for transforming data. Most of them lengthen the left tail and shorten the right tail. In order of increasing adjustment, they are square root, the 'natural' logarithm (to the base e, where $e = 2.7183$, and indicated by the letters 'ln' on a calculator), one divided by the square root (inverse square root) and one over the original value (inverse). Anything involving log or square root will not be practical with distributions which include zero or negative numbers, but you can add a fixed amount to every observation to make all the values positive. If a distribution is skewed to the left (e.g. skeletal muscle mass), the opposite effect (shortening the left tail in relation to the right tail) can be obtained by raising values to a power (such as 2 or e).

The graphs resulting from the first four transformations cited above are shown in Figure 4.6b–e. Again, the normal curve is superimposed on each graph. It is immediately apparent that the square root and natural log transformations give the best results (b) and (c), and that the inverse square root

and inverse transformations, for this set of data, are not helpful. But which of the obviously useful transformations is the best use?

Graphing the transformed data is useful for visualizing the impact of the transformations, but this approach falls short in two ways. First, it is rather laborious. Second, it does not tell us which transformation reduces the skewness most effectively (i.e. that brings the distribution closest to the normal). It would be far more useful if we had an index that helped us to see which transformation reduces skewness the most. The following approach will help [7].

Step 1. Carry out the transformations listed in Table 4.3. Find the standard deviation of x and of each of the four transformations.

TABLE 4.3　Transformations of Variable x

Square root	$\sqrt{x}$
Natural logarithm	$\ln(x)$
Inverse square root	$\dfrac{1}{\sqrt{x}}$
Inverse	$\dfrac{1}{x}$

TABLE 4.4　Coefficients of Variation of x and Transformed Variables

	Mean	Standard Deviation	Coefficient of Variation Formula	Value
Retinol (µg/d food only)	299.0407	345.147 92	$\dfrac{SD(x)}{\dot{x}}$	1.5422
Square root	16.0304	6.49 261	$\dfrac{2SD(\sqrt{x})}{\sqrt{\dot{x}}}$	0.8680
Natural log	5.4107	0.75 188	$SD(\ln(x))$	0.7519
Inverse square root	0.0723	0.03 808	$2\sqrt{\dot{x}}\,SD\left(\dfrac{1}{\sqrt{x}}\right)$	1.1395
Inverse	0.0067	0.01 647	$\dot{x}\,SD\left(\dfrac{1}{x}\right)$	3.6862

Step 2. Take the antilog of the mean of ln(x) and call it $\dot{x}$ (spoken 'x-dot'). $\dot{x}$ is, in fact, the geometric mean of the original observations. In the present case, $\dot{x} = 223.7966$.

Step 3. Calculate the five coefficients of variation using the formulae in Table 4.4.

The coefficient of variation with the smallest value tells you which transformation has removed the most amount of skewness. In our retinol example, the most effective transformation was obtained using the natural logarithm. This accords with the comparison of the histograms in Figure 4.6b–e, which suggests that natural log transformation (Figure 4.6c) fits most closely to the superimposed normal curve. The next smallest value (for the square root transformation) also accords with the next best fit, as shown in Figure 4.6b.

The last step is to test the transformed variable for normality using SPSS. If it can be regarded as a normally distributed variable, it is appropriate to use normal based statistics. If not, then nonnormal based statistics will be required (see Chapters 7–10). We will see how to test for normality in Chapter 6. Things are getting interesting.

4.5 EXERCISES

4.5.1

a. Give two formulae for the standard normal deviate
b. For a variable x which follows the normal distribution, what is the probability that x lies beyond the following values of u (a) in one direction and (b) in both directions?

1.645   1.96   2.326   2.576   2.88   3.291

4.5.2

For the calcium intake data on 100 Cambridge women aged 18–53 (see Chapter 2), assume that $\mu = 882$ and $\sigma = 300.3$. Using normal theory, determine:

a. The percentage of women with intakes below 700 mg/d, the UK Reference Nutrient Intake (RNI)
b. The percentage of women with intakes below 1000 mg/d, the US Dietary Reference Intake (DRI)
c. The percentage of women with intakes above 525 mg/d, the UK Estimated Average Requirement (EAR)

Compare your answers with the numbers obtained by direct counting of subjects in each of these ranges.

4.5.3

A dental epidemiologist wishes to estimate the mean weekly consumption of sweets among children of a given age in his area. After devising a scheme which enables him to determine the sweet consumption of a child during a week, he does a pilot survey and finds that the standard deviation of the weekly sweet consumption is about 3 ounces. He considers taking a random sample of either 25 children, or 100 children, or 625 children for the main survey. Estimate the standard error of the sample mean for each of these three sample sizes. How do these standard errors explain why large samples are more reliable than small samples?

REFERENCES

1. Carl Friedrich Gauss. https://en.wikipedia.org/wiki/Carl_Friedrich_Gauss#Algebra.
2. Online Statistics Education: A Multimedia Course of Study. http://onlinestatbook.com/.
3. Royal College of Paediatrics and Child Health. WHO-UK growth charts for children 2–18 years. https://www.rcpch.ac.uk/resources/growth-charts.
4. Nelson M, Erens B, Bates B, Church S, Boshier T. *Low Income Diet and Nutrition Survey. Volume 2:*

Food consumption and nutrient intake. TSO. London. 2007.

5. Committee on Medical Aspects of Food Policy. *Dietary Reference Values for Food Energy and Nutrients for the United Kingdom.* The Stationery Office. London. 1991.

6. Scientific Advisory Committee on Nutrition. *Iron and Health.* TSO. London. 2010.

7. Margetts B and Nelson M. *Design concepts in Nutritional Epidemiology.* 2nd edition. Oxford University Press. 1997. p. 77.

CHAPTER 5

Confidence Intervals and Significance Testing

5.1 INTRODUCTION

In Chapter 4, we looked at the probability distribution of sample means. This key concept will enable us to make decisions about whether what we observe in a sample is something that we are likely to see, or if it is a rare event.

The main aim of this chapter is twofold. First, we need to understand what is meant by a confidence interval, and how to calculate the limits of a confidence interval. Second, we will see how to apply that knowledge to help us decide whether to reject or accept a Null Hypothesis using two new concepts: *significance levels* and *test statistic*.

5.2 CONFIDENCE INTERVALS AND CONFIDENCE LIMITS

We now know from earlier chapters that statistics is an inexact science. It deals in the probabilities of events happening. There are, however, a few certainties. We know, for example, that for a given type of event (e.g. the throw of a die), the total probability of all possible outcomes is equal to 1.0. And for a given throw of the die, we can state the *average* probability of an event occurring (i.e. how often, over many throws, a four will come up). What we *cannot* say,

Statistics in Nutrition and Dietetics, First Edition. Michael Nelson.
© 2020 John Wiley & Sons Ltd. Published 2020 by John Wiley & Sons Ltd.
Companion website: www.wiley.com/go/nelson/statistics

with certainty, is what the outcome of a *particular* throw of a die will be. If I threw the die 10 times, I cannot predict for those 10 throws exactly how often a four would appear.

Statistics *can* help us decide whether the outcome that we observe is likely or not. Here is an example. If I throw a die once, I know that there is a one-in-six chance of the die showing a four. So, getting a four on one throw is not an unusual event. If I throw the die twice, what are the chances that both throws will yield a four? This is simple. If there is a one-in-six chance of throwing a four on the first occasion, there is an equal probability of throwing a four on the second occasion. (The two events are independent of one another.) So, the chance of throwing two fours in a row is $1/6 \times 1/6 = 1/36$. Not very likely, but certainly not highly improbable. The probability of throwing three fours in a row is $1/6 \times 1/6 \times 1/6 = 1/216$, or $P = 0.00463$. I would deem this to be a rare event; it would happen only 4.63 times (say, five times)[1] in 1000. So, if I throw a die three times, and it comes up with a four all three times, I might begin to suspect that my die is not straight – that it is weighted so that a four is likely to come up more often than one time in six. Of course, it is not impossible to throw a die three times and for it to come up with a four each time. But if I threw the die three more times, I know that the probability of seeing three fours again (six fours in a row) is infinitesimally small.

This kind of thinking applies widely in scientific investigation. If I see an event that is unlikely to occur, I might say to myself, 'Why did this occur? It is not what I was expecting'. But what do we mean by 'unlikely'? This is where confidence intervals play a role.

Let's go back to the example of the distribution of the height of 10–11-year-old boys that we looked at in Chapter 4. In that example, we asked ourselves 'What is the chance that a boy in this age group in England has a height less than 120 cm?' We found that the characteristics of a normal distribution (Figure 4.4c) allowed us to say where the cut-off points are that define the tails that contain 2.5% of observations.

Now we want to ask a similar question, but instead of concerning ourselves with an individual child, we want to know about groups of children. We might ask, 'Is the average height of a group of 30 boys attending school in a poor neighbourhood in Liverpool (128.5 cm) much lower than the average for the population as a whole (130.6 cm)?' If the answer is 'yes', we might want to investigate the problem from a socio-economic and nutritional perspective. If the answer is 'no', we might suggest that our observation was simply part of random sampling variation. But what do we mean by 'much lower'?

Put the question another way, and think about random sampling variation. If I draw 100 random samples of 30 boys from my population, I know that because of random sampling variation, the mean values for my 100 samples will in all probability not be equal to the population mean.[2] The key question is, what does the *distribution* of these sample means look like? Coming back to my original question about the boys from a poor neighbourhood in Liverpool, how far away from the *population* mean does a *sample* mean need to be before I class it as an unusual finding? Given the characteristics of the population, I could ask myself if a sample mean of 128.5 cm is something I am likely to observe, say, less than 5% of the time.

5.2.1 Specifying a Confidence Interval based on μ and σ

Start with the 1056 observations for height that we were looking at. These observations constitute all the possible observations in the *population* of

[1] I would usually round expressions like '4.63 times in 1000' to the nearest whole number, and say, for example, '5 times in 1000' for ease of understanding.

[2] Just by chance I might get one sample in which the mean *is* equal to the population mean, but that would be by luck rather than design.

10–11-year-old boys in England in 2015/2016.[3] Because this is population data, I know μ (130.5843 cm, the true population mean) and σ (4.34315 cm, the population standard deviation). I can then compute the standard error for a sample in which $n = 30$:

$$\text{SE} = \frac{\sigma}{\sqrt{n}} = \frac{4.34315}{\sqrt{30}} = \frac{4.34315}{5.4772} = 0.7929 \, \text{cm}$$

EQUATION 5.1   Calculation of the standard error based on σ and n

I said in Chapter 4 (Box 4.3) that the standard error (a measure of the distribution of sample means) relates to the normal distribution probability function in the same way as the standard deviation. This means that I can expect 2.5% of all possible sample *means* (for a given sample size n) to lie in each of the two tails of the distribution of sample means that are ±1.96 *standard errors* away from the population mean. This is analogous to my expectation that 2.5% of all the observations for height in the population will lie in each of the two tails that are ±1.96 *standard deviations* away from the population mean.

We can test this assumption by plotting the means of 100 simple random samples[4] in each of which there are 30 observations ($n = 30$). Figure 5.1a shows the distribution of the 1056 observations for height in the population. Figure 5.1b shows the distribution of the means of 100 samples of $n = 30$ randomly drawn from the population.

As expected, the mean of the 100 sample means, 130.3442 cm, is very close to the mean for all the individual observations in the population, $\mu = 130.4853$ cm. It is also evident that the distribution of the sample means closely follows the normal

curve (based in this case on the mean and the standard deviation of the sample means for my 100 values for $\bar{x}$). Indeed, the observed value for the standard deviation of our 100 sample means, 0.80095 cm, is very close to the standard error that we calculated above for a sample of $n = 30$, 0.7929 cm, based on σ and n (Equation 5.1). It looks as if the standard deviation of the *sample means* is a good approximation for the standard error.

Let's take this line of thought to its logical conclusion. If 2.5% of the *sample means* lie in each of the two tails that are ±1.96 standard errors *away* from the population mean, I can also say that 95% of the observations for sample means are likely to lie *within* ±1.96 standard errors either side of the population mean, that is:

$$\mu \pm 1.96 \times \text{SE}, \text{ or } 130.5843 \, \text{cm} \pm 1.96 \times 0.7929 \, \text{cm}$$

This yields two values, 129.0302 cm and 132.1384 cm.

My expectation is (I am 'confident') that 95% of the mean values for my 100 randomly drawn samples of $n = 30$ will lie between 129.0302 and 132.1384. If I count the number of random sample means (out of the 100 that I determined), I find that 93 of them lie within this range, and seven lie outside this range. I was expecting 95 out of 100 (95%) to be within the limits. Given random sampling variation, we seem to have a very good model to describe what is going on.

This is an application of the *central limit theorem*. This is one of the most important concepts in statistics. It says that if we take lots of samples of size n from an infinite (or very large) population,[5] the distribution of the sample means will tend toward normal with variance $= \sigma^2/n$ (the square of the standard error). The bigger the value for n, the closer the distribution of the sample means will be to the normal distribution. As a rough guide, we can say that once we have samples of 30 or more observations, the distribution of the sample means is likely to be close to normal.

[3]There may have been a few boys who were absent when the measurements were taken, but including their results will have a minimal impact on the average and the standard deviation.

[4]I have drawn the samples 'without replacement'. Why 'without replacement'? If you are not sure, go back to Chapter 2 and remind yourself of the differences between sampling 'with replacement' and 'without replacement'.

[5]Or samples that represent only a tiny fraction of the population from which they are drawn.

There is another very important characteristic of the central limit theorem: it applies to the distribution of sample means that are drawn from both normal *and* nonnormal distributions.[6] This is critical when we come to calculating confidence intervals and later when we start looking at statistical tests in Part 2.

5.2.2 The 95% Confidence Interval ($\bar{x}$ around μ)

In the previous section, we have (in fact) been setting out the concept of the *95% confidence interval*. In this instance, we are saying that we are *confident* that 95% of the sample means (for a given sample size) will lie between the two values that are ± 1.96 standard errors either side of the population mean μ, where $SE = \sigma/\sqrt{n}$, σ is the true population standard deviation, and n is the sample size. This assumes that we know μ (the true population mean) and σ (the true population standard deviation), and that the variable follows the normal distribution. Thus, we can define the 95% confidence interval for a normal distribution: the 95% confidence interval is defined by the two values between which, for a variable that follows the normal distribution, we are confident that we will find 95% of all possible sample means for a given sample size. The two values that we calculated above (129.0302 cm and 132.1384 cm) are the *confidence limits* that lie at either end of the 95% *confidence interval*.

Now we can answer our question about the average height of a sample of 30 boys from a poor neighbourhood in Liverpool. First, we made the assumption that this group of boys is drawn from a national population in which the mean height is 130.5843 cm and the population standard deviation is 4.34315 cm. There is then a 2.5% chance (or less) that the mean height of any group of 30 boys drawn from this population is less than 129.0302 cm, that is, outside lower limit of the 95% confidence interval.

I can reasonably conclude that the mean that I observed (128.5 cm) is an 'unusual' finding, in the sense that I would expect to see it less than 2.5% of the time in this population. Going back to the language that I used earlier, I can say that the sample mean is 'much lower' than I was expecting. I might conclude further that the cause of the short stature in this neighbourhood is worth investigating, as what I observed seems to be unusual.[7]

Before we leave this section, I want to consider the width of the distribution of the sample means shown in Figure 5.1b. Unsurprisingly, this is much narrower than the width of the distribution for the individual observations (compare the scales on the *x*-axis between Figures 5.1a and 5.1b). Indeed, if I plot the distribution from Figure 5.1b on the same *x*-axis that we used in Figure 5.1a, you can see how narrowly the values for $\bar{x}$ are distributed compared with the original distribution (Figure 5.1c). Common sense tells us that as the sample size n increases, the width of the distribution of the values for $\bar{x}$ gets narrower and narrower. This is consistent with the way in which the standard error, $SE = \sigma/\sqrt{n}$, is determined. As the sample size n increases, the value for SE gets smaller and smaller.

5.2.3 More than One Way to Define a Confidence Interval

In the example above, we assumed that we knew the population mean μ and standard deviation σ. We wanted to know whether it was 'likely' (95% or more of the time) or 'unlikely' (less than 5% of the time) that $\bar{x}$ would be within the 95% confidence interval around μ.

Most of the time, however, we don't know μ, we only know $\bar{x}$. We have said previously that $\bar{x}$ is our best estimate of μ. But where, exactly, do we think μ might lie? We know we cannot say exactly where μ lies. But it would be good to be able to say where we

---

[6]The central limit theorem holds true for most but not all distributions.

[7]Although before doing that, I might take a few more samples of boys from this same neighbourhood to make sure that my first finding wasn't just a fluke associated with random sampling variation.

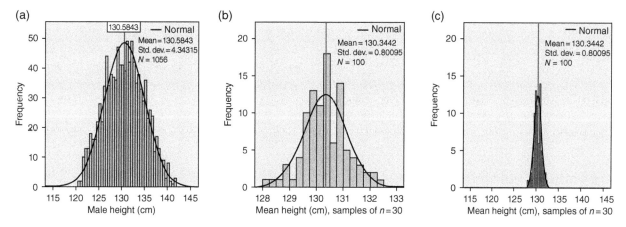

FIGURE 5.1 Distribution of (a) height (cm) in 1056 boys aged 10–11 years living in England in 2015–2016 and (b) mean height ($\bar{x}$) (cm) in 100 samples of $n = 30$, and (c) mean height in 100 samples of n=30 on the same x-axis scale as (a), all with normal curves superimposed.

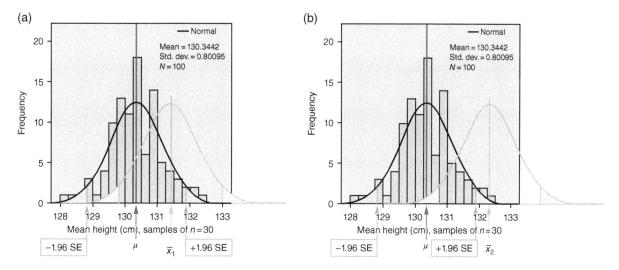

FIGURE 5.2 Relationship between μ, sample means, and 95% confidence intervals: (a) $\bar{x}_1$ within 95% confidence interval around μ; (b) $\bar{x}_2$ outside 95% confidence interval around μ.

thought μ lies and be right (say) 95% of the time. Can we create a 95% confidence interval for μ around $\bar{x}$?

Another leap of imagination is now required. Stop and think. If 95% of sample means lie within ± 1.96 standard errors of μ, it is also true that μ lies within ± 1.96 standard errors of $\bar{x}$ for the 95% of samples with mean values that lie inside the 95% confidence interval around μ. (Pause; take a deep breath; keep re-reading the previous sentence until

it makes sense; carry on.) This is illustrated in Figure 5.2a.[8]

The normal curve (in black) has been superimposed over the distribution of values for $\bar{x}$, centered

---

[8] I have assumed, for the purposes of these calculations, that the arithmetic mean of the 100 sample means is a good estimate of μ, and that the standard deviation of the *sample means* is a good estimate of the standard error based on σ and n.

BOX 5.1

The relationship between $\bar{x}$ and μ

For EVERY value of $\bar{x}$ that is within the 95% confidence interval around μ, the value for μ will be within the 95% confidence interval around $\bar{x}$.

around μ (the notional population mean). The 95% confidence interval around μ (based on $\mu \pm 1.96$ standard errors [see footnote 8]) is the unshaded area between the two shaded tails under the normal curve. I chose a value at random for one of the sample means that lies within the 95% confidence interval, and called it $\bar{x}_1$. Next, I copied the identical normal curve and confidence interval that I drew around μ, but centred it around $\bar{x}_1$ (the grey curve and shaded areas). As you can see, the value for μ is within the 95% confidence interval (the unshaded area) around $\bar{x}_1$ (Box 5.1).

Just to prove the point, in Figure 5.2b, I chose another value for $\bar{x}$ (I called it $\bar{x}_2$) that lay outside the 95% confidence interval around μ. As you can see, if I copy the normal curve and confidence interval and centre it around $\bar{x}_2$, the 95% confidence interval (unshaded area) around $\bar{x}_2$ does *NOT* contain μ (μ is in the grey shaded area to the left of the curve, outside the 95% confidence interval around $\bar{x}_2$). Point made.

What are the implications of this? For *every* sample that we draw from the population, there is a 95% chance that the true population mean μ will lie within the 95% confidence interval (± 1.96 SE) around $\bar{x}$ (assuming I know σ and n). I cannot say *exactly* where μ lies, but now I know *roughly* where it lies. The larger my sample, the smaller the standard error (because $SE = \sigma/\sqrt{n}$) and the better my estimate of where the true population mean lies.[9] I also have to accept that 5% of the time I am wrong. That is, for 5% of all possible values of $\bar{x}$, the true population mean will lie outside the 95% confidence

interval around $\bar{x}$. 'Tant pis', as they say in French. Never mind. I don't know which of the values for $\bar{x}$ will be in the 5% that don't include μ. I just have to accept that 5% of the time I will be wrong when I give the confidence intervals for μ. But it's the best we can do.

99% and 99.9% Confidence Intervals

Or is it? Maybe we *can* do better. One possibility would be to increase the level of confidence where we think μ lies. Instead of finding the limits of the 95% confidence interval, we could find the limits of the 99% confidence interval. I could then say that I am *99%* confident that I know where the true population mean lies. How do we do this?

If you remember from Chapter 4, if we multiplied σ by 2.576 instead of 1.96, the area under the curve around μ contained 99% of observations. By implication, if we multiply the standard error[10] by 2.576 instead of 1.96, 99% of sample means will lie within the 99% confidence interval either side of μ. Equally, if we calculate the 99% confidence interval around a sample mean, we can be confident that 99% of the time we will be right in saying that the true population mean μ lies within that interval. Of course, if we stop to think about it, we have sacrificed *precision* for *confidence*. The 99% confidence interval is wider than the 95% confidence interval (because we are multiplying SE by 2.576 rather than 1.96), but we are more confident (99% rather than 95%) that the value for μ lies inside the confidence interval around $\bar{x}$. If we cite the 99% confidence interval, we will be wrong about where the true population mean lies only 1% of the time. We could even calculate a 99.9% confidence interval (multiplying SE by 3.291), and be that much more confident about knowing where we think μ lies. The 99.9% confidence interval would be wider still, of course, and precision (knowing exactly where μ lies) would decrease further, but we would now be wrong about where we think the true population mean μ lies only 0.1% of the time.

---

[9]This helps to explain why larger samples provide better estimates of the true population mean than smaller samples.

[10]Based on σ and n

Now that we understand a confidence interval can be at different levels, we can define the confidence interval in more general terms using the *standard normal deviate* that we defined in Chapter 4. Just to review, we will express the standard normal deviate in terms of $\bar{x}$ and SE, the standard error.

When we established the limits of the 95% confidence interval, we used 1.96 as our multiplier for SE, because we saw from the normal distribution probability curve that 95% of values of $\bar{x}$ would lie ± 1.96 standard errors either side of the population mean μ. If we have values for $\bar{x}$, μ, σ, and n, we can define u, the standard normal deviate, as:

$$u = \frac{\bar{x} - \mu}{\sigma/\sqrt{n}} = \frac{\bar{x} - \mu}{SE}$$

EQUATION 5.2 Calculation of the standard normal deviate based on $\bar{x}$, μ, σ, and n

So, we can rearrange Equation 5.2 to say:

- the width of a confidence interval for $\bar{x}$ around μ can be defined as $\mu \pm u \times SE$.
- the width of the confidence interval for μ around $\bar{x}$ can be defined as $\bar{x} \pm u \times SE$.

If we say $u = 1.96$, that defines the 95% confidence interval. If $u = 2.576$, that defines the 99% confidence interval; and so on. These are the values for the standard normal deviate (given in Appendix A2) that relate to the areas under the curve in one tail ($\frac{1}{2}P$). Check Appendix A2 to make sure you grasp what is going on.

5.2.4 Deriving the Confidence Interval based on $\bar{x}$ and s

We usually don't know the values for μ and σ. More often, we know only the mean of one sample, ($\bar{x}$, our best estimate of the population mean μ) and s (our best estimate of the population standard deviation σ). Of course, for the purposes of testing our hypothesis, what we really want to know is, 'Where are we likely to find the true population mean'? That

is, can we define the confidence interval where we are likely to find μ based on our knowledge of $\bar{x}$ and s.

I want to approach this problem in two stages. For the moment, let's assume that we know the value of our sample mean, $\bar{x}$, and the true population standard deviation σ (for instance, based on previous research in this population). In the previous section, we saw that we were able to determine confidence intervals for μ around $\bar{x}$ because we knew the value for σ. But if we know only $\bar{x}$ and s, based on our sample observations, how do we calculate a 95% confidence interval when we don't know the value for σ? Can we just substitute s for σ when we calculate the limits of the confidence interval?

Sadly, the answer is no. 'Why not?' you ask grumpily. Because, as we have said before, s is our *best estimate* of σ. It might be exactly equal to σ, in which case all would be well. But of course, it could be greater than σ; or it could be less than σ. Let's think about what happens to the width of our confidence interval in each case.

- If s is greater than σ, the width of our confidence interval is wider than when we calculated it using σ (Figure 5.3a). As we can see in the figure, the 95% confidence interval includes the value for μ. Our assumption will be upheld that 95% of the time we will be right in saying that μ lies within the 95% confidence interval around $\bar{x}$.
- If s is less than σ, the width of our confidence interval is narrower than when we calculated the confidence interval using σ (Figure 5.3b). In this case, the value for μ lies *outside* the 95% confidence interval around $\bar{x}$. We would no longer be correct in saying that for a given sample mean $\bar{x}$, 95% of the time we will be right in saying that μ lies within the 95% confidence interval.

What is the solution to this problem?

When we determine s (based on our sample observations), we must accept that it may be an either an overestimate of σ or an underestimate.

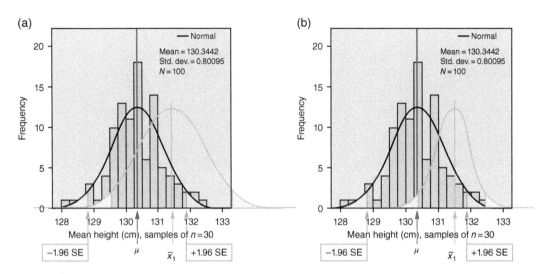

FIGURE 5.3   Relationship between μ, sample mean, and 95% confidence intervals according to value for s in relation to σ. (a) $s > \sigma$: μ within 95% confidence interval around $\bar{x}_1$; (b) $s < \sigma$: μ outside 95% confidence interval around $\bar{x}_1$.

We have no way of knowing. So, to be safe, we must *always* assume it is an underestimate. This may seem a bit over-cautious, but it is better to be conservative (over-cautious) in what we say about our findings than to come to a false conclusion because we made an incorrect assumption in our statistical model. If we always assume that s is an underestimate of σ, what can we do to ensure that the 95% confidence interval is wide enough to include μ for 95% of our sample means?

The simplest (and most obvious) thing to do is to increase the value by which we multiply the standard error to determine the width of the confidence interval. Bear in mind that we are now defining the standard error as $SE = s/\sqrt{n}$. So, instead of saying that the 95% confidence interval is ±1.96 SE either side of $\bar{x}$, we could say (for example) that it is ±2.0 SE either side of $\bar{x}$. But is 2.0 big enough? Should it be 2.1, or 2.2, or larger? By how much do we think s might be an underestimate of σ? Of course, we should bear in mind that as the sample size increases, the value for s will be closer and closer to σ. The bigger the sample, the closer our value for s will be to σ. Gradually, as our sample size gets bigger and bigger, the multiplier for the width of the 95% confidence interval will approach 1.96. Our choice of multiplier must therefore take sample size into account.

Happily, in 1908, an enterprising young analyst named William Sealy Gosset[11] worked out what the multipliers should be. He developed a new table for the multipliers for the confidence interval that took into account both the level of confidence that we want to achieve and the sample size. Think back to our discussion in Chapter 4 about the areas under the normal curve. We came up with the value of ±1.96 because normal theory tells us that (i) 95% of observations of a variable x lie within ±1.96 standard deviations of the true population mean, and (ii) 95% of values for sample means $\bar{x}$ lie within ±1.96 standard errors of the true population mean for a given sample size. We expressed these relationships in the concept of the standard normal deviate, u, using one of two expressions that we had looked at previously: $u = (x-\mu)/\sigma$ and $u = (\bar{x} - \mu)/(\sigma/\sqrt{n})$.

---

[11]William Sealy Gosset developed the '*t*-test' and published it under the pseudonym of 'Student' in 1908. It is often referred to as *Student's t-test*, not because it is just for students, nor because Gosset was being modest (a 'student' of mathematics), but because his employer, Guinness Brewery, did not allow their employees to publish in scientific journals under their own names (and so take the credit). The t statistic has become a foundation stone of modern statistical analysis.

Gosset came up with what he called the '*t*' distribution. It looks very much like the normal (bell-shaped) distribution, but it is wider. The smaller the sample size, the wider it gets. The bigger the sample size, the narrower it gets. Ultimately, if you measure every element in the population,[12] the *t* distribution converges with the normal distribution.

The definition of *t* looks very much like the definition of *u* based on the standard error. The only difference is the use of *s* instead of σ:

$$t = \frac{\bar{x} - \mu}{s/\sqrt{n}}$$

EQUATION 5.3 Definition of *t*

So, if we know $\bar{x}$, *s*, and *n*, we can rearrange Equation 5.3 to define the confidence limits for μ around $\bar{x}$ (Equation 5.4):

$$\bar{x} \pm t \times SE = \bar{x} \pm t \times \frac{s}{\sqrt{n}}$$

EQUATION 5.4 Limits of the confidence interval for μ around $\bar{x}$ if *s* and *n* are known

Even if I don't know σ, I can now come up with a reasonable estimate for where I think the true population mean lies either side of $\bar{x}$.

The next question is: how do I know which value of *t* to use? Gosset's tables of values for the *t* distribution are shown in Appendix A3. We said that the value we select for *t* will be determined by sample size and the width of the confidence interval that we want to establish. Looking in Appendix A3, we see three rows of values across the top of the table:

- values for *P* which relate to the areas in the tails of the *t* distribution
- the percentage of the areas in both tails under the curve
- the width of the confidence interval we want to determine

But if you look at the left-hand column of Appendix A3, instead of sample size *n*, you see a new term, *Degrees of freedom*, designated by ν (lower case Greek letter '*nu*').

Degrees of Freedom

Think back to our calculation of the standard deviation. Our aim was to estimate a measure of the variation of observations around the population mean, based on our sample observations. The first step was to find the sum of squares of the sample observations of variable *x*: $\sum (x - \bar{x})^2$. We expanded the numerator and found that $\sum (x - \bar{x})^2 = \sum x^2 - \left(\sum x\right)^2 / n$. We saw that the numerator for the standard deviation calculation is based on two sums: the sum of the squares of each sample observation (in the first term) and the square of the sum of the sample observations (in the second term). The purpose of finding $\sum x^2$ and $\sum x$ (in our 'short' method) is to help us estimate the standard deviation of the population.

Now, we need a 'pause and think' moment. There will be many samples of a given size *n* that yield the same result for $\sum x^2$ and $\sum x$. This is what we would hope and expect if we are using sample observations to help us estimate the population standard deviation. No one sample will give us the 'right' answer. It is possible, however, for many different samples to give us the *same* answer. The key concept here is that it is the values for $\sum x^2$ and $\sum x$, not one *particular* set of sample observations, that enable us to calculate *s*, our best estimate of σ.

Let's see what this means in practice. Say we have a sample where $n = 4$.[13] We have four observations: *a*, *b*, *c* and *d*. Say the sum of our four observations $a + b + c + d = \sum x$. When we have drawn our sample, three of the four observations could take any values for the variable in the population. But once we have drawn three observations, the

---

[12]If, going back to ideas put forward in Chapter 2, we say that we are dealing with samples drawn from an infinite population, we could also say that *t* will equal 1.96 when $n = \infty$.

[13]Yes, I know, this is a very small sample. But my point is easier to make.

value of the fourth observation will be fixed by $\sum x$.[14] The fourth value is effectively predetermined by the spread of observations in the population.[15] So, a, b, and c could take any value, but d would be determined by $\sum x$. Equally, I could have any valid values for a, b, and d for my sample observations, but then c would be fixed by $\sum x$. And so on. For a sample size of n, therefore, I have $n-1$ choices for the values of my sample observations before the value for $\sum x$ is reached.

Remember in Chapter 2 that we said that s would be a better estimate of σ if we divided the sum of squares by $n-1$ rather than n. Et voilà! Degrees of freedom has been with us all along, we just hadn't given it a name until now.

For the t distribution, $\nu = n-1$. We shall discover that degrees of freedom will be defined in different ways for different statistical tests.

5.2.5 Calculating the Confidence Interval based on $\bar{x}$ and s, using t

Suppose I now want to determine the 95% confidence interval for μ around $\bar{x}$ based on a set of sample observations. Say I have a sample of 30 boys aged 10–11 years with a mean height of $\bar{x} = 131.4133$ cm and standard deviation $s = 4.66275$ cm. I will use Equation 5.4, $\bar{x} \pm t \times s/\sqrt{n}$, to determine the limits of the confidence interval.

Let's just be clear about what we are doing. The 95% confidence interval for μ around $\bar{x}$ is shown by the limits to the unshaded area in the central part of the curve in the figure at the top of the t-table in Appendix A3. This area is equivalent to 100% (all possible observations) minus 5% (the area under the curve in the two shaded tails). We are confident that for 95% of samples that we draw ('95% of the time') we will be right in saying that μ lies inside this interval. For 5% of our samples, we will be wrong about where the true value for μ lies; μ will lie outside the 95% confidence interval that we determine.

First, we need to find the correct value for t in Appendix A3. I find the row for degrees of freedom where $\nu = n-1 = 30-1 = 29$. For the 95% confidence interval, I choose the column headed $P = 0.05$ which corresponds to 5% of the area under the curve in both shaded tails shown in the figure at the top of the t-table.

The value for t at the intersection of the row headed 29 and the column headed 0.05 is 2.045. As expected, it is larger than 1.96, the value that we would have used to determine the 95% confidence interval if we had known σ. We have allowed for the fact that s may be an underestimate of σ.

The first row of Table 5.1 shows the values for $\bar{x}$, s, n, ν, P, Confidence level, and t. In addition, I have computed the lower limit for the 95% confidence interval equal to 129.67 cm, and the upper limit equal to 133.15 cm. Because we are doing this as an exercise in a textbook on statistics, I know the value for $\mu = 130.3442$ cm. I can see that this falls within the 95% confidence interval.

If we had wanted to be more confident about where we would expect to find μ, we could have computed the limits for the 99% and 99.9% confidence intervals, also shown in Table 5.1. In order to have higher confidence levels, we use values for t which are 2.756 and 3.659, respectively. As a consequence of using larger and larger values for t, the interval gets wider and wider. As we said earlier, as the level of confidence concerning where we expect to find μ increases, the precision of our estimate decreases, that is, the confidence interval allows for greater error in where we think μ might be found.

In general terms, the *confidence interval* tells you one of two things:

1. where you can expect to find sample results a given proportion of the time, assuming you know the underlying probability function that governs the distribution of the variable and the value for the true population mean; and

2. if I have drawn a sample from a population with a known probability distribution, I can say where I would expect to find the true population mean with a given level of confidence.

---

[14]The same reasoning applies to $\sum x^2$.
[15]Given the probabilities for the values of x that underpin the population standard deviation.

TABLE 5.1 Values for the Upper and Lower Limits of the Confidence Interval for Three Levels of Confidence for a Sample in which $\bar{x} = 131.4133\,\text{cm}$ and $s = 4.66275\,\text{cm}$

$\bar{x}$	s	n	ν	P	Confidence Level	t	Confidence Interval	
							Lower Limit	Upper Limit
131.4133	4.66275	30	29	0.05	95%	2.045	129.67	133.15
131.4133	4.66275	30	29	0.01	99%	2.756	129.07	133.84
131.4133	4.66275	30	29	0.001	99.9%	3.659	128.30	134.56

BOX 5.2

General definitions of Confidence Interval and Confidence Limits

Confidence Interval

The interval within which, for a specified level of confidence and a given probability distribution, we would expect to find a parameter such as population mean or sample mean.

Confidence Limits

The pair of values at the upper and lower limits of a defined confidence interval.

The general definition of Confidence Interval is given in Box 5.2, together with a definition of *confidence limits*.

In this first exploration of the meaning of confidence interval, we have been talking about mean values (of populations or samples) for height, which follows the normal distribution. You can equally well determine confidence intervals for other types of distribution, such as Binomial or Poisson, where the outcome may be in terms of the average number of times that I might expect to see a particular outcome (think back to our example of the number of successful outcomes in our weight loss clinic, described in Chapter 4). As we shall see, the concept applies equally well to results that might be summarized as proportions, or odds ratios, or correlation coefficients.

5.3 LEVELS OF SIGNIFICANCE

In the scientific literature, you will come across phrases such as 'the finding was statistically

significant at the 5% level', or '$P < 0.05$'. This means that the authors of the article believe that if they assume the null hypothesis is true,[16] what they have observed was likely to occur less than 5% of the time. They might go on to say that they are 'rejecting the null hypothesis at the 5% level'.[17] It also indicates that the authors accept that there is a 5% chance that they could have observed what they observed even if the null hypothesis *is* true.

Assume the authors know the values for μ and σ. They can see if the observed value for a sample of size n and a mean of $\bar{x}$ falls outside the range given by the confidence interval defined as $\mu \pm 1.96\sigma/\sqrt{n}$ (Equation 5.2). If it does, they can say that the probability of that sample being drawn from the population with mean μ and standard deviation σ is less than 5%, or simply that $P < 0.05$. If the finding was statistically significant at the 1% level, the probability of observing a sample of size n and a mean of $\bar{x}$ from a population with mean μ and standard deviation σ is less than 1%, or simply that $P < 0.01$. And so on.

To summarize:

If $\bar{x}$ is outside the range $\mu \pm 1.96\,\sigma/\sqrt{n}$, then $P < 0.05$

If $\bar{x}$ is outside the range $\mu \pm 2.576\,\sigma/\sqrt{n}$, then $P < 0.01$

If $\bar{x}$ is outside the range $\mu \pm 3.291\,\sigma/\sqrt{n}$, then $P < 0.001$

The values are summarized in Table 5.2.

---

[16]Given caveats about the representativeness of their sample, the precision of the methodology, etc.

[17]We will have more to say about 'accepting' and 'rejecting' the null hypothesis in Chapter 6.

TABLE 5.2   Values for the Standard Normal Deviate Corresponding to Values for $\frac{1}{2}P$ and P in Appendix A2, and the Corresponding Confidence Intervals

u	$\frac{1}{2}P$	P	Confidence Level
1.96	0.025	0.05	95%
2.576	0.005	0.01	99%
3.291	0.0005	0.001	99.9%

These levels of significance are sometimes referred to as 'statistically significant', 'very statistically significant', and 'highly statistically significant', respectively, but to avoid ambiguity it is best to quote the P values directly. You may also see $P = 0.000$, especially in statistical summaries in tables produced by SPSS or other software. This means that $P < 0.0005$, but has been rounded to three decimal places. It does *NOT* mean that there is a 0% chance of the observation occurring.

5.4 A TEST STATISTIC

The culmination of this chapter is to explore how values for u and t can be used to interpret research findings. We have in effect done this already, but a different emphasis on the interpretation of the computed values for u and t will help us to see how levels of significance can be expressed.

First, what do we mean by a test statistic? In its narrowest sense, a test statistic is a computed value that helps us to decide whether to accept or reject a null hypothesis. In the wider sense, a test statistic helps us to understand:

- the probability that an observed sample was drawn from a defined population
- where we think the true population mean lies, given what we know about a sample mean and standard deviation or other statistical parameters (such as the proportions of observations in given categories, or the slope of a regression line)

Test statistics relate to the probability distributions that underlie the measurement that we are considering. We are going to explore the use of test statistics in this chapter using the normal and t distributions. We will see in Part 2 of the book that they can be computed for other statistical distributions as well.

5.4.1 Using u as a Test Statistic

If we go back to our statistical model, we are asking the question, 'What is the probability of drawing a sample with mean $\bar{x}$ from a population with mean μ?' More precisely, if we think in terms of the curve that shows the probability distribution of all possible sample means for samples of size n, I want to know the probability of drawing a sample with a mean of $\bar{x}$ that is a given distance (or further) away from μ, corresponding to the areas in the tails of the distribution. If my sample mean is in either of the tails that puts it a long way from μ, I can say that the probability of this occurring is very small. By 'a long way', I mean in either one of the tails that together correspond to 5% or less of the area under the curve.

Note that I have not said anything about whether the sample mean is above or below μ. When I draw a sample from the population, random sampling variation does not predict whether the value for the sample mean is greater than or less than μ. I am, in fact, more interested in how far *away* from μ my value for $\bar{x}$ lies than whether it is above or below the population mean. In the normal table (Appendix A2), the tabulated values are for $\frac{1}{2}P$, that is, the area under the curve in one tail of the probability distribution. If I want to know the probability of observing a sample with a mean a *given distance or more* from the population mean, I will have to double the tabulated value to determine P.

Let's return once more to the example of the 30 boys living in a poor neighbourhood in Liverpool. My question is, 'What is the probability of observing a mean value for height equal to 128.5 cm in a sample of 30 boys when I know μ and σ, such that μ

(the true population mean) is equal to 130.4853 cm and σ (the true population standard deviation) is equal to 4.343 15 cm'?

I have all the pieces of information I need to compute a value for the standard normal deviate: $\mu, \sigma, \bar{x}, and\ n$.[18] In this instance, I want to refer to the standard normal deviate u as my *test statistic*:

$$u = \frac{\bar{x} - \mu}{\sigma / \sqrt{n}} = \frac{128.5 - 130.5843}{4.343\,15 / \sqrt{30}} = \frac{-2.0843}{4.343\,15 / 5.47722}$$

$$= \frac{-2.0843}{4.343\,15 / 5.47722} = \frac{-2.0843}{0.793\,68} = -2.62612$$

EQUATION 5.5 Computed value for u (my *test statistic*) based on known population values for μ and σ and a chosen sample with mean of $\bar{x}$

Turn to the normal table in Appendix A2 and find this value for u (my test statistic). Because the values for u in the table are all positive, I will ignore the sign (for the moment), and look up $u = 2.62612$. Look down the first column and find the row headed 2.6 (the first two digits of my test statistic). The second digit after the decimal point is given by the columns headed 0.00, 0.01, and so on. Our computed value for u lies between 2.62 and 2.63. I find the corresponding values for $\frac{1}{2}P$ (the tabulated values in the body of the table) in the row headed 2.6 and the columns headed 0.02 and 0.03. These are 0.004 40 and 0.004 27, respectively.

The probability of drawing a sample of 30 boys with a mean this distance or further from the population mean is between 0.440% and 0.427% *in one direction*. Because the computed value for u was negative, I am looking at the tail below the population mean rather than the tail above the population mean (as shown in the illustration at the top of Appendix A2). As the normal distribution is symmetrical

around the population mean μ, the value for $\frac{1}{2}P$ will be the same in both tails.

There is one more issue to consider. Why do I need to double the value for $\frac{1}{2}P$ in the table when the sample mean was below the population mean? The answer is that when I drew my sample of 30 boys, I did not know if the sample mean would be above or below the population mean. I might have *expected* it to be lower because I was working in a part of town with many poor families. But random sampling variation does not predict where the sample mean will lie, regardless of the hypothesis I am working to. The Null Hypothesis says that if I draw a sample from this population, the observed sample mean could be anywhere in the distribution of sample means around the population mean. I am interested, therefore, in the probability of observing a sample mean *plus or minus* 2.626 12 standard errors away from the population mean. The probability of this occurring is P, not $\frac{1}{2}P$. To find P, therefore, I double the values in the table. Given the population characteristics, the probability of observing a sample mean of 128.5 cm is therefore between $2 \times 0.004\,40 = 0.008\,80$ and $2 \times 0.004\,27 = 0.008\,54$, or 0.880% and 0.854%.

If we express this in terms of significance levels, I could say that the probability of observing what we observed was between the 1% level and the 0.1% level of significance, or in numerical terms, $0.001 < P < 0.01$. I would deem this to be an unlikely event. There is only a small chance that the sample of 30 boys with a mean height of 128.5 cm came from the population with a mean of 130.5843 cm and a standard deviation of 4.343 15 cm. I could reasonably conclude that this sample of boys, in fact, came from a population with a lower mean height.

I can estimate an exact probability for P, of course, by using interpolation. How far does my calculated value for u (2.626 12) lie between 2.62 and 2.63? Linear interpolation says that 2.626 12 lies 61.2% of the way between 2.62 and 2.63:

---

[18]You will find, in this game of statistics, that the decision about which test statistic to compute is often a matter of finding the test statistic with the parameters that best match the information that you have available for the sample and the population.

$$\frac{2.626\,12 - 2.62}{2.62 - 2.63} = \frac{0.006\,12}{0.01} = 0.612$$

If I assume that the probabilities for P are linearly associated with the values for u,[19] then a good estimate of P would be to say that it lay 61.2% of the way between 0.008 80 and 0.008 54, that is:

$$P = 0.008\,80 - 0.612 \times (0.008\,80 - 0.008\,54)$$
$$= 0.008\,641$$

The probability of drawing a sample with the observed mean is thus 0.8641% – less than 1%, and therefore not very likely – so it is reasonable to conclude that this sample comes from a different population. Of course, there is a 0.8641% chance that I am wrong in drawing this conclusion, and that the sample really does come from the population of boys with a mean height of 130.5843.

I can go one step further and determine the 99% confidence limits for the true population mean around $\bar{x}$. I choose the 99% confidence interval because my calculations tell me there is a less than 1% probability that my sample came from the population with mean 130.5843 cm. Given that I know σ and n, I can say that the true population mean for this sample was somewhere between $\bar{x} \pm 2.576\,(\sigma/\sqrt{n})$, or $128.5 \pm 2.576\,(4.343\,15/\sqrt{30})$, which yields confidence limits of 128.5 ± 2.0426, or 126.4574 and 130.5426. This does not include the population mean for all 10–11-year-old boys, 130.5843 cm. I am right in concluding that, at the 1% level of confidence, this sample comes from a different population. To re-emphasize, there is a 1% chance that I am wrong in coming to this conclusion.

I could have used my computed value for $u = 2.626\,12$ and computed a 99.14% confidence interval (100%–0.8641%). When calculating findings for a confidence interval, this is what SPSS will do. There is no need to cling inflexibly to notions of 95% or 99% confidence intervals – they are simply convenient reference points for explaining ideas about the limits of our estimates for where we expect

to find the true population mean, given a sample mean.

Finally, I can decide whether to accept or reject the null hypothesis that my Liverpool sample was from the general population based on the computed test statistics. The null hypothesis says that my sample was drawn from the general population. By convention, if what I observed was likely to occur less than 5% of the time, I will reject the null hypothesis. I compare my computed test statistic with the value in the table for the normal distribution. I am interested in the two-tailed test. If my computed test statistic is greater than 1.96 or less than −1.96, I can conclude that the probability of that sample being drawn from the general population was less than 5%. My computed test statistic was −2.626 12, so I reject the null hypothesis at the 5% level. In fact, because my computed test statistic was less than −2.576, I can conclude that the probability of drawing that sample from the general population was less than 1%. I can therefore reject the null hypothesis at the 1% level and conclude that my sample was drawn from a different population.

5.4.2 Using t as A Test Statistic

The more likely scenario is that I will have only the sample data and know $\bar{x}$ and s on which to base my test statistic and estimates of confidence limits. I can do the same type of calculations as I have just done for u, but computing t instead. I will look up the result in the t-table (Appendix A3) rather than the table for the normal distribution.

I hope the following procedure will now seem wonderfully familiar. Given that I know $\bar{x}$, μ, s, and n (see footnote 15), I can calculate the value for t:

$$t = \frac{\bar{x} - \mu}{s/\sqrt{n}} = \frac{128.5 - 130.5843}{3.181\,43/\sqrt{30}}$$

$$= \frac{128.5 - 130.5843}{3.181\,43/\sqrt{30}} = \frac{-2.0843}{3.181\,43/5.477}$$

$$= \frac{-2.0843}{0.5808} = -3.588\,38$$

---

[19]A reasonable assumption, but not exactly right – if you were to do these computations using Excel or SPSS, you might get a value for P that differed in the second or third decimal place.

Ignore the sign, and look up 3.588 38 in the t-table[20] for $n - 1$ degrees of freedom, that is, $v = 30 - 1 = 29$. The calculated value for t falls between 2.756 and 3.659, that is, for values of t corresponding to probabilities of $P = 0.01$ and $P = 0.001$, respectively. (The values for P in the t-table include both tails of the distribution, so you don't need to double the values in the table as you did for the probabilities for u in Appendix A2.) As before, I can interpolate the value for P for the t statistic as I did for the u statistic:

$$\frac{3.659 - 3.58838}{3.659 - 2.756} = 0.078206$$

that is, 7.8206% of the way between 0.001 and 0.01, that is, $P = 0.001 + 0.078(0.01 - 0.001) = 0.001704$.

Now, you may want to complain. Why did we get one answer for P using u as a test statistic, and a different answer for P using t as a test statistic? The answers aren't a million miles away from each other – both values for P are between 1% and 0.1% – but they do differ: based on u, $P = 0.008641$; based on t, $P = 0.001704$. The similarity between the answers boosts our confidence that the values for P that we have estimated are probably not far from the truth. But random sampling variation means that every time we undertake the calculation for P based on t for a given sample, we are likely to come up with a value that will be slightly different from the value for P based on u. This highlights the impact of random sampling variation on statistical findings, and underlines the need to repeat studies with fresh samples to help make sure that what we have observed is not a fluke.

---

[20] As I did for the standard normal deviate, I ignore the sign when looking up the test statistic. I remember, of course, that a negative sign simply indicates that the value for the sample mean that I am considering is below the population mean. As the distributions of u and t are symmetrical, ignoring the sign won't affect my conclusions about the probabilities of observing what I have observed based on the areas under the curve.

5.5 EXERCISES

5.5.1

A computer was used to take 2000 random samples of 5 digits between 0 and 9. The mean value of the 2000 sample means was 4.5391. The sampling distribution of repeated sample means of 5 digits is shown theoretically to have a mean of 4.5 and standard deviation of 1.28.

a. What are the limits of the 95% confidence interval around μ for a sample of this size?
b. Is there any strong evidence to suggest that random digits generated by the computer do not have a mean of 4.5?
c. What is the exact value for P?

5.5.2

The mean level of prothrombin in the normal population is known to be 20.0 mg/100 ml of plasma and the standard deviation is 4 mg/100 ml. A sample of 40 patients showing vitamin K deficiency has a mean prothrombin level of 18.50 mg/100 ml.

a. How reasonable is it to conclude that the true mean for patients with vitamin K deficiency is the same as that for the normal population?
b. Within what limits would the mean prothrombin level be expected to lie for all patients with vitamin K deficiency? (i.e. give 95% confidence limits). Do the confidence limits include the mean for the population? What does this tell you about the relationship between values for probability and confidence limits?

(from Osborne [1])

5.5.3

A group of 30 women runs the 100 m sprint in an average of 11.5 seconds, with a standard deviation of 0.7 seconds.

a. Find the 95% confidence interval around $\bar{x}$.
b. What is the probability that this group of 30 athletes has been drawn from the group of world class runners in which the average sprint time for 100 m is 11.1 seconds?

REFERENCE

1. Osborne JF. *Statistical Exercises in Medical Research.* John Wiley. London. 1979.

STATISTICAL TESTS

Introduction

The previous chapters have explored issues concerning research methods and the design of studies. They have also laid the groundwork for understanding the ways in which statistical tests can be used to provide a better understanding of research results.

Part 2 deals with the practical application of statistical tests. Statistical tests are tools. When appropriately applied, they can reveal interesting and sometimes unexpected truths about the data. If they are misapplied, they can wreak havoc on scientific judgement, leading you to unjustified (and unjustifiable) conclusions. An important aim of this section of the book, therefore, is to identify the circumstances in which it is appropriate to use particular tests.

Creating a Model

Every time you carry out a statistical test, you must have in your mind a clear understanding of the hypothesis (or research question), the study design, and the nature of the variables that have been measured. This knowledge will lead you to an expectation concerning the way in which the data may behave. For example, suppose you want to know if eating breakfast influences children's grades at school. We could choose as our research model a two-sample unmatched design (Figure 1.3). The population would constitute all children attending schools in a particular area. The variable of interest would be school grades. We could define the 'active treatment' as 'eats breakfast regularly (5 or more days per week)', and the 'placebo' as 'does not eat breakfast regularly (2 or fewer days per week)'. We would need to define what we mean by 'breakfast'. You would not be in a position to measure the baseline characteristics because the 'intervention' in this experiment preceded your arrival. However, you would be in a position to select subjects who were similar in age, parental education, access to food, etc., and you could ensure that the proportion of boys and girls in the two groups was similar (using stratified or quota sampling). You could thus create a research model in which the principal difference in characteristics between the two groups was how regularly they ate breakfast. The hypothesis might be 'Eating breakfast regularly is associated with higher school grades' (at this stage we carefully avoid assuming that the association is necessarily causal). The null hypothesis (H_0) would be 'Eating breakfast regularly has no influence on school grades'. We need to make one more assumption, concerning the nature of the distribution of the variable we are measuring. Let us assume that the grades fall on a continuum from 1 to 100, and that in the population as a whole they follow a normal distribution. (We would need to assume also, for the purposes of this example, that the grades are standardized to take into account different levels of performance at different ages.)[1] Having made these assumptions, we would then find the statistical test which accords with our research design, which is appropriate for the data, and which allows us to determine if there are real differences in the average grades between the two groups of children.[2]

On first encounter, this process of making assumptions may seem artificial. How do we know which assumptions to make? How do we know that the assumptions are justified? We know, for example, that the grades are unlikely to be *exactly* normally distributed, and that the average age, level of parental education, and so on, may not be *exactly* the same in both groups of children. But if we can show that our assumptions are reasonable and justifiable (that is, that they approximate reality), then we can construct a *statistical model* which will predict the way in which we think our observations will behave. The model allows us to calculate probabilities relating to specific outcomes. If H_0 is true, for example, and there is no influence of breakfast on school grades, then we would expect the average grades in the two groups of children to be similar. If we get an answer very different from what we were expecting (i.e. if the average grades in the two groups are not similar), then we can reject the null hypothesis and say that eating breakfast is associated with higher school grades (assuming, here, that the outcome is in the direction we expected!). Exactly what we mean by 'very different from what we were expecting' or 'not similar' can be phrased in terms of the probabilities discussed in earlier chapters and revealed using appropriate statistical tests.

There may, of course, be other factors that influence this association (children who eat breakfast may also study harder, or read more). It would be up to us to think of all the other reasons (apart from eating breakfast) that might explain our findings, and to try and measure them or match for them in our study design. Ultimately, we might satisfy ourselves that eating breakfast really is the underlying reason for the differences in grades (or at least part of the reason).

Using Statistical Tests

The following chapters set out the assumptions and statistical models appropriate to a number of commonly used statistical tests. An example is provided for each test to show how the relevant formulae are manipulated. Each test yields a *test statistic*.[3] From the test statistic, it is possible to estimate the probability of the observed outcome occurring (assuming that the null hypothesis is true) by looking up the test statistic in a table of probabilities that takes into account the characteristics of the sample, for example, the number of degrees of freedom. If the probability of the observed outcome is high, we can accept the null hypothesis as being a reasonable expression of what actually occurs in the population. If the probability is low (and by convention our cut-off point is a probability of less than 5%), then we can reject the null hypothesis.

---

[1]You might discover, if you were to carry out a similar study, that the grading system used in the schools which participated was different from the one described here. You might need to alter your assumptions to accord with the data.

[2]The test, in fact, would be the unpaired *t*-test. Come back to this example when you have read Chapter 6 and see if you agree.

[3]The exception is Fisher's Exact Test, in which there is no test statistic because the probabilities of particular outcomes are calculated directly.

Each of the tests described in the chapters in Part 2 is presented using the same format

Fundamental principle. The basic assumption for virtually every test is that the null hypothesis is true.[4] We then see if the results which we have observed are different from what we were expecting. For each test there is an *expectation* (what we would expect to observe if the null hypothesis were true) and a *decision criterion* (how we decide whether to accept or reject H_0).

Assumptions. For every test, we will make a series of assumptions. These assumptions provide the basis for the statistical model which allows us to calculate the probabilities that will help us to decide whether to accept or reject the null hypothesis. If you cannot make *all* of the assumptions listed, (e.g. if the experimental design is different, or the variable does not conform to the required distribution) a different test *must* be chosen, or some specific limitations observed.

Example. A fully worked example is given for each test.

Model. For each example, the data are described in such a way as to find the statistical model which we think the data best fit. The description of the data set should reflect the assumptions for the model. In this way you can be sure that you are using the right test. If the model and the assumptions do not match, you should choose another test to undertake your analysis. The description will also be of help when using the Statistical Flow Chart (see Appendix A10). You should also state the hypothesis and the null hypothesis.

Test procedure. A detailed description is given of how to carry out the test and calculate the test statistic. This is followed by a worked example.

Decision and interpretation. Every test statistic is interpreted to decide whether or not to reject the null hypothesis. The interpretation of the test statistic usually requires reference to a table of probabilities which is given in the Appendices. You must make a clear statement about whether you accept or reject the null hypothesis. If you reject H_0, you must say at what level of statistical confidence it is rejected.

Conclusion. At the end of every statistical test, you must state in plain English your conclusion regarding the acceptability of your original hypothesis, with some useful supporting results which summarize your findings.

---

[4]Occasionally, the hypothesis is *null*, that is, we are not expecting to see an effect. In these cases, there is no need to formulate a null hypothesis.

CHAPTER 6

Two Sample Comparisons for Normal Distributions: The t-test

Learning Objectives

After studying this chapter, you should be able to:

- Identify data sets for which the t-test is the right test to use
- Carry out both the paired and unpaired t-test manually
- Use the table of values for the t distribution to determine the level of significance of the differences observed
- Use the statistical diagnostics from SPSS to know which type of unpaired t-test to use
- Interpret the output from SPSS to determine the level of significance of your findings

6.1 INTRODUCTION

One of the most common research aims is to find out if the values observed in two experimental groups are 'really' different, or if the observed differences could have arisen just by chance due to random sampling variation. For example, you may be interested in the differences in the rate of growth in two groups of children growing up in different circumstances. Or you may want to know if a drug is more effective than a placebo in a simple randomized trial.

The t-test is one of the most powerful tools in the repertoire of statistical tests.[1] In Chapter 5, we saw that the t distribution allows us to predict how observations in samples drawn from normally distributed

---

[1]The t-test is described as 'robust'. This means that the underlying data can deviate quite a bit from normal, and the t-test will still provide a good estimate of the level of significance of the finding. The tests described later in the chapter (like the beautifully mellifluous Kolmogorov–Smirnov test, and others available in SPSS) help you to find out the probability of a specific set of observations being derived from a normally distributed population. Statistical procedures such as Analysis of Variance (see Chapter 11), on the other hand, are not robust, in the sense that it will not provide a reliable estimate of significance if the underlying distribution of the variable in the population deviates very far from normal.

---

populations will behave.[2] In this chapter, we apply this knowledge to comparisons of sample data.

The *t*-test has two formats: paired and unpaired. We will work through these in turn.

6.2 PAIRED *t*-TEST

The paired *t*-test is used to compare two sets of observations which have been collected in a way that involves some form of matching. The matching can take two forms. First, you might collect repeat observations in the same subjects at two time points. For example, you might want to know if eating a diet with a low glycaemic index has a beneficial effect on fasting blood glucose levels. You would measure fasting blood glucose in each subject after an overnight fast, at the same time in the morning, at baseline; then give them the low glycaemic index diet for four weeks; and then measure their fasting blood glucose a second time, also fasting and at the same time in the morning as the first measurement. Schematically, the observations would look like those shown in Table 6.1.

TABLE 6.1 Observations of Fasting Blood Glucose Levels in 10 Subjects at Baseline and after Four Weeks

Subject	Time Point	
	Baseline	4 weeks
Subject 1	$x_{1,0}$	$x_{1,1}$
Subject 2	$x_{2,0}$	$x_{2,1}$
Subject 3	$x_{3,0}$	$x_{3,1}$
Subject 4	$x_{4,0}$	$x_{4,1}$
Subject 5	$x_{5,0}$	$x_{5,1}$
Subject 6	$x_{6,0}$	$x_{6,1}$
Subject 7	$x_{7,0}$	$x_{7,1}$
Subject 8	$x_{8,0}$	$x_{8,1}$
Subject 9	$x_{9,0}$	$x_{9,1}$
Subject 10	$x_{10,0}$	$x_{10,1}$

The observations are denoted by the variable *x*, and the subscripts denote the subject number (1 through 10) and the time of the observation (baseline = 0, 4 weeks = 1). Using this convention, every observation has a unique identifier.

You would use the same layout of data if you were comparing the impact of a drug and a placebo in one group of patients (see Figure 1.2). Each subject would take the drug for a specified period, and then take the placebo for the same length of time. Your protocol would need to allow for a suitable washout period between the drug and the placebo, randomization of the order in which the drug or placebo was administered, and an assurance that the subject was 'blind' to whether it was drug or placebo being taken.[3]

Alternately, instead of having one group of 10 subjects, you might have 10 pairs of subjects that have been matched for sex, age, body mass index, and fasting blood glucose levels. Group 1 is given the low glycaemic index diet for four weeks, and Group 2 simply follows their normal diet. Fasting blood glucose levels are measured at the end of four weeks.[4] The schematic for this would look similar to that for repeat observations and is shown in Table 6.2.

Again, the observations are denoted by the variable *x*, but this time the subscripts denote the pair number (1 through 10) and the group (1 or 2).

The paired *t*-test is used to see if there are statistically significant differences between the paired observations.

---

[2]In the next chapter we will work through tests for variables which are not normally distributed.

[3]We have already noted that it is not always possible to blind subjects, for example in experiments where the impact of different foods is being tested. Special care needs to be taken to ensure that subjects do not make changes in their dietary behaviour over and above the differences that you want to test.
[4]There is another model for this which would look at the 'differences between the differences'. where we include the baseline measures as part of the data set, but let's not get ahead of ourselves. We will come back to the 'differences between the differences' model later in the chapter.

TABLE 6.2 Observations of Fasting Blood Glucose Levels after Four Weeks of Intervention in 10 Matched Pairs of Subjects

Pair	Low GI Diet (Group 1)	Normal Diet (Group 2)
Pair 1	$x_{1,1}$	$x_{1,2}$
Pair 2	$x_{2,1}$	$x_{2,2}$
Pair 3	$x_{3,1}$	$x_{3,2}$
Pair 4	$x_{4,1}$	$x_{4,2}$
Pair 5	$x_{5,1}$	$x_{5,2}$
Pair 6	$x_{6,1}$	$x_{6,2}$
Pair 7	$x_{7,1}$	$x_{7,2}$
Pair 8	$x_{8,1}$	$x_{8,2}$
Pair 9	$x_{9,1}$	$x_{9,2}$
Pair 10	$x_{10,1}$	$x_{10,2}$

Fundamental principles

We start with the assumption that there is no difference between our two sets of observations, i.e. that the null hypothesis is true:

Expectation:	H_0: The average difference ($\bar{d}$) between *pairs* of observations in the population is zero. Mathematically: $\mu = 0$, so we expect $\bar{d} = 0$ (or something close to it).[5]
Decision criterion:	If the average difference is very different from zero, reject H_0. If the calculated value for **t** is greater *than* the tabulated value for a given number of degrees of freedom and $P = 0.05$, reject H_0.

[5]What we mean by 'or something close to it' is at the heart of how we make a decision about whether or not the observed difference is statistically significantly different from zero.

By 'very different', we are saying that the probability of the observed average difference ($\bar{d}$) occurring is less than 5%, that is $P < 0.05$.

For every statistical test that we want to carry out, it is important to set out the conditions and actions that will allow us to examine the data and come to a clear conclusion regarding the statistical significance of the findings. These steps are set out in Box 6.1.

Assumptions

The assumptions which underpin the paired *t*-test are shown in Box 6.2.

A few comments are appropriate concerning each of these assumptions.

BOX 6.1

The steps to carry out a statistical test

Assumptions – What are the criteria that must be met to apply the test?

Model – Make sure that the data fit the requirements to carry out the test

Test procedure – Step-by-step instructions to carry out the test

Decision and interpretation – How to interpret the test statistic, including the *rejection rule*

BOX 6.2

Assumptions for the paired t-test

1. Sample observations are drawn from normally distributed populations
2. The variance of the population is the same for both sets of observations
3. Samples are independent
4. Observations are paired between samples or repeated within experimental units

Sample observations are drawn from normally distributed populations. The probabilities which you calculate in the *t*-test are based on the assumption that the variable in the population from which the sample observations are drawn is normally distributed. If the population is *not* normally distributed, the probabilities will be wrong, and you may be led to the wrong conclusion when you assess the value for *P*. If the variable is not normally distributed, you can (i) try transforming it (see Chapter 4) and seeing if it then behaves like a normally distributed variable, or (ii) use a statistical test that makes no assumptions about the underlying normality of the distribution (see Chapter 7).

The variance of the population is the same for both sets of observations. The fundamental principal of the paired *t*-test is to see if the average of the differences between paired observations is zero. But we know that because of random sampling variation, the average difference will not be exactly zero. The amount of variation in the observed differences will help us to decide whether what we have observed is 'very different' from zero. For valid results from the paired *t*-test, it is important that the variation in both sets of observations is similar. Again, SPSS provides output to help you decide if this condition is met.

Samples are independent. This is an absolutely vital assumption. The null hypothesis assumes that any sample drawn from the population is a truly random sample. There must be no reason, therefore, that an observation in one sample should be related to the other – each one must be fully independent. This does not contradict the idea of matching between paired observations, because the requirement for independence of observations relates to the variable of interest, not the matching criteria.

Observations are paired between samples or repeated within experimental units. This is fundamental to the design of the study. Any other arrangement of data collection will require a different test.

Example 6.1 Paired t-test

In a study of nutrition education, 10 patients with diabetes were given programmed health education

TABLE 6.3   Patients with Diabetes: Healthy Eating Knowledge Scores Before and After Instruction

Patient	Before	After
1	65	85
2	81	69
3	69	92
4	42	69
5	77	88
6	69	88
7	69	92
8	69	77
9	77	88
10	58	96

about healthy eating. Patients were tested on their knowledge before and after instruction. The data are shown in Table 6.3.

An initial glance at the table shows that most of the patients appear to have increased their scores after education. You might ask 'Why bother to carry out a statistical test? Isn't it obvious that education improves the scores in this group of patients?' Well, yes, the answer probably is fairly obvious here. But there will be many circumstances where the answer is not obvious, and that is why statistical tests are needed.

Model

The model for the paired *t*-test is shown in Box 6.3.

This description matches the assumptions that we made, so we can carry out a paired *t*-test; these data appear to be appropriate to test using the paired *t*-test.[6]

For clarity about what we are testing, we need to state the hypothesis and the null hypothesis.

[6]This is not surprising. I would have to be a strange author indeed to choose an example that was not appropriate for the test I was trying to illustrate! In Chapter 13, however, you will have an opportunity to match descriptions of data sets to appropriate tests.

BOX 6.3

Model for the paired t-test

1. One variable, normally distributed. (We shall assume a normal distribution for now. Later, we will look more closely at how this assumption can be justified.)
2. One group of subjects, independently drawn from the population of patients with diabetes.
3. Repeat observations in each subject.
4. Test to see if the mean difference between repeat observations is different from zero.

H_1: Providing nutrition education to patients with diabetes will improve their knowledge of healthy eating.

H_0: Providing nutrition education to patients with diabetes will have no impact on their knowledge of healthy eating.

Test procedure: paired t-test[7]

The procedure for carrying out the paired *t*-test is shown in Box 6.4.

Step 1. Take the difference between each pair of observations.

The null hypothesis states that there is no effect of the intervention. In that case, the difference between the 'before' and 'after' scores should be zero. We know that the difference will not necessarily be zero for every subject – some scores will go up, and some will go down. In theory, however, if the null

---

[7]Throughout this book, I ask you to undertake the manual calculations for each test for two reasons. First, it helps you develop a firm grasp of how the test works. Second, when you look at the output from statistical software, I will ask you *NOT* to jump straight to the *P* value. Instead, pause to check that the values for the intermediate calculations given in the output (*n*, and the various sums computed on the way to calculating the test statistic) make sense in relation to your original data.

BOX 6.4

Test procedure for the paired t-test

1. Take the difference between each pair of observations.
   - **Note!!   Take the difference in the same direction for EVERY pair!**
   - **Note!!   The sign of the difference is important!**
2. Calculate the mean and standard deviation of the differences.
3. Calculate the value for *t*, where
   $t = \bar{d} / \text{SE} = \bar{d} / \left(s / \sqrt{n} \right)$.
4. Compare the calculated value for *t* with the value in Appendix A3. If the calculated value is greater than the value in the table when $P = 0.05$ at $n - 1$ degrees of freedom, reject H_0.
5. If the null hypothesis is rejected, decide the level at which to reject H_0.

hypothesis were true, we would expect the *average* difference in scores to be zero. Our first step, therefore, is to take the differences between paired observations and find the average difference.

Table 6.4 shows the differences calculated for each subject. It is vitally important to take the difference in the same direction for every subject. It does not matter whether you decide to take A − B or B − A, because our test is going to be 'two-tailed' (see Chapter 5). The important thing is that it must be possible for the average difference to equal zero, so the sign of the difference is important and must be retained.

When taking the difference, try and make the outcome meaningful. For example, if we want to demonstrate that the score goes up following education, it makes sense to subtract Before (B) from After (A) (that is, find A − B). This will yield a positive result when the score has gone up, and a negative result when the score has gone down. Even if you take the differences in the other direction, however, your conclusion based on the *t*-test will be the same.

TABLE 6.4   Patients with Diabetes: Healthy Eating Knowledge Scores Before and After Instruction: Differences and Differences Squared

Patient	Before (B)	After (A)	Difference (After–Before)	
			d	d²
1	65	85	20	400
2	81	69	−12	144
3	69	92	23	529
4	42	69	27	729
5	77	88	11	121
6	69	88	19	361
7	69	92	23	529
8	69	77	8	64
9	77	88	11	121
10	58	96	38	1444
			Σd = 168	**Σd² = 4442**

Step 2. Calculate the mean and standard deviation of the differences.

These are straightforward calculations. They will provide us with the information that we need to determine whether or not to reject the null hypothesis. Table 6.4 shows the difference d for each subject. If we find Σd, then we can divide by n to find the mean difference. In this example, $\Sigma d = 168$ and $n = 10$, so $\bar{d} = 168/10 = 16.8$.

The calculation for the standard deviation uses the 'short' formula:

$$s = \sqrt{\frac{\Sigma d^2 - \left(\Sigma d\right)^2 / n}{n-1}},$$

which relies on Σd and Σd^2, the values for which are shown at the bottom of the two right-hand columns of Table 6.4. And because there are 10 pairs of differences, $n = 10$.

The standard deviation of the difference $(d = A - B)$ is given by:

$$s = \sqrt{\frac{\Sigma d^2 - \left(\left(\Sigma d\right)^2 / n\right)}{n-1}} = \sqrt{\frac{4442 - \left(168^2 / 10\right)}{10-1}}$$

$$= \sqrt{\frac{4442 - 2822.4}{9}} = \sqrt{\frac{1619.6}{9}}$$

$$= \sqrt{179.96} = 13.415$$

Step 3. Calculate the value for t.

We assume under H_0 that if the health education programme has no effect, the average difference between the before and after scores should be zero, that is, $\mu = 0$. We know from Chapter 5[8] that $t = \left(\bar{d} - \mu\right) / \text{SE}$, but as $\mu = 0$ (assuming that the null hypothesis is true), we can say $t = \bar{d}/\text{SE}$. We know that $\text{SE} = s/\sqrt{n}$. So, our equation now says:

$$t = \frac{\bar{d}}{\text{SE}} = \frac{\bar{d}}{s / \sqrt{n}} = \frac{16.8}{13.415 / \sqrt{10}} = \frac{16.8}{4.24} = 3.96$$

Decision and interpretation

Our aim is to see if what we observed in our sample is close to what we would expect to observe when drawing a random sample of 10 observations from a population in which the average change in score was zero (i.e. accords with what we would have expected to see if the null hypothesis were true). To test the null hypothesis, we put this slightly differently: how far away from zero is our observed mean? By convention,[9] if what we have observed in that set of results is likely to have occurred less than 5% of the time (making the assumption that the

---

[8]In Chapter 5, we said $t = (\bar{x} - \mu)/\text{SE}$. In the paired *t*-test, our variable is d rather than x, but of course the relationship to the *t* distribution remains the same.

[9]When I say, 'by convention', I mean it has been agreed among statisticians that if what we have observed is likely to occur less often than one time in 20 (i.e. less than 5% of the time), then it is 'reasonable' to reject the null hypothesis. There is no hard and fast rule about this, but everyone (more or less) has signed up to the convention, so that when we say a finding is 'statistically significant', this is what we mean.

null hypothesis is true), then we reject the null hypothesis. The value for t that we have calculated is the distance (in standard errors) that our observed value lies from zero. If the distance is greater than what we would expect to see 5% of the time or less (i.e. we are in the tails of the t distribution corresponding to less than 5% of the total area under the curve in the figure at the top of Appendix A3), then we can reject the null hypothesis.

Step 4. Compare the calculated value for t with the value in Appendix A3.

The mechanics of this step are straightforward. Find the value in Appendix A3 appropriate for this data set and t-test. There were 10 pairs of observations and 10 differences, so degrees of freedom $\nu = n - 1 = 10 - 1 = 9$. The conventional cut-off point for deciding whether or not to reject the null hypothesis is $P = 0.05$ (that is, we want to reject the null hypothesis for all those answers whose chance of arising if the null hypothesis is true is less than 5%). Find the value in Appendix A3 for the column headed $P = 0.05$ and the row headed 9 (you should find the value 2.262).

Rejection rule: If the absolute value of the calculated value for t is *greater than* the value in the table, reject H_0.

In our example, the calculated value for $t = 3.96$. This is greater than 2.262, so we reject H_0.

If we had taken $B-A$ rather than $A-B$, the value for t would have been -3.96 because the average difference would have been negative. However, we are interested in the *distance* of t from zero, not its direction, so the sign of the difference (and hence the sign of t) are not important to the test. The null hypothesis did not make any prediction about whether the average difference observed was going to be positive or negative. (A researcher testing the efficacy of the learning package might want to see a positive outcome, but that is a different matter.) Thus, for the purposes of comparing our observed value for t with the values in Appendix A3, we should take the absolute value (or modulus) of the

calculated value for t to compare with the value in the table of the t distribution in Appendix A3.

The mechanics of the t-test thus appear to be quite simple. But it is important to return to the theoretical basis to understand how the test works.

Two-tailed or one-tailed test

The null hypothesis in this example did not predict whether the average difference observed was going to be greater than or less than zero. We are therefore interested in the 5% of the area under the curve in the figure at the top of Appendix A3 that lies in either direction away from zero (2.5% in either tail). Hence, the test is referred to as 'two-tailed'.

The null hypothesis predicts that there will be no change in score resulting from the intervention. We know that because of random sampling variation, even if the null hypothesis *is* true and the average difference in the population *is* zero, the average difference for every sample will *not* be zero. The question, therefore, is how far *away* from zero does the sample average need to be before we can reject the null hypothesis. (Note that we are not saying anything about whether the average is above or below zero – the null hypothesis does not predict a direction.)

Let us look at a graphical representation of what we would expect to see if the null hypothesis were true. Imagine that thousands of samples of $n = 10$ had been drawn from the population of patients with diabetes who received education and who took the tests. For each sample we could calculate a value for $\bar{d}$. Figure 6.1a shows the distribution of values for $\bar{d}$ for all these samples.

If the null hypothesis is true and $\mu = 0$, then we expect most of the values for $\bar{d}$ to be close to zero. Some values of $\bar{d}$ will be further away from zero than others. However, if the value for $\bar{d}$ for any *one* sample is a long way from zero (as in the present example), we could argue that there is only a very small probability that the sample that we were considering came from the population in which the null hypothesis is true. If the probability of what we observe has less than a 5% chance of happening

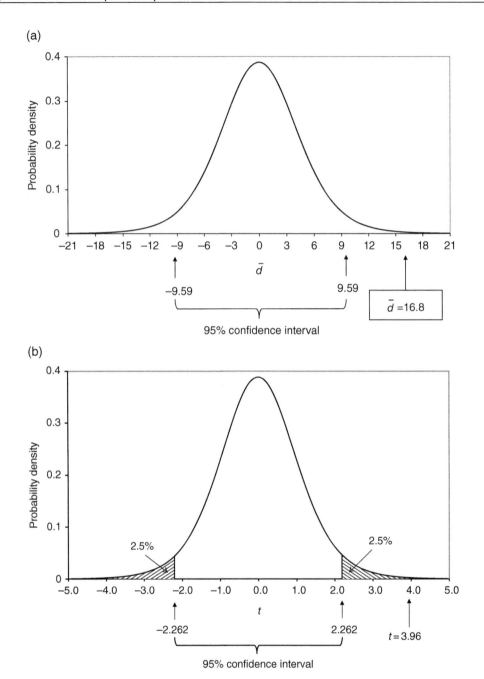

FIGURE 6.1   (a) Probability distribution of the values for $\bar{d}$, $\nu = 9$, if the null hypothesis is true. (b) Probability distribution of the values for t, $\nu = 9$, if the null hypothesis is true.

(that is, the observed value for $\bar{d}$ falls in either of the two tails in which only 2.5% of observations would be expected to fall), then we can say $P < 0.05$, and reject the null hypothesis. 95% of observations will be within the 95% confidence interval, and 5% will be outside the confidence interval.

The test statistic t is a standardized estimate of the distance of $\bar{d}$ from zero, expressed in terms of the number of standard errors. Figure 6.1b shows the distribution of values of t when $v = 9$.

If the value we calculate for t is within the 95% confidence interval for a population in which $\mu = 0$ (that is, $-2.262 < t < 2.262$), we can say that this value is within what we would expect to see 95% of the time if the null hypothesis were true. If the value for t lies outside the 95% confidence interval, we can argue that this finding is so unlikely (given a true null hypothesis) that it is reasonable to conclude that our observation comes from a different population in which μ does *not* equal zero. Thus, when we compare our calculated value for t (corresponding to the observed value for $\bar{d}$) with the value in the table, we are really seeing if the observed value for $\bar{d}$ is outside what we would expect to see 95% of the time if the null hypothesis were true. On that basis, when t is large[10] (greater than the value in the t table when $P = 0.05$ for a given value of v), we can reject H_0.

Step 5. If the null hypothesis is rejected, decide the level at which to reject H_0.

There is another decision that we need to make. It concerns the level of confidence that we have in rejecting the null hypothesis. Initially, if we have rejected the null hypothesis, we can say that our result is 'statistically significant at the 5% level'. But can we be more confident? Can we say that the probability of the observed result is less than 1%, or 0.1%? Our value for t, 3.96, is very much larger than 2.262. Is the probability of getting a value for t as large as this (that is, $\bar{d}$ being so far away from zero) very much less than 5%? The answer, if we look at Figure 6.1b, would appear to be 'Yes'. We are in very small areas of the tails of the distribution, and the sum of the areas under the curve beyond our observation (and in the other tail an equivalent distance away from zero) is much less than 5%.

Let us go back to Appendix A3. If we follow the row for nine degrees of freedom to the right, we come to columns headed 0.02, 0.01, and 0.001. The values

for t get larger as the probabilities get smaller: when $P = 0.02$, $t = 2.821$; when $P = 0.01$, $t = 3.250$; when $P = 0.001$, $t = 4.781$. This makes sense because the areas in the tail of the curve in Figure 6.1b get smaller as t gets larger. We can reject the null hypothesis with greater confidence: the probability of seeing what we have observed is substantially less than 5%. Our calculated value for t is greater than the value in the table when $P = 0.01$. Thus, we could say that $P < 0.01$, or that 'we can reject the null hypothesis at the 1% level'. The value does not allow us to reject the null hypothesis at the 0.1% level because our observed value for t is not greater than 4.781. We do not, however, *accept* the null hypothesis at this level. Once we have made the decision to reject the null hypothesis at the 5% level, it is gone, finished, caput, and we do not 're-accept' it at a different level of confidence.

Before we leave the issue of interpretation, there is a matter of semantics that we need to deal with. What exactly does the P value tell you? ***P is the probability of having found the observed result (or something further away from zero) if we assume that the null hypothesis is true.*** If the probability is very small (i.e. less than 5%), this suggests that the null hypothesis is not a very good representation of what goes on in the reality which gave rise to our particular sample, and we can reject H_0. This is not to say that we have 'proven' our hypothesis (remember that we can never 'prove' an exact hypothesis). There is the chance that the null hypothesis *is* true, and that although P is very small, we have observed one of those rare instances in which random sampling has led us to a result which is a long way from what we were expecting. This is the nature of statistical analysis. We can never be 100% sure that we have 'proved' our hypothesis.

More important, it is *incorrect* to say that P is the probability of the null hypothesis being true. The null hypothesis *is* either true *or* false.[11] But remember that the hypothesis (or the null hypothesis) is only

---

[10]Or strictly speaking, 'when the *absolute value* of t is large'.

[11]The probability of having made a mistake in rejecting the null hypothesis is, in fact, equal to the value of P at which we have rejected the null hypothesis. This is known as a 'Type I' error. We will come back to Type I (and indeed Type II) errors in Chapter 12.

an approximation of what we believe to be true (it is a *conjecture*). While the inability to be absolutely sure of anything may be a source of frustration, it leaves open the possibility that we can improve our models (there is room for *refutation*). We can incorporate more and more variables into our models (like our breakfast example in the Introduction to Part 2) that will give us a better approximation of reality. The model is thus only a tool to help us discover what we think is happening in reality, remembering (from Chapter 1) that we will never be able to observe reality directly. In the chapters in this section of the book, we will describe a number of very useful models that can help us to understand data collected in a wide variety of circumstances, and gradually work our way towards models which are increasingly complex.

Conclusion

Finally, we need to provide a brief summary and interpretation of our result in terms of the original hypothesis. In this example, we could say the following:

> *Giving nutrition education to a group of patients with diabetes improves their healthy eating knowledge scores. Average scores rose from 67.6 points before education to 84.4 points after education, an average increase of 16.8 points. We accept our hypothesis that the education program has had an effect on knowledge. This finding is statistically significant at the 1% level.*

It would be typical in a written report of your findings to give the mean together with either the standard deviation (if you want to tell your reader about the spread of values around the mean) or the standard error (if you want to tell your reader about the precision of the mean). In most instances, for normal data, you should report the mean and standard error.

In future examples, the results of the tests will not be presented in quite so detailed a fashion. But the basic elements (Fundamental principles, Assumptions,

Example, Model, Test procedure, Decision and interpretation, Rejection rule, Conclusion) will all be there.

6.3 UNPAIRED t-TEST

The unpaired *t*-test is appropriate for comparing the means of two groups of observations that are NOT paired and in which the variable of interest is normally distributed in the population from which the samples have been drawn. The groups must be similar regarding those characteristics that might have an influence on the variable of interest. For instance, if we were comparing growth in two groups of rats raised on different experimental diets, it would be important that they were from the same strain, of the same gender, and at the same stage of growth.

Fundamental principle

Expectation:	H_0: The means of the two populations from which the samples are drawn are the same, i.e. the difference between the population means is zero
	Mathematically: $\mu_1 = \mu_2$, or $\mu_1 - \mu_2 = 0$ Therefore, we expect $\bar{x}_1 - \bar{x}_2 = 0$ (or something close to it).
Decision criterion:	If the difference between sample means is very different from zero, reject H_0.
	If the calculated value for t is *greater than* the tabulated value for a given number of degrees of freedom and $P = 0.05$, reject H_0.

Assumptions

The assumptions which underpin the unpaired *t*-test are shown in Box 6.5.

A few comments are appropriate concerning each of these assumptions. As for the paired *t*-test, it

> **BOX 6.5**
>
> Assumptions for the unpaired t-test
>
> 1. Two groups of sample observations are drawn from normally distributed populations.
> 2. The samples are independent.
> 3. The variance of the population is the same for both sets of observations. (Equal variances assumption.)
> 4. Observations are not paired between samples. n_1 may or may not equal n_2.

TABLE 6.5 Mortality Ratio (MR) in 13 Hospitals with or without Intensive Care Unit (ICU) Staffing Problems

ICU with Staffing Problems		ICU without Staffing Problems	
Hospital Number	MR	Hospital Number	MR
1	0.84	9	0.59
2	0.88	10	0.90
3	0.93	11	0.92
4	1.00	12	0.96
5	1.04	13	1.10
6	1.13		
7	1.27		
8	1.58		

is important that the sample observations are drawn from a variable which is normally distributed in the population. We also need to assume that the variances of the variable of interest are the same in both populations. (This is known as the 'equal variances assumption'. If the variances are different [and there is a statistical test to help you decide if they *are* different], an alternative strategy is required for calculating the number of degrees of freedom – there is more on this below.) As before, we assume that the sample observations are randomly drawn from the populations and that they are independent of one another. Finally, we assume that the observations are *not* paired. If they were paired, we should be using the paired *t*-test.

Example 6.2 Unpaired t-test

A study looked at patient deaths in Intensive Care Units (ICUs). The mortality ratio (MR) of actual to predicted deaths was calculated for 13 ICUs. If MR < 1, there were fewer deaths than predicted; if MR > 1, there were more deaths than predicted. Table 6.5 shows the MR according to the presence or absence of staffing problems in the ICU in the 13 hospitals.

It looks as if the MR was higher more often in the ICU with staffing problems compared with the ICU without staffing problems. But there is an overlap between the two sets of observations. We need to carry out a statistical test to see if the

differences are 'real' or simply a product of sampling variation.

Model

The model for the unpaired *t*-test is shown in Box 6.6.

> **BOX 6.6**
>
> Model for the unpaired t-test
>
> 1. One variable, normally distributed. (As before, we shall assume that the variable is normally distributed without using a formal test for normality.)
> 2. Two groups of observations, independently drawn from the population of hospitals with Intensive Care Units.
> 3. The variances of the two populations (hospitals with or without ICU staffing problems) are the same.
> 4. Observations are *not* paired between samples.
> 5. Test to see if the difference between sample means of the two groups is different from zero.

This description matches the assumptions that we would need to carry out an unpaired t-test. The hypothesis and the null hypothesis are:

H_1: There is a higher MR in ICUs with staffing problems.

H_0: The MR in ICUs is not affected by staffing problems.

Test procedure: unpaired t-test

The procedure for carrying out the paired t-test is shown in Box 6.7.

Step 1. Calculate the mean and standard deviation for each set of observations.

Table 6.6 shows the sums of the observations and the sums of the squares of the observations.

Using these values, it is a simple matter to find the mean and standard deviation for each group using the formulae with which you by now should be familiar. We find the following values:

$$\overline{x}_1 = 1.084 \qquad s_1 = 0.244$$
$$\overline{x}_2 = 0.894 \qquad s_2 = 0.187$$

BOX 6.7

Test procedure for the unpaired t-test

1. Calculate the mean and standard deviation for each set of observations.
2. Calculate the difference between the means.
3. Calculate the value for the pooled standard deviation s_0.
4. Calculate the value for t, where
   $$t = \left(\overline{x}_1 - \overline{x}_2\right) / \left(s_0 \sqrt{\left(1/n_1\right) + \left(1/n_2\right)}\right).$$
5. Compare the calculated value for t with the value in Appendix A3. If the calculated value is greater than the value in the table when $P = 0.05$ at $n_1 + n_2 - 2$ degrees of freedom, reject H_0.
6. If the null hypothesis is rejected, decide the level at which to reject H_0.

Step 2. Calculate the difference between the means.

It appears that the MR in the ICU with staffing problems (MR = 1.084) is over 20% higher than the MR in ICU without staffing problems (0.894). The percentage difference is calculated as follows:

$$1.084 - 0.894 = 0.19$$
$$\frac{0.19}{0.894} \times 100 = 21.3\%$$

Is this a problem that needs to be tackled by the hospital administrations, or did the observed difference arise just by chance, and is not statistically significant?

Step 3. Calculate the value for the pooled standard deviation s_0.

We need to find out if the observed difference between the mean MRs (0.19) is statistically significantly different from zero (our expectation if the null hypothesis is true). To do this, we need to find a value for t, that is, to express the difference between the means in terms of the number of standard errors (this is exactly what we did for the paired t-test). To calculate the standard error, we will need a value for the standard deviation. But which standard deviation is it best to use: s_1 or s_2?

Let us go back to basic principles (such a comforting place). If the null hypothesis is true, then the two samples are from identical populations in which $\mu_1 = \mu_2$ and $\sigma_1 = \sigma_2$. We can say, therefore, $\sigma_1 = \sigma_2 = \sigma$. In theory, both s_1 and s_2 are equally good estimators of σ. They differ only because of random sampling variation. So, it makes sense to use all of the information that we have about the way in which observations vary around the mean and find a way to use both s_1 and s_2 in our calculations.

The simplest thing to do would be to take the average of the two values: $(s_1 + s_2)/2$

But s_1 is based on eight observations, while s_2 is based on only five. In theory, s_1 should be a better estimate of σ because it is based on more observations. It would make sense, therefore, to find a

TABLE 6.6   Mortality Ratio (MR) in 13 Hospitals with or without Intensive Care Unit (ICU) Staffing Problems

	ICU with Staffing Problems			ICU Without Staffing Problems		
Hospital Number	MR	MR²	Hospital Number	MR	MR²
1	0.84	0.7056	9	0.59	0.3481
2	0.88	0.7744	10	0.90	0.8100
3	0.93	0.8649	11	0.92	0.8464
4	1.00	1.0000	12	0.96	0.9216
5	1.04	1.0816	13	1.10	1.2100
6	1.13	1.2769			
7	1.27	1.6129			
8	1.58	2.4964			
$n_1 = 8$	$\Sigma_1 x = 8.67$	$\Sigma_1 x^2 = 9.8127$	$n_2 = 5$	$\Sigma_2 x = 4.47$	$\Sigma_2 x^2 = 4.1361$

weighted mean (see Chapter 2) which takes into account the number of observations in both samples[12]: $(n_1 s_1 + n_2 s_2)/(n_1 + n_2)$.

Statistics being what it is (confusing and difficult at times), this expression is not in fact the best estimator of σ. It is better to base s_0 on the variances of the groups rather than the standard deviations,[13] and to use the number of degrees of freedom for the 'weights' rather than n.

So, the final expression for the pooled variance looks like this:

$$s_0^2 = \frac{(n_1 - 1)s_1^2 + (n_2 - 1)s_2^2}{(n_1 - 1) + (n_2 - 1)}$$

---

[12]When you find a weighted mean, you must divide by the sum of the 'weights'; in this case $n_1 + n_2$. Also, as we have seen, the convention in mathematics is to leave out the 'times' sign when writing the formula for multiplying two numbers together. So, the expression $(n_1 \times s_1 + n_2 \times s_2)/(n_1 + n_2)$ is equivalent to $(n_1 s_1 + n_2 s_2)/(n_1 + n_2)$. We shall follow this convention for multiplication throughout the book. Of course, if you are writing a formula using numbers rather than symbols, the algebraic signs will be required for the expression to make sense.

[13]Variances behave better mathematically than standard deviations. That is why we keep coming back to them as the basis for our calculations. We will see this repeated in subsequent chapters in this section.

Remembering that the formulae for the variance for each set of observations are

$$s_1^2 = \frac{\Sigma_1 x^2 - \left(\Sigma_1 x\right)^2 / n_1}{n_1 - 1} \text{ and } s_2^2 = \frac{\Sigma_2 x^2 - \left(\Sigma_2 x\right)^2 / n_2}{n_2 - 1},$$

we can simplify our expression for s_0, save ourselves the trouble of calculating the standard deviations for both groups, and simply use Σx and Σx^2. The final expression for s_0^2 is therefore:

$$s_0^2 = \frac{\Sigma_1 x^2 - \left(\left(\Sigma_1 x\right)^2 / n_1\right) + \Sigma_2 x^2 - \left(\left(\Sigma_2 x\right)^2 / n_2\right)}{n_1 + n_2 - 2}$$

EQUATION 6.1   Pooled variance of the two sets of observations in an unpaired t-test.

In this example,

$$s_0^2 = \frac{9.8127 - \left(8.67^2 / 8\right) + 4.1361 - \left(4.47^2 / 5\right)}{8 + 5 - 2} = 0.0506$$

and $s_0 = \sqrt{0.0506} = 0.225$

Step 4. Calculate the value for t, where

$$t = \frac{\overline{x}_1 - \overline{x}_2}{\text{SE}} = \frac{\overline{x}_1 - \overline{x}_2}{s_0 \sqrt{\left(1/n_1\right) + \left(1/n_2\right)}}.$$

The value for t expresses the differences between the means in terms of the number of standard errors of the difference between the means. In this case, $SE = s_0\sqrt{(1/n_1)+(1/n_2)}$. This is analogous to the standard error that we calculated in Chapter 4, where we said that $SE = s/\sqrt{n} = s\sqrt{1/n}$. To find the standard error of the difference between the means, we need to take into account both n_1 and n_2; hence our new formula for the SE that takes the size of both samples into account. In this example,

$$SE = s_0\sqrt{\frac{1}{n_1}+\frac{1}{n_2}} = 0.225\sqrt{\frac{1}{8}+\frac{1}{5}} = 0.128,$$

so

$$t = \frac{\bar{x}_1 - \bar{x}_2}{SE} = \frac{1.084 - 0.894}{0.128} = \frac{0.19}{0.128} = 1.48$$

Decision and interpretation

Step 5. Compare the calculated value for t with the value in Appendix A3.

The procedure is essentially the same as for the paired t-test. Find the value in Appendix A3 appropriate for this data set and t-test. There were eight observations in one group and five in the other, so degrees of freedom $v = n_1 - 1 + n_2 - 1 = 8 - 1 + 5 - 1 = 7 + 4 = 11$. Keeping to the conventional cut-off point of $P = 0.05$ for rejecting H_0, we find the value in Appendix A3 for the column headed $P = 0.05$ and the row headed $v = 11$ (you should find 2.201).

> **Rejection rule**: If the absolute value of the calculated value for t is *greater than* the value in the table, reject H_0.

The calculated value for t, 1.48, is less than the tabulated value, 2.201. As our calculated value for t is *less than or equal to*[14] the value in the table, we

accept H_0 because the probability of the result which we observed arising just by chance if the null hypothesis is true is greater than 5%.

Again, a graphical representation may help you to understand the interpretation. Think of all the possible combinations of differences between values of $\bar{x}_1$ and $\bar{x}_2$ of sample sizes 8 and 5, respectively, which could be drawn from the two populations of hospitals (those with or those without staffing problems). Figure 6.2a shows the probability distribution of the values for $\bar{x}_1 - \bar{x}_2$ if the null hypothesis were true. Most of the values would be close to zero, but 5% of the differences would be a long way from zero (either <-0.282 or >0.282), given the size of the standard error. Figure 6.2b shows the same distribution, but expressed this time in relation to values for t for any set of observations in which there are 11 degrees of freedom.

It is quite clear that the difference which we have observed is well within the 95% confidence interval, whether we express it in terms of the difference between the means ($\bar{x}_1 - \bar{x}_2 = 0.19$, Figure 6.2a) or in terms of the calculated value for t ($t = 1.48$, the difference expressed in terms of the number of standard errors away from the expected mean of zero, as shown in Figure 6.2b).

Conclusion

The difference that we have observed is well within what would be expected if the null hypothesis were true, so we accept the null hypothesis. We could say:

The mean MR of ICUs with staffing problems (1.084) was higher than the MR in ICUs without staffing problems (0.894), but the difference failed to reach statistical significance ($p > 0.05$).[15]

Before we leave the unpaired t-test, however, we need to consider how to proceed if the equal variances assumption is not true.

---

[14]Technically, when the calculated value for t is *less than or equal to* the value in the table, we accept H_0. If the calculated value was exactly equal to the value in the table for $P = 0.05$, we would describe the result as being 'of borderline statistical significance'.

[15]In fact, according to the output from SPSS, $p = 0.17$. You could work this out for yourself by interpolating values within Appendix A3. If you feel like testing your interpolation skills, go ahead and do it for yourself.

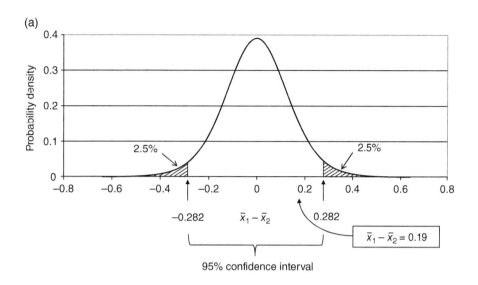

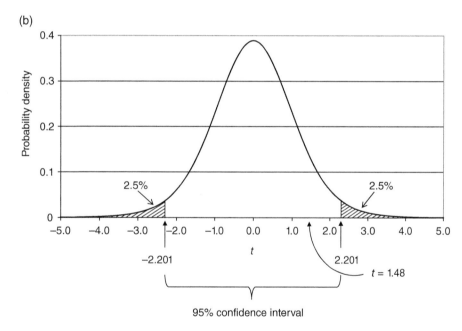

FIGURE 6.2 (a) Probability distribution of the values for $\bar{x}_1 - \bar{x}_2$, $\nu = 11$, if the null hypothesis is true. (b) Probability distribution of the values of t for $\bar{x}_1 - \bar{x}_2$, $\nu = 11$, if the null hypothesis is true.

The unequal variances assumption

There are many occasions when we cannot assume that the variances of the two populations are equal. If so, then the best estimate of the variance of the difference between two means with unequal vari-

ances is given by the expression: $\left(s_1^2 / n_1\right) + \left(s_2^2 / n_2\right)$. The standard error of the difference is then given by:
$SE = \sqrt{\left(s_1^2 / n_1\right) + \left(s_2^2 / n_2\right)}$, and t would be given as:
$t = \left(\bar{x}_1 - \bar{x}_2\right) / \sqrt{\left(s_1^2 / n_1\right) + \left(s_2^2 / n_2\right)}$.

Unfortunately, using this approach, the *smaller* sample is now contributing a greater weight to the standard error than the larger sample (because you are dividing the variance by a smaller number). In order to compensate, it is necessary to calculate the degrees of freedom in a way which reflects this. So instead of calculating $v = n_1 + n_2 - 2$, we calculate degrees of freedom using the Satterthwaite Formula:

$$df = \frac{\left(\dfrac{s_1^2}{n_1} + \dfrac{s_2^2}{n_2} \right)^2}{\dfrac{1}{n_1 - 1}\left(\dfrac{s_1^2}{n_1} \right)^2 + \dfrac{1}{n_2 - 1}\left(\dfrac{s_2^2}{n_2} \right)^2}$$

This reduces the value for degrees of freedom from 11 to 10.345. When $v = 11$ and $P = 0.05$, $t = 2.201$; when $v = 10$ and $P = 0.05$, $t = 2.228$. This means that you would need to achieve a larger value for t in order to be able to reject the null hypothesis at the 5% level.

In practice, SPSS will run the tests necessary to help you decide whether to accept or reject the equal variances assumption. If you reject the equal variances assumption, SPSS will undertake the Satterthwaite calculation and report the relevant values for t, v and P. See Section 6.4.5 for the relevant discussion and output.

6.4 EXERCISES

6.4.1

Ten patients with anorexia in the final stages of recovery were candidates for a trial of a new anti-anxiety drug. Patients received the drug over four weeks. Each patient was also given a placebo over four weeks. Anxiety scores were measured at the end of each treatment period. The order of administration of the active drug and the placebo was randomized for each patient. There was a washout period of four weeks between the administration of the drug and placebo (Table 6.7).

TABLE 6.7   Anxiety Scores of 10 Patients with Anorexia Given Drug or Placebo

Patient	Anxiety Score	
	Drug	Placebo
1	19	22
2	11	18
3	14	17
4	17	19
5	23	22
6	11	12
7	15	14
8	19	11
9	11	19
10	8	7

Was the new drug significantly more effective than the placebo in reducing patient anxiety?

6.4.2

Two groups of school children aged 14–15 years, matched for sex, were given anti-smoking teaching using either a video and discussion (Group A) or formal lecturing (Group B). Each group was tested, after teaching, for their knowledge relating to the hazards of smoking, and the results are shown in Table 6.8.

Is there evidence to suggest that one method of teaching is better than the other?

6.4.3

Weight gain (g) was measured between 4 and 12 weeks in two groups of infants in a village in Guatemala. One group was breast fed and the other bottle fed. The results are shown in Table 6.9.

Was there a significant difference in the rate of growth between the two groups of infants?

TABLE 6.8 Knowledge Scores Related to the Hazards of Smoking

Pair	Group A (Video)	Group B (Formal)
1	51	37
2	48	53
3	35	39
4	60	46
5	57	51
6	64	60
7	71	50
8	63	41
9	55	33
10	50	45

TABLE 6.9 Weight Gain (g) between 4 and 12 Weeks in Breast-fed or Bottle-fed Babies

Breast	Bottle
1600	600
1500	800
600	750
1000	700
1100	1000
1700	1200
900	
1500	
1400	
1600	

6.4.4

When you have read section 6.4.5, go back to the preceding three exercises and carry out the analyses using SPSS. The data sets are available online in the following SPSS.sav files:

- Ch06d01 (diabetes knowledge scores)
- Ch06d02 (ICU data)
- Ch06e01 (Anxiety data)

- Ch06e02 (Smoking data)
- Ch06e03 (Breast-feeding data

together with the related syntax (.sps) and output (.spv) files. When you run the analyses, don't forget to look at the syntax and ALL the output and make sure you understand it. If you don't, consult your tutor or friendly statistician.

6.4.5 SPSS Kolmogorov–Smirnov and Two–sample t-test

Once you have completed Exercise 6.4.3, have a look at the following approach to analysis using SPSS. I am not going to do this for every example in the text – this is a book about statistics and not a manual for SPSS. For each example in the text, I will put the data into an SPSS data set and include the syntax and output files. The output file shows the command syntax under the 'Log' entry immediately preceding the output. It can also be seen if you double click on the NOTES icon given for each test.

The first output (Figure 6.3) shows the results of a Kolmogorov–Smirnov one-sample test for normality. This is easy and quick to run and tells you straight away if the distribution of the observed values in your sample are likely to have come from a population in which the variable is normally distributed.

The command is under the nonparametric tests on the SPSS Analyze dropdown menu.

Analyze>Nonparametric Tests>One Sample. Click on 'Scan data'. Click on the FIELDS tab and select the data that you want to test. Click on the SETTINGS tab, click on Customize tests, then choose 'Test observed distribution against hypothesized (Kolmogorov–Smirnov test)'.

Click on OPTIONS, choose Normal, and click on Use Sample Data.

I have chosen the observations from Table 6.3 Patients with diabetes: healthy eating knowledge scores before and after instruction. I have looked at each data set separately. I have also combined them in to a single set of observations (VAR00003), as I am assuming that if the null hypothesis is true (both sets of observations come from the same population), they should be drawn from a similar distribution.

This is the syntax generate by the command:

NPTESTS
/ONESAMPLE TEST (Before After VAR00003)
    KOLMOGOROV_SMIRNOV(NORMAL=
    SAMPLE)
/MISSING SCOPE=ANALYSIS USERMISSING=
    EXCLUDE
/CRITERIA ALPHA=0.05 CILEVEL=95.

The output is shown in Figure 6.3.

The output is very easy to understand. The first column shows the name of the variable being tested, the mean, and standard deviation. It also tells you if it is normal! The second column tells you which test was run, and the third column shows you the P value. The null hypothesis in this case is that the observations were derived from a normally distributed population. If $P \geq 0.05$, we accept the null hypothesis. If $P < 0.05$, we reject the null hypothesis and assume that the data are derived from a population in which the distribution of the variable does not follow the normal distribution. Simple.

There is always a 'but', however. First, there are arguments about how small the sample should be in order to trust the result. We are using *very* small samples ($n < 30$). There is an alternate test,

Shapiro–Wilks, also available through SPSS, usually as a subcommand to other analyses. At least now you have a sense of how to interpret the output whichever test for normality you use. Second, for very large samples (e.g. $n > 1000$), both tests can be oversensitive: a normal-looking distribution needs to deviate only a little from the normal and K–S and S–W tests tell you it is not from a population in which the variable follows the normal distribution. Graphical inspection, testing for skewness and kurtosis, will give you further guidance. Again, getting help from your friendly statistician is the best way forward.

SPSS output: paired t-test

First, I am going to look at the SPSS output for the paired t-test. We will use the data set for the patients with diabetes.

Using the SPSS dropdown menus, I click on Analyze, then Compare Means, then Paired-samples T test. I then dragged the variable 'After' into the box labelled 'Variable 1' for 'Pair 1', and 'Before' in the box for 'Variable 2'. (I have done it in that order because SPSS subtracts the values for Variable 2 from the values for Variable 1, and I want to know in which direction the scores have changed, that is After−Before.) The result is shown in Figure 6.4.

Hypothesis test summary

	Null hypothesis	Test	Sig.	Decision
1	The distribution of before is normal with mean 68 and standard deviation 11.147	One-sample Kolmogorov–Smirnov test	0.077[a]	Retain the null hypothesis
2	The distribution of after is normal with mean 84 and standard deviation 9.536	One-sample Kolmogorov–Smirnov test	0.084[a]	Retain the null hypothesis
3	The distribution of VAR00003 is normal with mean 76.00 and standard deviation 13.274	One-sample Kolmogorov–Smirnov test	0.200[a,b]	Retain the null hypothesis

Asymptotic significances are displayed. The significance level is 0.05.

[a]Lilliefors corrected.

[b]This is a lower bound of the true significance.

FIGURE 6.3   SPSS output for Kolmogorov–Smirnov test for normality. *Source*: Reproduced with permission of International Business Machines Corporation.

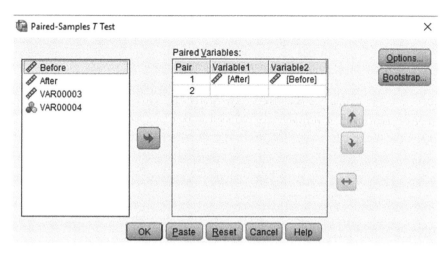

FIGURE 6.4 SPSS command screen for paired *t*-test. *Source*: Reproduced with permission of International Business Machines Corporation

You now have two choices. You can click on OK and produce output. Or you can click on PASTE and copy the syntax into an SPSS syntax file. I *always* do the latter. That way, I have a copy of the syntax. First, I can make sure I have carried out the command I wanted to carry out. Second, if I need to rerun the command, I can do so easily. (I might have revised the data, for example, by adding more observations, or I might want to run the same command with different variable names.) I strongly advise using the PASTE function whenever you use SPSS.

If you have pasted the syntax, go to the syntax file and run the command. Figure 6.5 shows the output.

SPSS gives you all you could possibly want by way of output. The mean value is the mean of $\bar{d}$, where $d =$ After$-$Before. The next two values show the standard deviation and standard error of $\bar{d}$. Then comes the limits of the 95% confidence interval for μ around $\bar{d}$ (i.e. where you would expect to find the true population mean μ and be right 95% of the time). As the 95% confidence interval does not include zero, you know already that the finding is statistically significant at the 5% level. The next value is for t, then degrees of freedom ($\nu = 9$), and finally P. The value for $P = 0.003$. We could have interpolated the value in Appendix A3 based on our calculated value for t. The

conclusion is the same: the finding is significant at the 1% level (that is, $0.01 > P > 0.001$).

SPSS output: unpaired *t*-test

Finally, we can look at the SPSS commands and output for an unpaired *t*-test. We will use the ICU data from Table 6.5. This time, you need to put all the data in one column, and in a second column identify the group from which each observation came (I used '0' for the ICU with staffing problems and '1' for the ICU without staffing problems.

First, I checked that the data were probably derived from a normally distributed population using the Kolmogorov–Smirnov test.[16] All was well.

Second, I clicked on Analyze, then Compare Means, then Independent-samples T test to produce the following syntax:

```
T-TEST GROUPS=ICUgroup(0 1)
/MISSING=ANALYSIS
/VARIABLES=ICUboth
/CRITERIA=CI(.95).
```

---

[16]NPTESTS
/ONESAMPLE TEST (ICU1 ICU2 ICUboth) KOLMOGOROV_
    SMIRNOV(NORMAL=SAMPLE)
/MISSING SCOPE=ANALYSIS USERMISSING=EXCLUDE
/CRITERIA ALPHA=0.05 CILEVEL=95.

Paired samples test

| | | | | Paired differences | | | | |
| | | | | | 95% confidence interval of the difference | | | | |
	Mean	Std. deviation	Std. error mean	Lower	Upper	t	df	Sig. (2-tailed)
Pair 1 After − Before	16.800	13.415	4.242	7.204	26.396	3.960	9	0.003

FIGURE 6.5   SPSS output for paired t-test. *Source*: Reproduced with permission of International Business Machines Corporation.

Group statistics

ICU group		N	Mean	Std. deviation	Std. error mean
ICU both	0.00	8	1.0838	0.24395	0.08625
	1.00	5	0.8940	0.18703	0.08364

Independent samples test

| | | Levene's test for equality of variances | | t-test for equality of means | | | | | | | |
| | | | | | | | | | | 95% confidence interval of the difference | |
		F	Sig.	t	df	Sig. (2-tailed)	Mean difference	Std. error difference	Lower	Upper
ICU both	Equal variances assumed	0.572	0.465	1.480	11	0.167	0.18975	0.12823	−0.09248	0.47198
	Equal variances not assumed			1.579	10.345	0.144	0.18975	0.12015	−0.07675	0.45625

FIGURE 6.6   SPSS output for unpaired t-test. *Source*: Reproduced with permission of International Business Machines Corporation.

I ran this to produce the output shown in Figure 6.6. The first table in Figure 6.6 shows n, mean, SD, and SE for each group. All very helpful, showing that the mean for the ICU units without staffing problems is lower than for the ICU with staffing problems. Is the difference statistically significant?

The second table in Figure 6.6 has two rows of output. The first two values in the first row show the results for Levene's test for equal variance: an F statistic and a P value (in SPSS speak, the P value is denoted by 'Sig.'). The null hypothesis for Levene's test is that both sets of observations come from populations with equal variances (that is, $\sigma_1^2 = \sigma_2^2$). As $P > 0.05$, we accept the null hypothesis that both variances are derived from the same or equivalent populations.

As we accepted the null hypothesis for Levene's test, we look at the results from the statistical analysis in the first row ('Equal variances assumed').[17] The SPSS output accords with the one we did manually: $t = 1.48$, $P > 0.05$, and we accept the null hypothesis. The other useful piece of information is the limits to the 95% confidence interval. These include zero, a further indication that the mean difference (0.18975) might well have been derived from populations between which the mean difference was zero. Our observed difference is not exactly equal to zero because of random sampling variation.

---

[17]If we had rejected the null hypothesis for Levene's test, we would have assumed that the variances for the two samples were not equal, and used the results for the unpaired t-test in the second row of output.

CHAPTER 7

Nonparametric Two-Sample Tests

Learning Objectives

After studying this chapter you should be able to:

- Know when to use nonparametric two-sample tests rather than the t-test
- Understand when and how to use the Mann–Whitney test for unmatched two-sample data
- Understand when and how to use the Wilcoxon signed-rank test for matched two-sample data
- Know when and how to use the Wilcoxon sign test

7.1 INTRODUCTION

In Chapter 6, we looked at when and how to use the t-test to understand when observations from two samples, whether matched or unmatched, differed from each other statistically. The limitation of the t-test is that the sample data should be derived from populations in which the variable of interest follows the normal distribution.

This chapter looks at the equivalent of the t-test for nonnormally distributed data. For unpaired data, we will use the Mann–Whitney test. For paired data, we will use the Wilcoxon signed-rank test. We will also have a look at the Sign test for data which have only two outcomes – Yes or No, up or down, etc.

The reason for using the *t-test* was twofold. First, it meant that we could use all the information available for interval or ratio variables in the statistical analysis, and for ordinal variables which follow a normal distribution. Also, in Chapter 4, we looked at how to transform data, so that even if our original observations were not from a normally distributed population, we could try and create a distribution of observations that was normal in character so that we could use the t-test for our analyses. Second, we said that the t-test was *powerful*: this means it is very good at returning a value for P which is likely to reflect the true probability of observing what we observed assuming the null hypothesis is true.

Statistics in Nutrition and Dietetics, First Edition. Michael Nelson.
© 2020 John Wiley & Sons Ltd. Published 2020 by John Wiley & Sons Ltd.
Companion website: www.wiley.com/go/nelson/statistics

There comes a point, however, when the *t*-test is not the right test to use:

- The data are from a variable that is not normally distributed.
- The data cannot be transformed to something approximating the normal distribution. Measurements of alcoholic beverage consumption or Vitamin B_{12} intake, for example, do not lend themselves to transformation into a normally distributed variable.
- The sample size is too small to determine whether or not the observations are drawn from a normally distributed population.[1]

The tests that we will look at in this chapter rely on the *position* of an observation in a set of observations. We will use the *ranks* of observations to carry out the statistical tests. Ordinal measurements (first, second, third, etc.) already conform to this requirement. Interval or ratio scale variables need to be put in rank order and the values of the ranks used to carry out the test. In the latter case, we have lost some data: an interval or ratio scale variable has had to be transformed into an ordinal variable, and information about the distance from one measurement to the next will have been lost.

7.2 UNPAIRED NONNORMAL DATA: THE MANN–WHITNEY TEST

This test is for *unpaired* data drawn from a population of observations in which the variable is not normally distributed. It assumes that there are two independent samples. It is the nonparametric equivalent of the unpaired *t*-test. It also goes by the name of Wilcoxon rank-sum test (because it is based on the sums of the ranks).

As we did for the *t*-test, we will set out the conditions and actions that will allow us to examine the data and come to a clear conclusion regarding the

statistical significance of the findings. These steps are set out in Box 7.1.

Assumptions

The assumptions which underpin the Mann–Whitney test are shown in Box 7.2.

Example

In a study of the impact of chemotherapy on taste sensation, subjects were asked to score the extent to which taste sensation was adversely affected after three months of chemotherapy. Scores were recorded for two different chemotherapy regimens on a scale from 0 to 20. Larger scores indicated greater adverse impact on overall taste sensation.

Look at the data in Table 7.1 and see if it fits the required assumptions.

BOX 7.1

The steps to carry out a statistical test

Assumptions – What are the criteria that must be met to apply the test?

Model – Make sure that the data fit the requirements to carry out the test

Test procedure – Step-by-step instructions to carry out the test

Decision and interpretation – How to interpret the test statistic, including the *rejection rule*

BOX 7.2

Assumptions for the Mann–Whitney test

1. Two groups of sample observations are drawn from a population in which the variable is not normally distributed
2. The samples are independent
3. Observations are *not* paired between samples. n_1 may or may not be equal to n_2

---

[1] We touched on this in Chapter 6 when we introduced the Kolmogorov–Smirnov and Shapiro–Wilks tests.

TABLE 7.1 Overall Adverse Taste Impact Score Following Three Months of Chemotherapy: Higher Score Indicates Greater Impact

Regimen A		Regimen B	
Patient Number	Score	Patient Number	Score
1	7	13	15
2	6	14	14
3	4	15	17
4	11	16	16
5	16	17	16
6	4	18	16
7	10	19	14
8	6	20	12
9	9	21	14
10	3	22	17
11	13	23	16
12	5		

Model

The model for the *Mann-Whitney* test is shown in Box 7.3.

The data fit. Let's look at the test procedure.

Test procedure

The test procedure for the *Mann-Whitney* test is shown in Box 7.4.

First, find the median scores of the two groups: Regimen A = 6.5; Regimen B = 16.0

Our next task is to assign ranks to the original observations. We put the scores in numerical order and assign a *rank* to each value. This should be really straight forward. The lowest score is assigned a rank of 1, and the highest score a rank of 23 (as we have 23 observations from 23 patients). The lowest score is 3, which we assign a value of 1. But when we look in Table 7.2 at the highest score (17) we see it has been assigned a rank of 22.5. What is going on?

BOX 7.3

Model for the Mann–Whitney test

1. One variable, not normally distributed.
2. Two groups of observations, independently drawn from patients receiving chemotherapy.
3. Observations are *not* paired between samples.
4. Variable may be ordinal (ranks) or interval or ratio (continuous or discrete)
5. Test to see if the difference between the sample medians in the two groups is different from zero.

BOX 7.4

Test procedure for the Mann–Whitney test

1. Combine results for both groups and rank, keeping note of which result (and rank) belongs to which group (see Table 7.2)
2. Calculate the sum of the ranks for each group separately (R_1 and R_2)
3. Check your sums
4. Calculate the Wilcoxon U statistic
5. Compare the calculated value for U with the tabulated value in Appendix A4 for n_1 and n_2. If the calculated value for U is *less than or equal to* the value in the table, reject the null hypothesis.

When the scores have equal values (what are call 'tied' values), *we assign ranks that are the average of the ranks that we would have assigned if the values had not been tied.* So, the second and third observations are both scores of 4. We could arbitrarily assign one score a rank of 2 and the other score a rank of 3. But to be statistically correct, we assign both scores the average of the ranks that we would have assigned had they not been tied: $(2+3)/2 = 5/2 = 2.5$. Simple enough. Of course, you could argue that this does not affect the sum of ranks within a group and think it does not matter. It does matter, however, when scores are tied *between* groups.

TABLE 7.2   Overall Adverse Taste Impact Score Following Three Months of Chemotherapy, Ranked by Intervention Group: Higher Score Indicates Greater Impact

Regimen A	Rank	Regimen B	Rank
3	1		
4	2.5		
4	2.5		
5	4		
6	5.5		
6	5.5		
7	7		
9	8		
10	9		
11	10		
		12	11
13	12		
		14	14
		14	14
		14	14
		15	16
16	19		
		16	19
		16	19
		16	19
		16	19
		17	22.5
		17	22.5
	86		190

In our example, five patients have a score of 16, one in Regimen A and four in Regimen B. The ranks that we need to assign have values of 17, 18, 19, 20, and 21. It would be wrong to arbitrarily assign any one of these values to the score in Regimen A, as it would have an impact on the sum of ranks for both groups. The safest thing to do, as we did before, is to assign the average of the ranks for all five scores to

all five values: $(17+18+19+20+21)/5 = 95/5 = 19$. All of the observations are assigned a rank of 19. The two highest scores are also tied, so they are assigned a rank of 22.5, the average of the ranks 22 and 23.

When you have assigned ranks and added up the sums of the ranks for the two groups, it is a good idea to check your sums. Ensure that:

$$R_1 + R_2 = \tfrac{1}{2}(n_1 + n_2)(n_1 + n_2 + 1)$$

$$86 + 190 = \tfrac{1}{2}(12+11)(12+11+1) = \tfrac{1}{2}(23)(24)$$

$$276 = 276$$

Then calculate the test statistic, Wilcoxon's U. This is a measure of overlap between the two samples.[2]

$$U_1 = n_1 n_2 + \frac{n_2(n_2+1)}{2} - R_2 = 8$$

$$U_2 = n_1 n_2 + \frac{n_1(n_1+1)}{2} - R_1 = 124$$

Again, it is important check your maths by seeing that:

$$U_1 + U_2 = n_1 \times n_2$$

$$8 + 124 = 11 \times 12 = 132$$

The test statistic is then the *minimum* of the two values, that is:

$$U = \min(U_1, U_2) = 8$$

Decision and interpretation

If H_0 is true, that is, both sets of observations were drawn from the same or identical populations, the median values would be similar and we would expect

---

[2]The Mann–Whitney test is also known as the Wilcoxon rank-sum test. It uses the Wilcoxon U statistic to find P.

to see a lot of overlap between the two samples. We can think of U as a measure of overlap between the two samples. The expectation is that U_1 and U_2 would be similar. If there is little overlap, the values for U will be very different, and $\min(U_1, U_2)$ will be small. We can reject H_0 if the calculated value for U is *less than or equal to*[3] the relevant value in the table in Appendix A4 (the values for the Wilcoxon U statistic).

The values for U are shown in the body of the table. n_1 is given down the left-hand side and n_2 in the top row. There are two tables: one for $P = 0.05$ and one for $P = 0.01$.

In this example, the value in Appendix A4 for sample sizes of $n_1 = 12$ and $n_2 = 11$ and $P = 0.05$ is $U_{12,11} = 33$. As our calculated value (8) is *less than* the tabulated value, we can reject H_0 at $P < 0.05$ (small values are statistically significant). Can we reject H_0 at the 1% level ($P < 0.01$)? As the calculated value for U is less than the value in the table for $U_{P=0.01, n1 = 12, \text{and } n2 = 11} = 24$, we can reject the null hypothesis at the 1% level. Stop to think about it, and you will understand why the values for U when $P = 0.01$ are smaller than the values for U when $P = 0.05$. It indicates that there is less overlap between the samples, and therefore a greater probability that the two sets of observations came from different populations.

The table is symmetrical, so it doesn't matter which way round you originally assigned the labels for observations in group 1 and group 2. For example, you will see that at $P = 0.05$, the U value when $n_1 = 11$ and $n_2 = 12$ ($U = 33$) is the same as the value when $n_1 = 12$ and $n_2 = 11$. The main thing is to keep track of which sums of ranks (R), values for U and values for n relate to which set of observations.

> **Rejection rule:** If the calculated value for $U_{n1,n2}$ is *less than or equal to* the value in the table for $U_{n1,n2}$ when $P = 0.05$, reject H_0.

---

[3] This rule is different from the t-test, where statistical significance ($P < 0.05$) was likely if the calculated test statistic was *greater than* the value in the t table. One of the purposes of going into a lot of detail about how the test statistics are derived is to help you make sense of the rules that govern when to accept or reject the null hypothesis.

There are three points to note. First, we are using n rather than $n - 1$ when we look up the values in the table. This is because the basis for the calculation of the test statistic does not rely on the degrees of freedom but on the actual number of observations. Second, the rejection rule says that the finding is of statistical significance if the calculated value for the test statistic is less than *or equal to* the value in the table. Because the table is based on directly calculated probabilities relating to discrete observations, the tabulated values are selected to be below the cut-off probabilities. For example, the probability of $U_{P=0.01, n1,n2}$ occurring is *already* less than 1%. So, if the calculated value for the test statistic is equal to the tabulated value, the probability of that outcome is already below the stated probability (not equal to it, as was the case for the values for t in Appendix A3). Third, the number of ties has an impact on the calculated value of U. A statistical technique is available to take into account the number of ties. The impact is small, but it is important to apply the correction if you can.[4]

Conclusion

We said at the outset (Box 7.3) that the aim was to 'Test to see if the difference between the sample medians in the two groups is different from zero'. We can conclude that the impact of chemotherapy Regimen A on taste sensation (median impact score = 6.5) was less than the impact of Regimen B (median impact score = 16), and that the two medians are statistically significantly different at the 1% level, i.e. that the difference between the sample medians *is* different from zero.

---

[4] I have not applied the correction in our present calculation because the technique is fiddly and in the present example, we are well within the confidence level for rejecting the null hypothesis. Most of the time you will be determining the significance of the test using statistical software. SPSS, for example, accounts for ties in the Mann–Whitney U Test (and other nonparametric tests that rely on ranks) if you have the Exact Tests module installed when using the NPAR tests in SPSS. For further details on how to cope with ties, see: https://www.ibm.com/support/pages/how-does-spss-account-ties-mann-whitney-u-test

7.3 WILCOXON SIGNED-RANK TEST

This test is used for paired samples. It is the non-parametric equivalent of the paired *t*-test.

Assumptions

The assumptions which underpin the Wilcoxon signed-rank test are shown in Box 7.5.

Example

Two strains of wheat for use in a famine relief programme were tested for crop yield under controlled conditions in a randomized block design. Does one strain give a higher yield than the other?

Look at the yield data in Table 7.3 to see if it fits the required assumptions.

Model

The model for the Wilcoxon signed-rank test is shown in Box 7.6.

The data fit. We have no previous experience of these crops in the present circumstances, so we are assuming that the data are not normal in character. Let us look at the test procedure.

Test procedure

The test procedure for the Wilcoxon signed-rank test is shown in Box 7.7.

TABLE 7.3   Yields of Two Strains of Wheat in a Randomized Block Design (Bushels per Acre)

Block	Type A	Type B
1	36.9	36.8
2	35.2	37.1
3	31.2	31.4
4	34.1	34.1
5	36.1	35.9
6	34.1	35.2
7	37.2	37.9
8	36.8	37.2
9	29.6	30.2
10	35.4	36.5

BOX 7.6

Model for the Wilcoxon signed-rank test

1. Two sets of observations that are paired
2. One variable, not normally distributed
3. Variable is interval or ratio (not rank [ordinal])
4. Test to see if the differences between the yields is different from zero

---

BOX 7.7

Test procedure for the Wilcoxon signed-rank test

1. Find the differences between the yields in each block
2. Rank the differences, *ignoring* the sign, and *ignoring* the zeros
3. Find the sum of the ranks of the positive differences $(R+)$ and the sum of the ranks of the negative differences $(R-)$
4. Find $T = \min(R+, R-)$
5. Compare calculated test statistic T with tabulated value in Appendix A5 for $n =$ number of nonzero differences

---

BOX 7.5

Assumptions for the Wilcoxon signed-rank test

1. Two samples or sets of observations are randomly drawn in pairs
2. The variable in the population is *not* normally distributed
3. Variables must be interval or ratio (not rank [ordinal])

The steps of the test procedure are set out in Table 7.4.

We find that $R+ = 3.5$ $R- = 41.5$. $T = \min(R+, R-) = 3.5$, and there were 9 nonzero differences.

If we had taken the difference in the opposite direction (B−A), $R+$ and $R-$ would have taken the opposite values, but T (the minimum value) would be the same.

Decision and interpretation

From the table for the Wilcoxon T statistic (Appendix A5), we see that $T_{n=9, P=0.05} = 6$. As the calculated value $T = 3.5$ is *less than or equal to* the tabulated value, we can reject H_0 at $P < 0.05$. If the calculated value had been less than or equal to 3, we would have been able to reject the H_0 at the 2% level.

Because we were not making any predictions about which strain would have the higher yield (the null hypothesis is that the two yields would have been the same), our expectation is that the values for $R+$ and $R-$ would have been similar. The bigger the difference between $R+$ and $R-$, the more likely it is that the yields are different. It is a two-tailed test. Also, the consideration regarding the cut-off values in the Wilcoxon signed-rank test (less than or *equal to*) is the same as in the Mann−Whitney test: calculated values that are *equal* to the tabulated values are statistically significant at the designated level because the probability of the tabulated values arising is less than the designated level of statistical significance.

Rejection rule: If the calculated value for $T_{n,P}$ is *less than or equal to* the value in the table for $T_{n,P}$ when $P = 0.05$, reject H_0

Conclusion

We conclude that the yield from Strain B was greater than the yield from Strain A, statistically significant at the 5% level. The median yields were 35.3 bushels per acre for Strain A and 36.2 bushels per acre for Strain B, a difference of 2.5%.

TABLE 7.4 Yields of Two Strains of Wheat in a Randomized Block Design (Bushels per Acre), with Computations

Block	Type A	Type B	Difference	Modulus of Difference	Rank of Modulus (Ignore Zeros)	Ranks	
						Positive Differences	Negative Differences
1	36.9	36.8	0.1	0.1	1.0	1	
2	35.2	37.1	−1.9	1.9	9.0		9
3	31.2	31.4	−0.2	0.2	2.5		2.5
4	34.1	34.1	0				
5	36.1	35.9	0.2	0.2	2.5	2.5	
6	34.1	35.2	−1.1	1.1	7.5		7.5
7	37.2	37.9	−0.7	0.7	6.0		6
8	36.8	37.2	−0.4	0.4	4.0		4
9	29.6	30.2	−0.6	0.6	5.0		5
10	35.4	36.5	−1.1	1.1	7.5		7.5
					Sum of ranks	3.5	41.5

7.4 WILCOXON SIGN TEST

This test is for paired samples where there is a binary outcome.

The Wilcoxon sign test was most famously used in 1950s ads for washing powder. 'Scientific tests have proven that SUDSO washes whiter than its nearest rival brand!' Two piles of laundry were presented to the lucky housewife (always a housewife). She was asked to say which pile was whiter. In the ad, she pointed the SUDSO pile. Shock, surprise, wonder! In reality, she might have pointed to either pile. How could the advertisers (short of outright lying) say that 'scientific tests have proved' that SUDSO washes whiter?

The Wilcoxon sign test is a simple test for binary outcomes. The expectation is that if the null hypothesis is true, both outcomes are equally likely. How discrepant do the outcomes need to be before the null hypothesis can be rejected?

Assumptions

The assumptions which underpin the Wilcoxon sign test are shown in Box 7.8.

Let us use the wheat yield data again. We want to know simply if, in each pair of observations, one strain out-performed the other.

Model

The model for the Wilcoxon sign test is shown in Box 7.9.

BOX 7.8

Assumptions for the Wilcoxon sign test

1. Two samples or sets of observations are randomly drawn in pairs
2. The variable in the population is *not* normally distributed
3. One value (treatment, response, etc.) can be said to be 'greater' or 'better' than the other

---

BOX 7.9

Model for the Wilcoxon sign test

1. Two sets of paired observations (yield of wheat)
2. One variable with binary outcomes (Strain A or Strain B is greater)
3. Test to see if there is a preference for one outcome over the other

---

This time, rather than rank the differences according to their size, we simply determine the sign of the differences in yield. We count the number of positive and the number of negative differences (again, ignoring the zeros). In this example, there were two instances in which Strain A outperformed Strain B; for the remainder of the seven nonzero comparisons, B outperformed A.

We can say: $\Sigma+ = 2$, $\Sigma- = 7$. This is the basis for the test statistic for the sign test, R:

$R = \min(\Sigma+, \Sigma-) = \min(7, 2) = 2$. There were 9 nonzero differences.

From the table in Appendix A6, we see that for 9 sets of observations and $P = 0.05$, the cut-off for $R_{n=9, P=0.05} = 1$. As the calculated value was *greater than* the value in the table, we accept H_0.

Rejection rule: If the calculated value for $R_{n,P}$ is *less than or equal to* the value in the table for $R_{n,P}$ when $P = 0.05$, reject H_0.

Conclusion

Why is the conclusion from the sign test different from that based on the Wilcoxon signed-rank test? We are using less information in the sign test than in the signed-rank test. We are relying only on the *direction* of the difference and ignoring the *size* of the difference. As a consequence, the test is less sensitive.

In order to give yourself the greatest chance of demonstrating a statistically significant outcome, always use the maximum amount of information available and select the statistical test that is appropriate. We will look at our options in the flow chart when we get to Chapter 13.

7.5 SPSS

SPSS provides useful and easy-to-interpret output for the nonparametric tests. The command sequence is Analyze>Nonparametric Tests and then One sample, Independent Samples (unpaired), or Related Samples (paired). It then decides which test best fits your data! It is better to have your own thoughts on this, of course, as computers make mistakes. The SPSS files for the examples from this chapter are on the book website:

- Data: ch07d01.sav
- Data: ch07d02.sav
- Syntax: ch07d01.sps

- Syntax: ch07d02.sps
- Output: ch07d01.spv
- Output: ch07d02.spv

The SPSS output for the Mann–Whitney test for the unpaired data on loss of taste sensation is shown in Figure 7.1.

It reported P (Sig.) $= 0.000$ (i.e. $P < 0.0005$) and tells you to reject the null hypothesis. A bit too simple for my liking. It reminds me of driverless cars. You still need to satisfy yourself that it is taking you where you wanted to go and analysed the right data in the way that you thought it should.

For the wheat yield data, the output for the two sets of results (Wilcoxon signed-rank test and Wilcoxon sign test) is shown in Figure 7.2.

Hypothesis test summary

	Null hypothesis	Test	Sig.	Decision
1	The distribution of score is the same across categories of group.	Independent-samples Mann–Whitney U test	0.000[a]	Reject the null hypothesis.

Asymptotic significances are displayed. The significance level is 0.05.

[a]Exact significance is displayed for this test.

FIGURE 7.1 SPSS output for Mann–Whitney analysis. *Source*: Reproduced with permission of International Business Machines Corporation.

Hypothesis test summary

	Null hypothesis	Test	Sig.	Decision
1	The median of differences between TypeA and TypeB equals 0.	Related-samples sign test	0.180[a]	Retain the null hypothesis.
2	The median of differences between TypeA and TypeB equals 0.	Related-samples Wilcoxon signed rank test	0.024	Reject the null hypothesis.

Asymptotic significances are displayed. The significance level is 0.05.

[a]Exact significance is displayed for this test.

FIGURE 7.2 SPSS output for Wilcoxon sign test and Wilcoxon signed-rank test. *Source*: Reproduced with permission of International Business Machines Corporation.

The results accord with our manual calculations. Using the Wilcoxon signed-rank test, we reject the null hypothesis. Using the sign test, we accept the null hypothesis. SPSS makes your life easier by giving you the exact values for *P*. But it is only because you now know the backgrounds to the tests that you would be able to understand why one result was statistically significant at the 5% level and the other was not.

7.6 EXERCISES

7.6.1

In a study comparing two treatments for pressure areas (bed sores), patients were given a healing score derived from reported pain, appearance, size, etc. (Table 7.5). Is there a difference in the outcome using the two treatments?

TABLE 7.5   Scores for Pressure Scores in Two Groups of Hospital Patients Given Two Different Treatments

Treatment A		Treatment B	
Patient Number	Score	Patient Number	Score
1	7	13	8
2	9	14	1
3	6	15	3
4	8	16	8
5	8	17	7
6	9	18	4
7	6		
8	7		
9	8		
10	2		
11	7		
12	7		

State the null hypothesis.

Describe the model. Decide which test to carry out to see if there is a difference in scores between the two treatment groups.

7.6.2

Two standard procedures for measuring children's height in the field were compared. In the first (A), gentle traction was applied on the mastoid process (resulting in slight lifting) and in the second (B), the child was standing free. Results for 20 children are given in Table 7.6 (from Osborne [1]).

TABLE 7.6   Estimates of Child Height Using Two Different Assessment Methods

Child	A	B
1	108.4	108.2
2	109.0	109.0
3	111.0	110.0
4	110.3	110.5
5	109.8	108.6
6	113.1	111.9
7	115.2	114.8
8	112.5	112.6
9	106.3	106.3
10	109.9	109.7
11	108.8	108.6
12	110.7	110.0
13	112.0	112.4
14	111.6	111.7
15	109.9	108.9
16	106.7	106.0
17	113.5	113.3
18	110.0	109.9
19	111.2	110.3
20	109.7	109.3

a. State the null hypothesis.
b. The field director of the refugee camp where you are working wants to know if it is worth taking additional time to train field workers to use method A (requiring traction to be applied to the mastoid process) or if height can be measured using the slightly quicker method with the children free-standing (method B).
c. Carry out a *quick* test to investigate any systematic difference between the two methods.

d. Tell the field director that you will confirm the result later that day.

Test the data using the Wilcoxon signed-rank test (T).

REFERENCE

1. Osborne JF. *Statistical Exercises in Medical Research*. Wiley. London. 1979.

CHAPTER 8

Contingency Tables, Chi-Squared Test, and Fisher's Exact Test

Learning Objectives

After studying this chapter, you should be able to:

- Identify data sets for which the chi-squared test and Fisher's Exact Test are the right tests to use
- Carry out the chi-squared test manually for a table with p rows and q columns (a p × q contingency table) and determine levels of statistical significance using the chi-squared table
- Learn to use Yates' correction for small numbers of observations or expected values
- Carry out Fisher's Exact Test manually for 2 × 2 contingency tables
- Interpret SPSS output to determine the level of significance of your findings

8.1 INTRODUCTION

We often want to know if there is an association between observations in categories. Its simplest form is a comparison in which each variable has two categories. Is there an association, for example, between gender (boy or girl) and the number of children who meet the minimum recommendation for physical activity (60 minutes or more per day)? Or we might have multiple categories. In a comparison of five towns in Northamptonshire, is there an association between the town a child lives in and the number of children with none, 1–3, or 4 or more decayed, missing or filled teeth? The Chi-squared (χ^2)[1] test helps us establish if the associations that we observe are statistically significant, or if apparent differences in the numbers that we observe in different categories have arisen just by chance. The word *contingency* reflects the relationship between variables – the outcome for one variable (the dependent variable) can be said to be

[1]The lower-case Greek letter χ (chi) is pronounced 'ky', to rhyme with 'sky'.

Statistics in Nutrition and Dietetics, First Edition. Michael Nelson.
© 2020 John Wiley & Sons Ltd. Published 2020 by John Wiley & Sons Ltd.
Companion website: www.wiley.com/go/nelson/statistics

contingent on the value for the other variable (the independent variable). In the examples above, we might argue that observed physical activity level is dependent on gender, or that the number of decayed, missing, and filled teeth is dependent (in part, at least) on the town where you live. Sometimes the direction of the association between the variables may not be immediately obvious – which variable is dependent, and which is independent – but an association may exist, and we want to determine the statistical significance of the association.

Observations must be *counts*. Data are arranged in a table with rows and columns. The smallest contingency table you can have is one in which each variable has two categories (a *fourfold*, or *2 × 2 contingency table*). The chi-squared test calculates the difference between what is observed and what would be expected if the null hypothesis were true (i.e. that there is no association between the two variables, or that the samples do not differ from one another with respect to the variable of interest). If the difference is large, we can reject the null hypothesis. The distribution of the χ^2 statistic enables us to say how large the difference must be before we can reject H_0.

8.2 THE FOUR-FOLD OR 2 × 2 CONTINGENCY TABLE

Fundamental principles

Expectation:	H_0: There are no differences in the relative proportions of the number of observations in each column in each of the two rows in the table
	Mathematically: χ^2 (chi-squared) $= \sum [(O - E)^2/E] = 0$
Decision criterion:	If the relative proportions of the numbers of observations in each column are very different in the two rows, reject the null hypothesis. If the calculated value for the test statistic χ^2 (chi-squared) is **greater than** the tabulated value for one degree of freedom at $P = 0.05$, reject H_0.

BOX 8.1

Assumptions for a 2 × 2 contingency table

1. There are two variables, each with two categories
2. Samples are random and independent
3. The values in tables must be counts
4. Values are arranged in a table with two rows and two columns
5. The total number of observations (N) must be at least 20
6. No expected value (E) is less than 5

Let's break this down into something more intelligible.

Assumptions for the 2 × 2 table

Assumptions for a 2 × 2 contingency table are shown in Box 8.1.

In the next section, you will see how to carry out the chi-squared test and find out exactly what we mean by and how to compute 'expected' (E) values. If $N < 20$ or values for $E < 5$, you can still test the significance of the association by using Yate's correction for small samples, or by carrying out Fisher's Exact Test. These options are described in Section 8.4.

Every 2 × 2 contingency table is set out as shown in Table 8.1.

By convention, the number of observations (the *counts*) are labelled **a, b, c,** and **d**. These are known as the *inner cells*. We need to know the sum of the counts for each row (r_1 and r_2) and for each column (c_1 and c_2). We can therefore say:

$$r_1 = \mathbf{a} + \mathbf{b}$$
$$r_2 = \mathbf{c} + \mathbf{d}$$
$$c_1 = \mathbf{a} + \mathbf{c}$$
$$c_2 = \mathbf{b} + \mathbf{d}$$

TABLE 8.1   General Layout of Data for a Four-Fold[a] or 2×2 Contingency Table

	Variable 2		Row Total
	Column 1	Column 2	
Variable 1			
Row 1	a	b	r_1
	(inner cells)		(marginals)
Row 2	c	d	r_2
Column total	c_1	c_2	N
	(marginals)		

[a] I was curious to know the origin of the term 'four-fold'. I thought it might be a quaint and archaic expression invented by Fisher or one of the early Twentieth Century statisticians to describe this particular type of table, retained in the literature for its legacy value. It is much more prosaic – it refers simply to anything with four units or members. Like the Mitroff–Kilmann Four-fold Way of Knowing, which is not (as I had hoped) a mystical path to insight into why (for example) you are taking a course in statistics, but instead has to do with the social psychology of science (equally interesting). Kilmann is also famous for his work on conflict resolution, which I thought might be useful if you got into a tussle with your statistics lecturer.

These are referred to as the *marginal values*, or *marginals*. Finally, we need to know the total number of observations in the table, $N = \mathbf{a} + \mathbf{b} + \mathbf{c} + \mathbf{d}$.[2]

The calculations for the chi-squared test are straightforward if rather tedious (especially for large contingency tables). First, it will be clearer if we change the labels that we have used for the observed counts (the letters **a, b, c**, and **d** in Table 8.1) to ones that indicate the position of the cell in the table in terms of the row and column numbers. For a 2×2 table, for example, these would be O_{11}, O_{12}, O_{21}, and O_{22}, respectively, where the upper-case letter O is used to indicate the observed count in each cell. In general terms, O_{ij} indicates the count in the cell in row i and column j. Pure laziness means I don't bother putting a comma between the row and column numbers in the subscripts.

Now, stop and think for a moment. If H_0 were true, there would be no association between the variables in the rows and the columns. If there were no association, the counts in the cells in each row would be in the same proportion as the counts in the column totals. To carry out the chi-squared test, we need to find the value for each cell that we would *expect* to see if the null hypothesis were true. These are the values for E that I mentioned above.[3]

Let's return to our example at the start of the chapter about the relative proportions of boys and girls meeting the daily recommendation for physical activity [1]. Say roughly one-fifth of the children in our survey met the recommendation. If there were no association between gender and meeting the recommendation for physical activity, then we would expect one-fifth of the boys and one-fifth of the girls to have met the requirement. If the proportion meeting the recommendation was different in girls compared with boys (say 18% in one and 24% in the other), then we might say there was a gender effect. Of course, what we observed may simply be due to random sampling variation. How big does the difference between boys and girls need to be before we can reject the null hypothesis and say that there really *are* differences in levels of physical activity between boys and girls? Is the difference between what we expected to see (one-fifth in both boys

[2] You will notice that $N = r_1 + r_2$ and $N = c_1 + c_2$. Checking that the sum of row totals and the sum of the column totals are the same is an effective way to check that your row totals and column totals have been added up correctly.

[3] Pause. Take a deep breath. Reread this paragraph. This is at the heart of the test, so it needs to make sense to you at this point.

TABLE 8.2   General Layout of Data for a Four-Fold or 2×2 Table, with Statistical Annotation for Completion of the Chi-Squared Test

			Variable 2		Row Total
			Column 1	Column 2	
Variable 1					
Row 1		Observed	O_{11}	O_{12}	r_1
		Expected	$E_{11} = \dfrac{r_1 c_1}{N}$	$E_{12} = \dfrac{r_1 c_2}{N}$	
		Difference	$O_{11} - E_{11}$	$O_{12} - E_{12}$	
		Difference squared	$(O_{11} - E_{11})^2$	$(O_{12} - E_{12})^2$	
		Taking E into account	$\dfrac{(O_{11} - E_{11})^2}{E_{11}}$	$\dfrac{(O_{12} - E_{12})^2}{E_{12}}$	
Row 2		Observed	O_{21}	O_{22}	r_2
		Expected	$E_{21} = \dfrac{r_2 c_1}{N}$	$E_{22} = \dfrac{r_2 c_2}{N}$	
		Difference	$O_{21} - E_{21}$	$O_{22} - E_{22}$	
		Difference squared	$(O_{21} - E_{21})^2$	$(O_{22} - E_{22})^2$	
		Taking E into account	$\dfrac{(O_{21} - E_{21})^2}{E_{21}}$	$\dfrac{(O_{22} - E_{22})^2}{E_{22}}$	
Column total			c_1	c_2	N

and girls) and what we observed (18% and 24%) big enough to say that it is statistically unlikely ($P < 0.05$, assuming that the null hypothesis is true) and so reject the null hypothesis? This is what the chi-squared test will help us to determine.

We have already used O_{ij} to denote the *observed* value in each cell. Surprise, surprise, we use the upper-case letter E to denote the *expected* values, and the subscripts i and j to denote the cell, that is, E_{ij}. How do we find the expected values (what we would expect to see if the null hypothesis were true)? The *expected* count in the first cell (the intersection of row 1 and column 1), E_{11}, would be the total number of observations in the row total (r_1) times the proportion of the observations in the first column (c_1) out of the total, N. That is: $E_{11} = r_1(c_1/N)$. A simple algebraic rearrangement of the formula makes it easier to remember: $r_1(c_1/N) = r_1 c_1/N$. In English, we would say that $E_{11} = r_1 c_1/N$ (the *expected* value in each cell) is equal to the row total times the column total divided by N. The observed count and the formula to compute the expected value for each cell are shown in Table 8.2. Don't be put off by all the

formulae in the table – the next sections will take us through their meaning and calculation step-by-step as we work out how to compute the χ^2 test statistic.

Our aim is to find the total amount of difference in the table between what we observed and what we expected to see if the null hypothesis were true. We *could* do this by adding together the differences for all four cells. For the first cell (row 1, column 1), the difference is $O_{11} - E_{11}$; for the next cell, it is $O_{12} - E_{12}$; and so on. There is a problem, however. If you do the maths, you find that total of the four values for $O - E$ is equal to zero. Now, we have had this problem before. Think back to the calculation of the standard deviation. Remember that if we found the difference between each value of variable x (x_i) and the mean of all the observations ($\bar{x}$), and then added all the differences together, the total came to zero (that is $\Sigma(x_i - \bar{x}) = 0$). We got around this problem by squaring the differences $(x_i - \bar{x})^2$ to get rid of the sign of the difference.[4] The same

_____

[4]This proved to be a better solution, mathematically, than taking the absolute value, or modulus – effectively just ignoring the sign.

solution works for the chi-squared test. So instead of simply calculating $O - E$ for each cell, we are going to find $(O - E)^2$ (Table 8.2). You might think that if we added *these* values together, we would have a measure of the total amount of deviation between what we observed and what we expected if the null hypothesis were true. But there is another issue.

This one relates to sample size. We need to allow for the fact that larger samples have the potential to produce larger values for the differences (and hence the squares of the differences) between O and E. We can take this into account by dividing the square of the difference in each cell by E, the expected value for the cell. Thus, for the cell in the first row and first column, $(O_{11} - E_{11})^2/E_{11}$ gives us the best measure of the difference between O_{11} and E_{11} because it takes sample size into account. I can generalize the expression for every cell in the table and write $(O_{ij} - E_{ij})^2/E_{ij}$. This looks a bit cumbersome with all the subscripts, so if I want a general term for the expression, I just write $(O - E)^2/E$.

Finally, I want to know for the entire table the *total* amount of deviance between what we observed and what we expected to see if the null hypothesis were true, taking into account the size of the difference in each cell and the sample size. We can now add together the values for $(O - E)^2/E$ for all four cells in our 2 × 2 table. The sum of these four measures of deviance gives us our test statistic, chi-squared, denoted by χ^2. This is the lower case Greek letter chi, χ, raised to the power of 2. To express it mathematically, we say:

$$\chi^2 = \Sigma \left[\frac{(O - E)^2}{E} \right]$$

EQUATION 8.1.   Mathematical expression for the calculation of the chi-squared (χ^2) test statistic

$(O - E)^2/E$ is calculated for *every* cell in the table.

There is one more issue to consider: degrees of freedom. Think back to the t-test. We saw that

the value for our cut-off to determine statistical significance varied with sample size. We also saw that sample size, n, was not the best value to use when looking up significant values for t. We looked instead at degrees of freedom. In relation to the t-test, we saw that, ultimately, the value for t was dependent not on the individual values for x but on Σx and Σx^2. For a sample with n observations, $n - 1$ of those observations could take any value that was valid for the variable x. The value for the nth observation, however, was determined by all the other values in the sample and Σx and Σx^2. So, we said that there were $n - 1$ degrees of freedom, which we labelled ν (lower-case Greek letter *nu*).

The same logic applies to the chi-squared calculations. For the purposes of the calculation of χ^2, the row and column totals r_1, r_2, c_1, and c_2 (together with the value for N) determine the computed values for E and hence the value of the chi-squared test statistic. Now think about how much freedom of choice we have in assigning values for O in a 2 × 2 table. Once we have an observed value for one cell in the table, the remaining three values are determined by the row and column totals. So, in a 2 × 2 contingency table, there is only one degree of freedom.[5] We use the same symbol, ν, to denote degrees of freedom in relation to χ^2.

After that rather long theoretical introduction, let's go back to our example relating to differences in the numbers of boys and girls meeting the recommended levels of physical activity that I mentioned earlier. Results are shown in Table 8.3. It appears that there is a slightly higher percentage of boys meeting the standard for physical activity level (24.2%) compared to girls (18.3%). Is the difference between boys and girls statistically significant, or is the apparent difference a results of random sampling variation?

---

[5]We shall see in the next section how to determine the number of degrees of freedom for tables bigger than 2 × 2.

Fundamental principle

Expectation:	H_0: There is no difference in the proportion of boys and girls meeting the standard for physical activity.
Decision criterion:	If there is a difference in the proportion of boys and girls meeting the standard for physical activity statistically significant at the 5% level, reject H_0. If the calculated value for the test statistic χ^2 (chi-squared) is **greater than** the tabulated value for one degree of freedom at $P = 0.05$, reject H_0.

Model

The model for a 2×2 contingency table is shown in Box 8.2.

BOX 8.2

Model for a 2×2 contingency table[6]

1. Two variables – gender and physical activity – each with two categories: boy, girl; meeting or not meeting physical activity requirements
2. Random sample of children aged 5–15 years in England
3. The values in the table are counts
4. Values are arranged in a table with two rows and two columns (see footnote 6)
5. The total number of observations $N = 3220$ (N must be greater than 20)
6. No expected value (E) is less than 5

---

[6]In Table 8.3, I have added two additional columns showing the percentages of boys and girls meeting or not meeting the recommended physical activity level. These are not needed to carry out the chi-squared test but make it easier to understand the findings. I have omitted the columns with percentages in Table 8.4 when we set out the calculations to determine the test statistic.

TABLE 8.3 Physical Activity Level versus Gender in Children Living in England, 2015

	Physical Activity Level			
	Meeting Standard[a]		Not Meeting Standard	
	n	%	n	%
Gender				
Boys	384	24.2%	1206	75.8%
Girls	298	18.3%	1332	81.7%

[a] At least 60 minutes (1 hour) of moderate to vigorous intensity physical activity (MVPA) on all seven days in the last week.

First, we must satisfy ourselves that the data fit the model.

It looks as if the data fit the minimum requirements for undertaking a chi-squared analysis (we'll deal with the question about values for E in a minute).

Now let's undertake the calculations needed for the chi-squared test (Table 8.4). I have put the formulae in the table, to make it easy to follow.

Test procedure

The test procedure for a 2×2 contingency table is shown in Box 8.3.

- *Find the values for E for every cell (row total times column total divided by N).* When we carry out the first set of calculations for E, we see that our data satisfy the last criterion in the model for the chi-squared analysis (all values for E in a 2×2 table are greater than 5.0). I have retained three decimal places for E, even though the observed values are whole numbers. This helps to improve the precision of the calculation of the test statistic. Very important in terms of manual calculation is to note that the sum of the values for E in every row and every column equal the corresponding marginal values (sum of the observed values) for the row and column.

BOX 8.3

Test procedure for a 2 × 2 contingency table

1. Find the values for E for every cell (row total times column total divided by N)
2. Take the difference between O and E for every cell
3. Square the values for $O - E$ in every cell
4. Divide the square of $O - E$ by E: $(O-E)^2/E$
5. Add together the values for the standardized deviations for all cells in the table:

$$\chi^2 = \Sigma \left[\frac{(O-E)^2}{E} \right]$$

6. Find the value for χ^2 in Appendix A7 for $\nu = 1$ and $P = 0.05$

- *Take the difference between O and E for every cell.* Now you can see the problem about simply adding together the total deviance in the table: in a 2×2 table, all the values for $O - E$ are the same size, but two are positive and two are negative. If we add them all together, we get zero. Also note that in a 2×2 table, the size of the difference for $O - E$ is the same for every cell – it is only the sign that differs.
- *Square the values for O – E in every cell.* Again, in a 2×2 table, the size of the squares of the difference of $O - E$ is the same in every cell. Now, however, all the values are positive. Again, I have retained three decimal places to improve the precision of the estimate for chi-squared.
- *Divide the square of O – E by E: $(O-E)^2/E$.* We have now calculated a measure of deviation for each cell that takes sample size into account.
- *Add together the values for the standardized deviations for all cells in the table.* This gives us our chi-squared test statistic:

$$\chi^2 = \Sigma \left[\frac{(O-E)^2}{E} \right]$$

Again, out of laziness, I have not bothered to put in all the subscripts – but you know where they belong. In the present example, $\chi^2 = 6.626 + 1.780 + 6.463 + 1.737 = 16.606$

- *Find the value for χ^2 in Appendix A7 for $\nu = 1$ and $P = 0.05$.* The value for $\chi^2_{1,0.05} = 3.841$. Compare this with the calculated value for chi-squared, 16.606.

Decision and interpretation

Now, the fun part. At the outset, we assumed that the null hypothesis is true. If that were the case, equal proportions of boys and girls in our sample would be meeting the standards for physical activity levels. We further assumed that any deviation from that assumption in our observations arose simply because of random sampling variation.

Now, ask yourself a question: 'What value would we expect for χ^2 if the null hypothesis were true?' Stop and think. If the value for E (the *expected* value) is what we expect to see if the null hypothesis is true, then (in theory) the observed values should be very close the values for E in each cell. If that were the case, then $O - E$ in each cell would be close to zero. So, the values for $(O-E)^2/E$ would be close to zero. And the sum of all those values (the calculated chi-squared test statistic) would be close to zero. So, if the null hypothesis were true, the calculated value for the chi-squared test statistic should be zero or very close to zero.

Our next question, therefore, is 'How far away from zero does the calculated value for chi-squared need to be before we can say it is an unlikely result (assuming the null hypothesis is true), and reject the null hypothesis?' In previous chapters, we said that if what we observed (assuming the null hypothesis was true) was likely to occur less than 5% of the time, we would reject the null hypothesis at the 5% level. The same logic applies with the chi-squared test.

Let's look at the distribution of the values for χ^2 in the table in Appendix A7 and the graph at the top of the table. First, regarding the table, we can see that it is arranged like the one for the t distribution in Appendix A3. The χ^2 values are in the body of the table. Degrees of freedom are shown down the left-hand side. The values for P (the probability of observing what we observe assuming the null hypothesis is true) are given in the top row. As the values for P get smaller and smaller, the values for the test statistic get larger and larger.[7] This is consistent with what we said above: our expectation is that if the null hypothesis were true, the value for chi-squared would be close to zero.

If we look at the graph above the table, zero corresponds to the origin (the extreme left of the x-axis). The total area under the curve (the probability of all possible outcomes) is equal to 1.0. The shaded area to the right of the value for the test statistic, $\chi^2_{\nu,P}$, is the percentage of the area under the curve.[8] The cut-off point specifies both degrees of freedom (ν) and the value for P that we regard as statistically significant. The larger the computed value for chi-squared (as shown in the graph and in the table), the smaller the shaded area, and the less likely it is that what we observed occurred simply because of random sampling variation.

> **Rejection rule**: If the calculated value for χ^2 is *greater than* the value in the table for $\chi^2_{\nu,P}$ when *P = 0.05*, reject H_0.

In our current example, if the calculated value for chi-squared is greater than the value in the table for $\nu = 1$ and $P = 0.05$, we can reject the null hypothesis at the 5% level. The calculated value for chi-squared for our given set of observations equals 16.606. The value in the table for $\chi^2_{\nu\ =\ 1, P\ =\ 0.05} = 3.841$. Because the calculated test statistic is *larger* than the χ^2 value in the table for $\nu = 1$ and $P = 0.05$, we can reject the null hypothesis at the 5% level. This means there is less than a 5% chance of observing what we observed if the null hypothesis is true: $P < 0.05$. What we observed is, in fact, well to the right of the 5% cut-off point.

Conclusion

We accept the Hypothesis (H_1) and conclude that there really is a difference between the percentage of boys and girls meeting the recommended physical activity levels. Moreover, given the evidence, it is reasonable to conclude that boys are more likely to meet the standard for physical activity than girls.

We can now take a step further. Let's compare our calculated value for chi-squared with values in the table for values of P less than 0.05. We may be able to reject the null hypothesis with a greater degree of confidence. The values in the table for $\chi^2_{\nu\ =\ 1, P\ =\ 0.01} = 6.635$ (the 1% level) and for $\chi^2_{\nu\ =\ 1, P\ =\ 0.001} = 10.828$ (the 0.1% level). Our calculated value for $\chi^2 = 16.606$. We can therefore say that the probability of observing what we observed (assuming the null hypothesis is true) is not only less than 1.0%, it is less than 0.1% ($P < 0.001$). Thus, we can be very confident in rejecting the null hypothesis that we have made the right decision and conclude with a high degree of confidence that our findings show a real difference between boys and girls. We must remember, of course, that there is a probability of something under 1 in 1000 ($P < 0.001$) that we are making a mistake in rejecting the null hypothesis, and that this result *could* have occurred by chance even if the null hypothesis were true, but something less than 1 in 1000 times.

8.2.1 Standardized Residual

Before we leave this section, there is one more useful concept to explore that provides further insight into the chi-squared analysis. When we computed the chi-squared test statistic, we squared the difference between O and E (to get rid of the sign) and divided by E (to standardize for sample size). Summing these values for all the cells in the table yielded a test

---

[7]They also get larger as the number of degrees of freedom increases. We'll come back to this in Section 8.3.

[8]The curve for chi-squared is one-tailed, whereas the curve for the t distribution was two-tailed. This is because, given the way in which the test statistic is calculated, the values for the chi-squared distribution cannot be less than zero. Values for t, on the other hand, could be positive or negative. The null hypothesis for the t-test said that the difference should be zero, but for most hypotheses did not specify the direction of the difference. Hence the probabilities for the t distribution needed to include both tails, and were described as 'two-tailed', whereas the chi-squared distribution is 'one-tailed'.

TABLE 8.4   Physical Activity Level versus Gender in Children Living in England, 2015

Gender			Physical Activity Level		Row Total
			Meeting Standard[a]	Not Meeting Standard[a]	
Boys	Observed		384	1206	$r_1 = 1590$
	Expected	$E_{ij} = \dfrac{r_i c_j}{N}$	336.764	1253.236	$E_{11} + E_{12} = 1590$
	Difference	$O_{ij} - E_{ij}$	47.236	−47.236	
	Difference squared	$(O_{ij} - E_{ij})^2$	2231.242	2231.242	
	Taking E into account	$\dfrac{(O_{ij} - E_{ij})^2}{E_{ij}}$	6.626	1.780	
	Standardized residual	$\dfrac{O_{ij} - E_{ij}}{\sqrt{E_{ij}}}$	2.574	−1.334	
Girls	Observed		298	1332	$r_2 = 1630$
	Expected	$E_{ij} = \dfrac{r_i c_j}{N}$	345.236	1284.764	$E_{21} + E_{22} = 1630$
	Difference	$O_{ij} - E_{ij}$	−47.236	47.236	
	Difference squared	$(O_{ij} - E_{ij})^2$	2231.242	2231.242	
	Taking E into account	$\dfrac{(O_{ij} - E_{ij})^2}{E_{ij}}$	6.463	1.737	
	Standardized residual	$\dfrac{O_{ij} - E_{ij}}{\sqrt{E_{ij}}}$	−2.542	1.318	
Column total			$c_1 = 682$	$c_2 = 2538$	$N = 3220$
			$E_{11} + E_{21} = 682$	$E_{12} + E_{22} = 2538$	

[a] At least 60 minutes (1 hour) of moderate to vigorous intensity physical activity (MVPA) on all 7 days in the last week.

statistic that we could compare with the chi-squared distribution. The test statistic told us the probability of observing what we observed over the entire table (assuming the null hypothesis is true). But is it possible to say which cell (or cells) contributed most to the statistical significance of the finding?

We can see from Table 8.4 that some of the values for $(O - E)^2/E$ are larger than others. It would be reasonable to assume that the cells with the larger values contributed more to the 'significance' of the

finding. But surely some of the variation between what we observed and what we expected (I hear you protest) must be due in part to random sampling variation. To put it another way, can we identify those cells that contributed most to the significance of the finding; and which cells, in fact, are more likely to reflect random sampling variation?

The concept of the *standardized residual* helps us to address this question. In statistical parlance, the *residual* is the difference between what we observed and what we expected. Instead of squaring it (to get rid of the sign), we take the difference, *keep* the sign and, as before, standardize the difference (to take sample size into account) using the value for E. This time, however, instead of dividing by E, we divide by the square root of E, giving us the expression for the standardized residual: $(O_{ij} - E_{ij})/\sqrt{E_{ij}}$. The value for the standardized residual is shown in the last row in each section for boys and girls in Table 8.4.

Now, between you and me, we like this a lot. As a useful rule of thumb, if the value is 2.0 or greater, we can argue that these cells in particular are the ones that contributed most to the statistical significance of our finding. The sign is helpful because it tells us about the *direction* of the difference between what we observed and what we expected. If the value for the standardized residual is less than 2.0, we can say that the difference between O and E may, in fact, have arisen because of random sampling variation (allowing, of course, for the fact that the total χ^2 sum tells you that the associations across the table as a whole are not likely to have arisen by chance, i.e. $P < 0.05$).

So, let's go back to our conclusion about the results. We said that boys and girls are not equally likely to meet the standards for physical activity (because more boys than girls appeared to meet the standards, and our value for chi-squared was greater than what we expected to see just by chance). Looking at the table, we now see that the biggest standardized residual was in the cell for the percentage of boys exceeding our expectation about meeting the standards. We can legitimately focus on this one cell, pinpointing the key finding. So, we can now state our conclusion with statistical reference to the table by saying:

Boys are highly statistically significantly[9] more likely to meet the minimum standard for physical activity (24.2%) compared with girls (18.3%) (P < 0.001).

---

[9]The language plays on the convention that the level of significance of the statistical finding is reflected in key words:
   • 'Statistically significant': $P < 0.05$
   • 'Very statistically significant': $P < 0.01$
   • 'Highly statistically significant': $P < 0.001$

This is a concise way of summarizing the observations in the table. We do not really need to mention the deviations between what was observed and what was expected in any of the other cells in the table unless there is a particular point you want to make. Lastly, it is always useful (and clearer) to include the value for P in any description of your findings.

8.3 p × q TABLES

In the previous section, we dealt with a specific case for contingency tables: the 2×2 table. We will come back to the 2×2 table before we leave this chapter to see how to deal with small samples, and how to deal with small values for E. Now we can expand our horizons and see how to undertake statistical analysis of more complex data where there are more than two rows or two columns. Instead of looking at the special example of the 2×2 table, we are going to consider the general model: the $p \times q$ table.

First, we need to set out the assumptions for the $p \times q$ table (as we did for the 2×2 table), and then check that the data fit the model to ensure that we are using the right test for the data.

Assumptions

Assumptions for a $p \times q$ contingency table are shown in Box 8.4.

BOX 8.4

Assumptions for a p × q contingency table

1. There are two variables, each with two or more categories
2. Samples are random and independent
3. The values in tables must be counts
4. Values are arranged in a table with p rows and q columns
5. The total number of observations (N) must be at least 20
6. Not more than 20% of expected values (E) can be less than 5.0
7. No expected value (E) can be less than 1.0

TABLE 8.5   Labelling of Data for a Table with Three Rows and Four Columns

Variable 1	Column 1	Column 2	Column 3	Column 4	Row Total
	Variable 2				
Row 1	a	b	c	d	r_1
Row 2	e	f	g	h	r_2
Row 3	k	l	m	n	r_3
Column total	c_1	c_2	c_3	c_4	**N**

You will notice a variation in the criterion for the expected values (E) compared with the assumptions for the 2×2 table. For the $p \times q$ table, we *may* have values for $E < 5$, provided the total number of values for $E < 5$ does not exceed 20% of values for E in the table. For example, in a 3×4 table (12 cells), two values for $E < 5$ would be allowed, as it would represent 2/12 or 17% of the total number of values for E. None of the values for E should be less than 1.0, however.

A note on small values for E

These rules of thumb for small values for E safeguard the validity of the statistical model that underpins the chi-squared test. If there are more than 20% of values for $E < 5$ in a $p \times q$ table, or E is less than 1.0, (or less than 5.0 in a 2×2 table), you are inflating the value for $(O-E)^2/E$ for those cells by dividing by a small value for E. When you compared your calculated test statistic with the value in Appendix A7, you might end up rejecting the null hypothesis because your calculated value for χ^2 exceeded the value in the table at $P = 0.05$. If the calculated value for χ^2 was inflated because of small values of E, however, it may be that the true probability of observing what you observed was in fact greater than 5%. Choosing to reject the null hypothesis when you should in fact be accepting it is known as a Type I Error – the incorrect rejection of a true null hypothesis.[10]

Of course, you can (and should) apply a little common sense concerning these rules in practice.

For example, if you had a value for $E = 4.99$ in a 2×2 table (or 4.9, or even 4.8), and a calculated value for χ^2 that comfortably exceeded the cut-off point in the chi-squared table at $P = 0.05$, it would not be unreasonable to reject the null hypothesis at the 5% level.[11] If the calculated value for χ^2 were only just above the 5% cut-off level, or you had computed a value for $E = 3.5$, you would be wise to exercise caution. We will explore how to deal with these issues later in the chapter.

Labelling the cells in a p × q table

In the 2×2 table, we used lower-case letters for the observed values (number of counts). We could use the same approach for a $p \times q$ table. Starting as before with the letter **a** to denote the count in the upper left-hand corner of the table (the intersection of row 1 and column 1), we can move to the next cell in the row, label the count with the letter **b**, then the letter **c** for the next cell, then (for a table with four columns) the letter **d** (Table 8.5). The first cell in the second row would use the next letter in the alphabet (in this case **e**), and so on. This quickly runs into a problem, however, as the cell in the start of the third row should, by rights, be denoted using the letter **i**. But we have already used the letter **i** to denote a specific row, and the letter **j** to denote a specific column. So, we would have to skip **i** and **j**, and go to the next letter, **k**.

[10]We will talk more about this in Chapter 12.

[11]When we look at the output from SPSS, you will see that the interpretation of a statistical test relies on the interpretation of the intermediary values, not just the P value.

This is getting very messy. Instead, let's stick to our more general labels for each cell: O_{11}, O_{12}, O_{13}, O_{14} for the observed values in the first row, O_{21}, O_{22}, O_{23}, O_{24} for the second row, and so on. Then there is no ambiguity. We use the same approach to label the expected values: E_{11}, E_{12}, E_{13}, E_{14}, etc.

Let's go back to the physical activity data. We looked at the results for all boys and girls of age 5–15 years, and whether or not they met the standard. But there are more aspects to consider in the data. Are there some children who do moderate amounts of activity but do not reach the recommended level? Do the results differ by age group? There are lots of other things we might consider (region, income group, ethnic group, changes over time), but let's stick with age and physical activity level for the moment.

The survey [1] reported three levels of activity[12]:

1. Meets recommendations: Physically active for at least 60 minutes on all 7 days a week

2. Some activity: Physically active for 30–59 minutes on all 7 days or 60 minutes or more on 3–6 days

3. Low activity: Lower levels of activity

The survey reported results in four age groups: 5–7 years, 8–10 years, 11–12 years, and 13–15 years.

Let's see if there is an association between physical activity level and age group. First, we need to check that the data fit the model underpinning the assumptions for a $p \times q$ table.

_____

[12]Reporting on physical activity is a complicated business. Just for clarity, the results:
- Include the amount of time spent in activities such as walking, sports, exercise, or other active things done in the last week while in a lesson at school
- Exclude activities such as walking, sports, or exercise done during school breaks
- Include only those children who attended school on at least one day in the previous week
- Exclude walking and cycling to school (which was assessed under modes and use of transport).

Model

The model for a $p \times q$ contingency table is shown in Box 8.5.

The data appear to fit the model. The results are set out in Table 8.6. We will check the values for E shortly to make sure they comply with the model.

It appears that as children get older, they are less and less likely to meet the recommendations for physical activity. It also looks as if most of the change is related to a decrease in the percentage of children meeting the requirements and an increase in low activity levels at age 13–15; the 'some activity' level goes up with age until 13–15, when it drops again. A chi-squared analysis will help us to find out if the apparent changes are statistically significant and help us to understand the key characteristics of the way in which physical activity levels change with age.

Test procedure

The test procedure for a $p \times q$ contingency table is shown in Box 8.6.

We carry out the chi-squared test exactly as we did before for the 2×2 table (Box 8.3), but this time we carry out our calculations for 12 cells rather than

---

BOX 8.5

Model for a p × q contingency table

1. Two variables – age and physical activity level. Physical activity has three levels, and age has four levels
2. Random sample of children aged 5–15 years in England
3. The values in the table are counts
4. Values are arranged in a table with three rows and four columns
5. The total number of observations $N = 3220$ (N must be greater than 20)
6. Not more than 20% of values for (E) are less than 5.0
7. No value for E is less than 1.0

TABLE 8.6   Physical Activity Level versus Age Group in Children Living in England, 2015

Age Group	5–7		8–10		11–12		13–15		Total	
Physical Activity Level	n	%	n	%	n	%	n	%	n	%
Meets recommendations	279	28.1%	218	24.5%	92	15.7%	93	12.4%	682	21.2%
Some activity	455	45.9%	453	50.9%	344	58.6%	372	49.5%	1624	50.4%
Low activity	258	26.0%	219	24.6%	151	25.7%	286	38.1%	914	28.4%
All children	992	100%	890	100%	587	100%	751	100%	3220	100%

BOX 8.6

Test procedure for a p × q contingency table

1. Find the value for E for every cell (row total times column total divided by N)
2. Take the difference between O and E for every cell
3. Square the values for $O - E$ in every cell
4. Divide the square of $O - E$ by E: $(O-E)^2/E$
5. Add together the values for the standardized deviations for all cells in the table:

$$\chi^2 = \Sigma \left[\frac{(O-E)^2}{E} \right]$$

6. Find the value for χ^2 in Appendix A7 for $\nu = (p-1)(q-1)$ and $P = 0.05$, where p is the number of rows and q is the number of columns

$$\chi^2 = \sum_{i=1}^{p} \sum_{j=1}^{q} \left[\frac{(O_{ij} - E_{ij})^2}{E_{ij}} \right]$$

EQUATION 8.2.   Mathematical formula for χ^2 for any $p \times q$ table

where p is the number of rows, q is the number of columns, and the letters i and j the labels for each row number and column number, where i ranges from 1 to p, and j ranges from 1 to q. 'Simply Glorious!' as Toad would say.[13]

Before we can look up the comparable value for χ^2 in Appendix A7, we need to determine the number of degrees of freedom for a $p \times q$ table. The same principle applies as that which we followed in determining the number of degrees of freedom for the 2×2 table. The expected values for each cell (E_{ij}, where i refers to the ith row and j to the jth column), are effectively determined by the row and column totals and the total number of observations N, that is $E_{ij} = r_i c_j / N$.

In the current example, there are four observations in each row. Following our previous argument, three of the observations could take any value, but the fourth value in the row will be determined by the row total. Thus, there are potentially three degrees of freedom in each row. You might think, therefore, that there are nine degrees of freedom. However, we also need to take into account that there are three

four (Box 8.6). The results are set out in Table 8.7. First, we find the values for E for each cell: row total times column total divided by N, that is $E_{ij} = r_i c_j / N$. None of the values for E is less than 5.0, so we are safe to carry out the test without breaking the rules about small values for E. We calculate $O - E$ for each cell, square it, and divide by E. We add together the 12 results for $(O_{ij} - E_{ij})^2/E_{ij}$ to find $\chi^2 = \Sigma [(O - E^2)/E]$. In this case, $\chi^2 = 107.87$.

To share with you the beauty of concision that is a mathematical formula, here is the full-fat expression for χ^2 for any $p \times q$ table:

[13]From *Wind in the Willows* by Kenneth Grahame. If you haven't read it, it is right up there with *The Phantom Tollbooth*. Keep it by your bedside for times when the study of statistics is getting you down. The wealthy, aristocratic, incorrigible Toad will always cheer you up.

TABLE 8.7   Physical Activity Level versus Age Group in Children Living in England, 2015

			Age group				Row Total
			5–7	8–10	11–12	13–15	
Physical activity level							
Meets recommendations	Observed		279	218	92	93	$r_1 = 682$
	Expected	$E_{ij} = \dfrac{r_i c_j}{N}$	210.11	188.50	124.33	159.06	
	Difference	$O_{ij} - E_{ij}$	68.89	29.50	−32.33	−66.06	
	Difference squared	$(O_{ij} - E_{ij})^2$	4746.27	870.07	1045.06	4364.28	
	Taking E into account	$\dfrac{(O_{ij} - E_{ij})^2}{E_{ij}}$	22.59	4.62	8.41	27.44	
	Standardized residual	$\dfrac{O_{ij} - E_{ij}}{\sqrt{E_{ij}}}$	4.75	2.15	−2.90	−5.24	
Some activity	Observed		455	453	344	372	$r_2 = 1624$
	Expected	$E_{ij} = \dfrac{r_i c_j}{N}$	500.31	448.87	296.05	378.77	
	Difference	$O_{ij} - E_{ij}$	−45.31	4.13	47.95	−6.77	
	Difference squared	$(O_{ij} - E_{ij})^2$	2053.27	17.06	2298.99	45.77	
	Taking E into account	$\dfrac{(O_{ij} - E_{ij})^2}{E_{ij}}$	4.10	0.04	7.77	0.12	
	Standardized residual	$\dfrac{O_{ij} - E_{ij}}{\sqrt{E_{ij}}}$	−2.03	0.19	2.79	−0.35	
Low activity	Observed		258	219	151	286	$r_3 = 914$
	Expected	$E_{ij} = \dfrac{r_i c_j}{N}$	281.58	252.63	166.62	213.17	
	Difference	$O_{ij} - E_{ij}$	−23.58	−33.63	−15.62	72.83	
	Difference squared	$(O_{ij} - E_{ij})^2$	556.02	1130.80	244.00	5303.91	
	Taking E into account	$\dfrac{(O_{ij} - E_{ij})^2}{E_{ij}}$	1.97	4.48	1.46	24.88	
	Standardized residual	$\dfrac{O_{ij} - E_{ij}}{\sqrt{E_{ij}}}$	−1.41	−2.12	−1.21	4.99	
Column total			$c_1 = 992$	$c_2 = 890$	$c_3 = 587$	$c_4 = 751$	$N = 3220$

observed values in each column. Two of them can take any value, but the third value will be determined by the column total. So, in a table with p rows and q columns, there are $p-1$ degrees of freedom in each row, and $q-1$ degrees of freedom in each column. Thus, there are $(p-1)\times(q-1)$ degrees of freedom in a $p \times q$ table. Or to use mathematical parlance, degrees of freedom (ν) in a $p \times q$ contingency table is:

$$\nu = (p-1)(q-1)$$

EQUATION 8.3. Number of degrees of freedom (ν) in a $p \times q$ contingency table

In the present example, $\nu = (4-1)(3-1) = 3 \times 2 = 6$. In a 4×3 table, there are, therefore, six degrees of freedom.

> **Rejection rule**: If the calculated value for χ^2 is *greater than* the value in the table for $\chi^2_{\nu,P}$ when $P = 0.05$, reject H_0.

Decision and interpretation

The value for χ^2 in Appendix A7 for $\nu = 6$ and $P = 0.05$ is 12.592. Our calculated value, 107.87, far exceeds the value in the table. Thus, as our calculated value is greater than the value in the table for $\chi^2_{\nu=6,P=0.05}$, we can reject the null hypothesis at the 5% level. We conclude that there is a statistically significant association between age group and the proportions of children meeting different levels of the recommendation for physical activity. As before, we can go further with our analysis. We see that not only is our calculated value greater than the tabulated value for $\chi^2_{\nu=6,P=0.05}$, it is also greater than the value for chi-squared with 6 degrees of freedom and $P = 0.001$, $\chi^2_{\nu=6,P=0.001} = 22.458$. We can therefore confidently reject the null hypothesis at the 0.1% level.

Conclusion

Now we need to ask ourselves two questions. First, what is the nature of the association between age and physical activity. We have already answered this question above when we looked at the percentages in Table 8.6: by the time they reach the 11–12 age group, their physical activity levels appear to be in decline. Second, we need to ask ourselves where the strength of the association lies. Look at the values for the standardize residuals in Table 8.7. There are three values much larger than the rest: 4.75 (children age 5–7 years meeting the recommendations for physical activity); −5.24 (children age 13–15 years meeting the recommendations for physical activity); and 4.99 (children age 13–15 years with low levels of physical activity). Not wishing to insult teenagers, but really this comes as no surprise. The positive values indicate that what we observed (O) is above what we were expecting (E), and the negative value indicates that what we observed was below what we were expecting. In research terms, I might summarize this by saying, 'Young children age 5–7 years are the most likely to have physical activity levels at or above the recommendation (28.1%). Children in the oldest age group (13–15 years) are least likely to achieve the recommended levels (12.4%) and most likely to have low activity levels (38.1%) compared with other children in the 5–15 year age range ($P < 0.001$)'. There are some other values for the standardized residual which are greater than 2.0 or less than −2.0 (our rule of thumb for the observations that we can regard as contributing most to the significance of the association between the two variables), but they contribute much less to the overall significance than the three that I have cited. In the interests of being concise, it is best to report those findings that give the audience a clear sense of what is going on and spare them excessive detail. We will talk more about this in Chapter 15.

8.4 SMALL SAMPLE SIZE

At the beginning of the chapter, and in **A Note on small values for E**, I said that there are some useful alternate approaches when the conditions of the chi-squared test are not met, either because of small sample size or because there are too many small values for E. Let's use an example of the association

TABLE 8.8   Number of Children Aged 13–14 Years Whose Fruit and Vegetable Consumption Met Recommendations, by Sex

	Meeting Recommendation for Fruit and Vegetable Consumption				Total
	Yes		No		
	n	%	n	%	
Boys	2	13.3%	13	86.7%	15
Girls	7	46.7%	8	53.3%	15
Total	9		21		30

BOX 8.7

Model for a 2 × 2 contingency table with small sample

1. Two variables – gender and fruit and vegetable consumption – each with two categories: boy, girl; meeting or not meeting the 5-a-day recommendation
2. Random sample of children aged 13–14 years
3. The values in the table are counts
4. Values are arranged in a table with two rows and two columns
5. The total number of observations $N = 30$ (N must be greater than 20)
6. No expected value (E) is less than 5

between gender and the number of portions of fruit and vegetables consumed by children in a fictional classroom survey of children's eating habits.[14]

As part of his teaching about healthy lifestyle, a class teacher is keen to find out if his Year 9 pupils are meeting the recommendations for fruit and vegetable consumption (five portions per day) [2, 3]. He devises a simple checklist to ask his pupils how often they ate a portion of fruit or vegetables or drank fruit juice or smoothies in the previous week. He wants to test the hypothesis that girls are more likely to meet the recommendations than boys. The results are shown in Table 8.8.

It looks as if the girls in this class are much more likely to meet the recommendations for fruit and vegetable consumption. Although the difference between boys and girls looks large in percentage terms, numerically the difference between 2 out of 9 (boys) and 7 out of 9 (girls) is something that might have arisen just by chance. He wants to know if the findings are statistically significant, and we agree to help him.

The first thing we need to do is see if the data fit the model to carry out a chi-squared test for (in this instance) a 2 × 2 table.

Model

The model for a 2 × 2 contingency table with a small sample is shown in Box 8.7.

You might think that from these results it was screamingly obvious that the boys are less likely than the girls to meet the recommendations for fruit and vegetable consumption. Certainly, these findings confirm social stereotypes about teenage eating habits. But the sample size is quite small. It may be that these differences have arisen just by chance, due to random sampling variation,[15] and there really are no differences in the percentages of boys and girls meeting the recommendations for fruit and vegetable consumption. One of the purposes of statistical analysis is to provide a means whereby we can test our prejudices against an objective measure to see if what we believe to be true is confirmed when we collect evidence.

Now, in terms of the model, we have a problem. When we compute the values for E (Table 8.9), we see that two of them are less than 5. This violates one of the criteria that need to be met if we are to carry out a chi-squared test and expect a valid result

---

[14]I made up these results to illustrate what happens statistically when the numbers in an evaluation are small. But they are probably not a million miles from reality.

[15]The population, in this case, is all pupils aged 13–14 years attending school in this part of England.

TABLE 8.9 Number of Children Aged 13–14 Years Whose Fruit and Vegetable Consumption Met Recommendations, by Sex, Showing Values for Observed and Expected

		Meeting Recommendation for Fruit and Vegetable Consumption				
		Yes		No		Total
		n	%	n	%	
Boys	O	2	13.3%	13	86.7%	15
	E	4.5		10.5		
Girls	O	7	46.7%	8	53.3%	15
	E	4.5		10.5		
Total		9		21		30

for both χ^2 and P. You might say, 'Well, 4.5 is only a little bit less than 5.0, so let's cross our fingers, carry out the chi-squared test, and hope for the best!' If we do that (not cross our fingers, but carry out the chi-squared test), we find that $\chi^2 = 3.9683$. The value in Appendix A7 for χ^2 for $P = 0.05$ and one degree of freedom is 3.841 (this is a 2×2 table, remember, so there is one degree of freedom). Our calculated value (3.9683) is greater than the value in the chi-squared table. We might therefore conclude that we should reject the null hypothesis, accept the hypothesis, and say that girls are more likely than boys to meet the recommendation for fruit and vegetable consumption. But! We said above (**A note on small values for E**), even if the miscreant value for E is only just below 5.0 (as in this case), we needed to be cautious, especially if the value for P is borderline. In our present example, $P = 0.0464$[16] is only just below the 5% cut-off point, $P < 0.05$. There is a danger that because we have violated one of the rules for the chi-squared model, we might be making a Type I error (incorrect rejection of a true null hypothesis). So, we cannot safely reject the null hypothesis.

Fortunately, there is a solution to this problem. In fact, there are two commonly used solutions.

8.4.1 Yates' Correction for Continuity

The first solution was developed in the 1930s by Frank Yates, an English statistician. He argued that there was a way to correct for the possibility that small values of E could result in an overestimate of the calculated value for χ^2 and hence the statistical significance of one's findings. His solution was to reduce the size of the numerator in the expression $(O - E)^2/E$ *before* squaring it. His 'correction for continuity',[17] as it is known, yields the following equation:

$$\chi^2_{Yates} = \Sigma \frac{\left(\left|O - E\right| - 0.5\right)^2}{E}$$

EQUATION 8.4. Calculation of the χ^2 test statistic with Yates' correction for continuity

The first step is to take the modulus (absolute value) of the difference between the observed and expected values in each cell, $|O - E|$. This gets rid of the sign of the difference.[18] When we subtract 0.5 from the modulus, we reduce the size of the difference for *every* cell before we square it.[19] *Then*

---

[16]I used the Excel function '=CHISQ.DIST.RT' to find P. For a given number of degrees of freedom, the Excel function computes P, the area under the curve to the right of the test statistic (the shaded area in the figure at the top of Appendix A7).

[17]'Continuity of what?' you may ask. The chi-squared distribution is a continuous distribution that approximates the binomial distribution, which is based on discrete observations. The chi-squared distribution provides a good approximation of the probabilities associated with the binomial distribution for larger numbers of observations ($N \geq 20$, $E \geq 5$). Below these values for N and E, it begins to lose precision, hence the limits set out in the assumptions that govern the use of the test.

[18]Earlier, we got rid of the sign by squaring the difference. Now, we want to get rid of the sign so that we can reduce the *size* of the difference and *then* square it.

[19]If we didn't take the modulus, the size of the positive values would be reduced (e.g. 4.5 − 0.5 = 4.0), but the size of the negative values would be increased (−4.5 − 0.5 = −5.0) before squaring. This would defeat the purpose of the adjustment and not correct the estimate of χ^2 in a useful way. Our aim is to reduce the size of the numerator in the expression $(O - E)^2/E$ for *every* cell.

we square the result, divide by E, and add the results for all four cells together to give the corrected value, χ^2_{Yates}. For our present example, $\chi^2_{Yates}=2.5397$. This is very much lower than the uncorrected value for chi-squared that we calculated above, 3.9683. Moreover, when we compare 2.5397 with the cut-off value 3.841 for chi-squared with one degree of freedom and $P=0.05$ in Appendix A7, we see that the value is well below the cut-off. On this basis, with Yates' correction, we would accept the null hypothesis, and avoid a Type I error. Indeed, using the Excel '=CHISQ.DIST.RT' function, we find that the value for P corresponding to $\chi^2_{Yates}=2.5397$ is $P=0.1110$, well above the 5% level. So, using Yates' correction, there really is no question that we should accept the null hypothesis.

Yates himself suggested that his correction might be an over-correction, and statistically very conservative. But it is better to be conservative (statistically speaking) than to make false claims for one's findings and risk making a Type I error.[20,21]

Yates' correction is not limited to 2×2 tables. It can be applied to any $p\times q$ table in which

---

[20]It is human nature to want to find results from our research that fit in with our ideas and support our hypothesis. The whole point of undertaking statistical analysis is to protect ourselves from such tendencies, and to be as objective as we can in describing our research findings. It is also important in research to report findings that do *not* support our hypothesis, so that we develop a clearer understanding of which factors are genuinely associated with the outcome that we are interested in.

[21]**For the nerds:** One of the most annoying discoveries for students first learning about statistical analysis is that, for all its apparent rigour, there remain arguments at the most fundamental level about the right approach to something as seemingly straightforward as the chi-squared analysis. As recently as 2007, Campbell wrote an article [4], which sets out the many approaches to the analysis of a 2×2 table and the resultant variations in the computed values for P. He also proposes an alternate approach, using $N-1$ rather than N as the divisor for finding E. The jury is still out, apparently, and more modelling is needed. Campbell's arguments were cogently summarized by Bruce Weaver in 2017 (https://sites.google.com/a/lakeheadu.ca/bweaver/Home/statistics/notes/chisqr_assumptions).

(for example) more than 20% of values for $E<5$. But a word of caution is needed. It is unwise to use Yates' correction to compute a value for P where all the values of $E<5$, or in any table where values for $E<1$. Because it is a *correction* for small values, there is a limit to which the correction yields a valid result for the χ^2 test statistic. Common sense must prevail if one is to find a valid estimate of P. Findings of borderline significance always warrant caution in their interpretation.

One final word about Yates' correction. For a 2×2 table, χ^2_{Yates} can be calculated using an algebraic simplification of Equation 8.4, using the notation set out in Table 8.1:

$$\chi^2_{Yates,2\times2}=\frac{N\left(|ad-bc|-N/2\right)^2}{r_1r_2c_1c_2}$$

EQUATION 8.5.   Simplification of the mathematical expression for the calculation of the χ^2 test statistic with Yates' correction for a 2×2 table

8.5 FISHER'S EXACT TEST

Yates worked with Sir Ronald Aylmer Fisher FRS in the early 1930s. Fisher was a biologist, geneticist, and without doubt, one of the great geniuses of statistical science in the 20th century. We will have more to say about his work in Chapter 11 (Analysis of Variance).

Fisher's Exact Test is exactly that: it yields a value for P that is the *exact* probability of observing a table with a given set of observations, given the marginal values. It applies to 2×2 contingency tables. Because the test yields an exact and directly calculated value for P, there is no Appendix with a table of probabilities associated with a calculated test statistic.

Look again at Table 8.8. Recall that there is one degree of freedom. Let's focus on three values: the observed value in the upper left-hand corner, the one we have called **a** in Table 8.1. In the set of observations that we are considering (Table 8.8), **a** $=2$. Given the marginal value $c_1=9$, the corresponding observed value in the lower left-hand corner (**c**, again, using the labels in Table 8.1) is **c** = 7.

Given that there is one degree of freedom, there are nine other tables that could have arisen (been drawn randomly from a population of 13–14 year-old pupils) with these same marginal values but different values for **a**. Suppose that when the teacher carried out his survey, he found that none of the boys and 9 of the girls met the recommendations (**a** = 0 and **c** = 9). Or one boy and 8 girls met the recommendations (**a** = 1 and **c** = 8). Or any other combination up to **a** = 9 and **c** = 0 (where 9 is the upper limit consistent with the marginal value for the first column). All these possible tables are valid sets of observations consistent with the marginal values.

Now think about the probability of each of these tables occurring. If the null hypothesis is true (there is no association between gender and meeting the recommended level of fruit and vegetable consumption) and there are equal numbers of boys and girls in the class ($r_1 = 15$ and $r_2 = 15$), it would be reasonable to expect that of the pupils that met the recommendation ($c_1 = 9$), roughly half would be boys and half would be girls (say 4 boys and 5 girls, or 5 boys and 4 girls). Next most likely to be observed would be 3 boys and 6 girls, or 6 boys and 3 girls. Least likely would be 0 boys and 9 girls, or 9 boys and 0 girls. The equal probability scenario is, in fact, reflected in the values for E in the first column: $E_{11} = 4.5$ and $E_{12} = 4.5$.

Fisher's brilliance was to work out how to determine the value for P for every possible table that could occur given the marginal values in a 2×2 table. These are shown in Table 8.10.

As we predicted, the highest probabilities were associated with tables in which **a** = 4 or **a** = 5. The next highest probabilities were associated with tables in which **a** = 3 or **a** = 6. The smallest probabilities were associated with the tables in which **a** = 0 or **a** = 9.

The calculation of P is straightforward:

$$P = \frac{r_1!\, r_2!\, c_1!\, c_2!}{N!\, a!\, b!\, c!\, d!},$$

EQUATION 8.6. Fisher's formula for the calculation of P for a 2×2 table with a given set of observed values and marginals

TABLE 8.10 The Probabilities Based on Fisher's Exact Test of the Possible Tables Relating to Gender and Meeting the Recommendations for Fruit and Vegetable Consumption, Given the Marginal Values in TABLE 8.8

If a=	P=
0	0.000 35
1	0.006 75
2	0.047 23
3	0.159 17
4	0.286 51
5	0.286 51
6	0.159 17
7	0.047 23
8	0.006 75
9	0.000 35

where $r_1!\, r_2!\, c_1!\, c_2!$ is equal to the factorials[22] of the marginal values all multiplied together, and $N!\, a!\, b!\, c!\, d!$ is equal to the factorials of the observed values multiplied together, all multiplied by the factorial value for N. The values generated are very large, so if you are doing the calculations manually, you will need a good calculator (better than the one on your phone) or access to a spreadsheet like Excel.[23]

The probabilities generated for each value of **a** are shown in Table 8.10. As we discussed above, the highest probabilities are for the tables in which **a** = 4 or **a** = 5 ($P = 0.286 51$). The next lowest are for the tables in which **a** = 3 or **a** = 6 ($P = 0.159 17$). And the lowest probabilities are for tables where **a** = 0 or **a** = 9 ($P = 0.000 35$). All these values for P added together equals 1.0.

---

[22]Where $n! = 1 \times 2 \times 3 \times \ldots \times (n - 1) \times n$. So $5! = 1 \times 2 \times 3 \times 4 \times 5 = 120$. By convention, $0! = 1$.

[23]You may find that your calculator or even Excel struggle to cope with the potentially very large values generated by the factorial function. In practice, therefore, you may need to alternate the multiplications and divisions, that is divide $r_1!$ by $N!$, then multiply by $r_2!$, then divide by $a!$, and so on.

For the results that we observed in Table 8.8, $\mathbf{a} = 2$, so $P = 0.04723$. You might therefore say, 'Hurrah!, the result is statistically significant at the 5% level'. But! (there's always a 'but'). When we looked at the results in the chi-squared test, we asked ourselves, 'What is the probability of observing the calculated value for χ^2 *or greater*?', that is, what is the area under the curve that lies to the right of the value for χ^2? Following the same principle, we need to add together the probabilities for the corresponding tail of the values for $\mathbf{a}$, that is, for $\mathbf{a} = 2$ and $\mathbf{a} = 1$ and $\mathbf{a} = 0$. If we add these three probabilities together, we get a value equal to 0.0 5432. But wait! There is a second 'but'! This value for P relates only to one tail of possible outcomes for our null hypothesis. We should say that the value we have calculated is $\frac{1}{2}P = 0.05432$. If we want to make our test two-tailed (to make it equivalent to our previous tests), we need to double this value, and say $P = 0.10864$. So, based on the two-tailed version of Fisher's Exact Test, we should again (as with Yates' correction) accept the null hypothesis.[24]

Let's review. When we calculated the value for chi-squared without any correction, we got a value for $P = 0.0464$. When we used Yates' correction, the value for $P = 0.111$. Now, using Fisher's Exact Test, we get a value for $P = 0.109$. While the uncorrected chi-squared calculation would lead us to reject the null hypothesis, either of the two alternatives would lead us to accept the null hypothesis. Given that our aim is to be statistically conservative and avoid a Type I error, Yates' correction and Fisher's Exact Test lead us to the safer decision. The conclusion? If the values for E or N break the rules for using the chi-squared test, it is essential to use the methods that will generate a reliable value for P and minimize the risk of making a Type I error.

8.6 USING ALL YOUR DATA

When examining the results in a contingency table, two features frequently arise that need a cool head to address correctly. Let's look at an example.

Our teacher (who was concerned about the low levels of fruit and vegetable consumption in the boys in his class[25]) has now corralled the entire school into using his method to assess fruit and vegetable consumption. He wants to test a new hypothesis, namely that as children grow older, their fruit and vegetable consumption is less and less likely to meet the recommendations. He has a comprehensive set of results for children aged 5–15 years in a small rural school with 193 pupils. When presenting the results, however, he gets rather carried away. He thinks that the more detail he provides, the more useful the results will be to his fellow teachers to motivate them to encourage more fruit and vegetable consumption. His table of results is shown in Table 8.11.

The first impression one has is that the level of consumption declines as pupils get older. And while it is encouraging that many children appear to eat four or five portions of fruit and vegetables every day (46.6% + 21.8% = 68.4%), almost a third of children are eating three portions per day or less, and some (it would appear) are eating virtually none. Having been stung by his disappointment at failing to demonstrate the truth of his previous hypothesis (that girls were more likely to meet the recommendations than boys), the teacher again asks for our help with the analysis of the data to see if the obvious trends bear up under closer, statistical scrutiny. Again, we agree to help. The model is shown in Box 8.8.

The results in Table 8.11 are presented in a 6×4 contingency table, and appear to conform to the first five elements of a model for a $p \times q$ table.

---

[24]I am sorry there are so many interpretations of P in this section. The P in Equation 8.6 is the probability of observing a table with a particular value for $\mathbf{a}$, given the marginal values. $\frac{1}{2}P$ is the sum of the probabilities in the 'tail' of the distribution of the possible values for $\mathbf{a}$. It relates to the P that we have used to define the area under the curve for our two-tailed distributions, where the total area under the curve is equal to $P = 1.0$. (Indeed, if you add up all the values for P in Table 8.10, you get 1.0000.) So, the statistical interpretation of the final calculated value for P for Fisher's Exact Test is the two-tailed equivalent of the other statistical tests that we have been looking at, like t and Wilcoxon U.

[25]Even though he failed to show statistically that girls were more likely to meet the recommendations than boys.

BOX 8.8

Model for a 6 × 4 contingency table with small sample

1. Two variables – age and levels of fruit consumption. Fruit consumption has six levels, and age has four levels
2. Random sample of children aged 5–15 years in a region in England
3. The values in the table are counts
4. Values are arranged in a table with six rows and four columns
5. The total number of observations $N = 193$ (N must be greater than 20)
6. Not more than 20% of values for (E) are less than 5.0
7. No value for E is less than 1.0

So far so good. The results appear ripe for a chi-squared analysis. The next step is to find the values for E, remembering that in a $p \times q$ table, not more than 20% of values for E can be less than 5.0, and no value can be less than 1.0. The results for E are shown in Table 8.12.

Immediately, we see a problem. With all this detail in results from a small school, some categories have very small numbers of children. In consequence, there are many values for $E < 5$ (10 out of 24, or 42%), and one value for $E < 1$. We have violated two of the criteria for carrying out a chi-squared analysis.

Now, when the teacher learned of the problem and looked at the data, he said, 'Why don't we just ignore the bottom two rows? After all, less than 10% of children have either one or zero portions of fruit and vegetables per day, and my real concern is to boost intake generally and stop the decline in consumption as children get older (if we find there really is one, statistically speaking). This would get over the rule that says we can't have more than 20% of values for E less than 5.0 – we would only have 2 out of 16 values – that's 12.5% – and we lose the value for $E < 1.0$!'

I laughed quietly to myself. 'Sadly', I say, 'that breaks a fundamental rule relating to chi-squared analysis: NEVER OMIT ROWS OR COLUMNS FROM A TABLE IN A CHI-SQUARED ANALYSIS'. He looked annoyed. 'Why not?' he said. I explained, patiently, and paraphrase my arguments below.

The rules for the statistical tests that we are exploring in this book assume that samples are drawn in such a way as to be representative of a defined population. Any omission of data is likely to invalidate the representativeness of the sample and

TABLE 8.11 Number (and Percentage) of Children Aged 5–15 Years Attending a Small Rural School Consuming Between Zero and Five or More Portions of Fruit and Vegetables per Day, by Age Group

Number of portions eaten per day	Age Group (Years)									
	5–7		8–10		11–12		13–15		Total	
	n	%	n	%	n	%	n	%	n	%
5 or more	34	63.0%	31	52.5%	10	38.5%	15	27.8%	90	46.6%
4	10	18.5%	17	28.8%	3	11.5%	12	22.2%	42	21.8%
3	2	3.7%	2	3.4%	6	23.1%	9	16.7%	19	9.8%
2	5	9.3%	5	8.5%	4	15.4%	10	18.5%	24	12.4%
1	3	5.6%	1	1.7%	2	7.7%	5	9.3%	11	5.7%
0	0	0.0%	3	5.1%	1	3.8%	3	5.6%	7	3.6%
All pupils	54	100.0%	59	100.0%	26	100.0%	54	100.0%	193	100.0%

TABLE 8.12   Number (Observed and Expected) of Children Aged 5–15 Years Attending a Small Rural School Consuming Between Zero and Five or More Portions of Fruit and Vegetables per Day, by Age Group

| Number of portions eaten per day | Age Group (Years) | | | | | | | | | |
| | 5–7 | | 8–10 | | 11–12 | | 13–15 | | Total | |
	O	E	O	E	O	E	O	E	O	E
5 or more	34	25.18	31	27.51	10	12.12	15	25.18	90	90
4	10	11.75	17	12.84	3	5.66	12	11.75	42	42
3	2	5.32	2	5.81	6	2.56	9	5.32	19	19
2	5	6.72	5	7.34	4	3.23	10	6.72	24	24
1	3	3.08	1	3.36	2	1.48	5	3.08	11	11
0	0	1.96	3	2.14	1	0.94	3	1.96	7	7
All pupils	54	54	59	59	26	26	54	54	193	193

the generalizability of the findings, and undermine the validity of the statistical test and the P value derived. Two considerations:

- *Omitting outlying values from the analysis.* Outliers often provide important information about the true variability of the observations made. Outliers should be omitted from analyses only in exceptional circumstances and based on clearly defined rules established before data collection begins, or because there is a genuine reason to think that the measurement is not valid.
- *Omitting rows or columns from a chi-squared analysis.* **Never** omit rows or columns from a contingency table in a chi-squared analysis. If values for E or N in a contingency table do not meet the conditions for chi-squared analysis, there are three possible solutions:
  - Combine rows or columns in such a way as to (i) yield a meaningful interpretation of the findings and (ii) meet the conditions for analysis. If this is not successful,
  - Reduce the table to a 2×2 contingency table (the minimum needed for a chi-squared analysis) and check values for E and N. If the conditions for a chi-squared analysis are still not met,
  - Use Yates' correction or Fisher's Exact Test to undertake the analysis.

Rule Number 1 for chi-squared analysis is shown in Box 8.9.

Rule Number 2 for chi-squared analysis is shown in Box 8.10.

BOX 8.9

CHI-SQUARED ANALYSIS:

RULE NUMBER 1

NEVER OMIT ROWS OR COLUMNS FROM A TABLE IN A CHI-SQUARED ANALYSIS

BOX 8.10

CHI-SQUARED ANALYSIS:

RULE NUMBER 2

COMBINE ROWS OR COLUMNS IN A WAY THAT YIELDS MEANINGFUL INTERPRETATION OF THE FINDINGS

TABLE 8.13 Number (Observed and Expected) of Children Aged 5–15 Years Attending a Small Rural School Consuming Between Zero and Five or More Portions of Fruit and Vegetables per Day, by Age Group

Number of portions eaten per day	Age group (years)										
	5–7		8–10		11–12		13–15		Total		
	O	E	O	E	O	E	O	E	O	E	%
5 or more	34	25.18	31	27.51	10	12.12	15	25.18	90	90	46.6%
4	10	11.75	17	12.84	3	5.66	12	11.75	42	42	21.8%
2–3	7	12.03	7	13.15	10	5.79	19	12.03	43	43	22.3%
0–1	3	5.04	4	5.50	3	2.42	8	5.04	18	18	9.3%
All pupils	54	54	59	59	26	26	54	54	193	193	100.0%

Let's get back to our results in Table 8.11. Using the guidance above, the most sensible approach would be to combine rows or columns to ensure that the values for E did not violate the criteria for the chi-squared test. Given that we are particularly interested in the relationship between age and consumption, it would make sense to combine rows rather than columns. If we combine the bottom two rows (for pupils eating 1 or zero portions of fruit and vegetables per week), we lose the value for $E < 1.0$, but still end up with too many values for $E < 5.0$ (5 out of 20, or 25%). So, let's go one step further and combine the bottom three rows. Or we could combine the bottom two rows, and the middle two rows. The result is shown in Table 8.13. Note (as we said earlier in the chapter) that in each row and column, the sum of the values for E is the same as the sum of the observed values.

The results are still interpretable, give us a better-balanced set of results, and we have overcome the problem of small values for E (no values for $E < 1$, and only 1 out of 16 values [6.25%] for $E < 5$). If we carry out the chi-squared analysis, and show the resulting table with the standardized residuals, we can provide a meaningful interpretation of the findings (Table 8.14).

First, we find that the calculated value for $\chi^2 = 26.065$. We compare this with the tabulated value for χ^2 in Appendix A7 for $\nu = 9$ (we now have a 4×4 table, so $\nu = (4-1)(4-1) = 3 \times 3 = 9$). We find

that our calculated value for χ^2 lies between 23.589 (when $P = 0.005$) and 27.877 (when $P = 0.001$). With a simple interpolation in the table, we find $P = 0.002$. We can confidently reject the null hypothesis and tell our (now) happy teacher that there is a very statistically significant association between age group and fruit and vegetable consumption.

To put it succinctly, and following the guidance about the use of the standardized residuals to help us interpret the findings, we see that pupils aged 13–15 are the least likely to meet the recommendations for eating five portions of fruit and vegetables per day (28% compared with 47% averaged across all pupils, standardized residual $= -2.03$) and most likely to be in the group consuming only 2–3 portions per day (35% compared with 22% across all pupils, standardized residual $= 2.01$). In contrast, younger pupils aged 5–7 years are the most likely to achieve the recommended level of consumption (63% compared with 47% overall, standardized residual $= 1.76$[26]) in part because of access to a free fruit and vegetable scheme operated in the school for Infant pupils. Children aged 11–12 years were similar to children age 13–15 years and were more likely than the average (38% compared with 22%, standardized residual $= 1.75$) to consume only 2–3 portions of fruit and vegetables per day.

---

[26]Not quite at our 2.0 cut-off, but helpful in guiding us to the cells contributing the most to the significance of the findings.

TABLE 8.14   Number Observed and Percentage Within Age Group Consuming Specified Number of Portions of Fruit and Vegetables per Day Among Children Aged 5–15 Years Attending a Small Rural School by Age Group, together with Standardized Residuals

Number of portions eaten per day		Age Group (Years)				All Pupils
		5–7	8–10	11–12	13–15	
5 or more	n	34	31	10	15	90
	%	63.0%	52.5%	38.5%	27.8%	46.6%
	Std resid[a]	1.76	0.66	−0.61	−2.03	
4	n	10	17	3	12	42
	%	18.5%	28.8%	11.5%	22.2%	21.8%
	Std resid	−0.51	1.16	−1.12	0.07	
2–3	n	7	7	10	19	43
	%	13.0%	11.9%	38.5%	35.2%	22.3%
	Std resid	−1.45	−1.69	1.75	2.01	
0–1	n	3	4	3	8	18
	%	5.6%	6.8%	11.5%	14.8%	9.3%
	Std resid	−0.91	−0.64	0.37	1.32	
All pupils		54	59	26	54	193

[a]Std resid: Standardized residual.

8.7 SPSS

Access to chi-squared, Yates' correction and Fisher Exact Test in SPSS is through the **Crosstabs** function. For purposes of analysis in SPSS, the expectation is that each row of the data sheet is a 'case' with observations of the relevant variables.

I will illustrate the function and statistical options using the SPSS data files 'ch08d01.sav' and 'ch08d02.sav' on the website. For the analysis of the data in Table 8.3, my SPSS data file has $N = 3220$ lines which show, for each case (line by line), the sex of the subject (Boy = 1 and Girl = 2) and whether or not they meet the standard for physical activity (Yes = 1 and No = 2). In the old days, you could not carry out a chi-squared test in SPSS using the summarized data as it appears in Table 8.3 (whereas you can in Excel). A modified procedure now allows the tabulated data to be analyzed directly.

Click on Analyze>Descriptives>Crosstabs> Statistics, click on the Chi-square box, and click Continue. Now click on Cells to generate the most helpful output. In the box labelled Counts, Observed will already be ticked. Click on Expected. In the Percentages box, click Row. In the box labelled Residuals, click on Standardized. Click Continue to go back to the main Crosstabs screen.

Now click Paste to save the syntax to a syntax file ('ch08d01.sps') or click OK to run. The output on the website ('ch08d01.spv') contains the same pieces of information as in Tables 8.3 and 8.4. The SPSS table of analysis is shown in Figure 8.1. It shows the counts, expected values, percentages, and standardized residuals, as requested. These match the values in Table 8.4.

Figure 8.2 shows SPSS output for chi-squared analysis in **Crosstabs**. In the first row, you see the calculated Pearson chi-squared test statistic ($\chi^2 = 16.606$). This is identical to the value we

Sex * Meets standards Crosstabulation

			Meets standards		
			Meets standard	Does not meet standard	Total
Sex	Boy	Count	384	1206	1590
		Expected count	336.8	1253.2	1590.0
		% within sex	24.2%	75.8%	100.0%
		Standardized residual	2.6	−1.3	
	Girl	Count	298	1332	1630
		Expected count	345.2	1284.8	1630.0
		% within sex	18.3%	81.7%	100.0%
		Standardized residual	−2.5	1.3	
Total		Count	682	2538	3220
		Expected count	682.0	2538.0	3220.0
		% within sex	21.2%	78.8%	100.0%

FIGURE 8.1 SPSS output for Crosstabs for sex and physical activity data. *Source*: Reproduced with permission of International Business Machines Corporation.

Chi-square tests

	Value	df	Asymptotic significance (2-sided)	Exact sig. (2-sided)	Exact sig. (1-sided)
Pearson chi-square	16.606[a]	1	0.000		
Continuity correction[b]	16.256	1	0.000		
Likelihood ratio	16.634	1	0.000		
Fisher's exact test				0.000	0.000
Linear-by-linear association	16.600	1	0.000		
N of valid cases	3220				

[a]0 cells (0.0%) have expected count less than 5. The minimum expected count is 336.76.

[b]Computed only for a 2x2 table.

FIGURE 8.2 SPSS output for chi-squared analysis in **Crosstabs** for sex and physical activity data. *Source*: Reproduced with permission of International Business Machines Corporation.

calculated earlier. Second, you will see Asymptotic Significance (two-sided), the P value computed directly (rather than requiring us to look up the cut-off points for the test statistic in a table). The test is 2-sided because we make no assumptions about the direction of deviance from what we expect to see if the null hypothesis is true. The value $P = 0.000$ means that $P < 0.0005$, not that there is a zero chance of observing this outcome if the null hypothesis is true. There is also a helpful footnote regarding values for E, telling us there are no values for $E < 5$.

The chi-squared test statistic computed with Yates' Continuity Correction and probability based on Fisher's Exact Test are also shown. These are not relevant here, but they are for smaller data sets.

Chi-square tests

	Value	df	Asymptotic significance (2-sided)	Exact sig. (2-sided)	Exact sig. (1-sided)
Pearson chi-square	3.968[a]	1	0.046		
Continuity correction[b]	2.540	1	0.111		
Likelihood ratio	4.144	1	0.42		
Fisher's exact test				0.109	0.054
Linear-by-linear association	3.836	1	0.50		
N of valid cases	30				

[a]2 cells (50.0%) have expected count less than 5. The minimum expected count is 4.50.

[b]Computed only for a 2x2 table.

FIGURE 8.3   SPSS output for chi-squared analysis in **Crosstabs** for sex and fruit and vegetable consumption data. *Source*: Reproduced with permission of International Business Machines Corporation.

Let's go back to the results for pupils meeting the recommendations for fruit and vegetable consumption (Table 8.8). Using the same syntax in SPSS as before, the output for fruit and vegetable data is shown in Figure 8.3. The footnote to the chi-squared analysis tells us that 50% of the values for E are less than 5. As wise students of statistics, you now know that this means the chi-squared P value ($P=0.046$) is not reliable, and that two-tailed P values based on Yates' correction or Fisher's Exact Test will yield a safer result. Hence my warnings about not just reaching for the P value in SPSS output. You need to know *which P* value to use.

8.8 EXERCISES

8.8.1

Men and women were quizzed about the likely need for changes in dietary habits as they grew older (Table 8.15). Was gender significantly associated with a difference in response?

TABLE 8.15   Numbers of Women and Men who Thought Changes in Dietary Habits Would be Necessary as They Grew Older

	Women	Men
Yes	125	52
No	35	35

8.8.2

Following surgery in hospital, patients were offered nutritional support from a dietitian at home as part of their follow-up. Table 8.16 shows nutritional status assessed three months post-discharge. Is the provision of dietetic support at home associated with improved nutritional status three months post-discharge?

TABLE 8.16   Number of Patients Who Had Nutritional Status Assessed Three Months Post-discharge: Nutritional Status versus Accepting or Declining Nutritional Support at Home Post-surgery

	Nutritional status			
	Good	Moderate	Poor	Malnourished
Dietetic support				
Accepted	19	10	8	5
Declined	6	5	12	15

8.8.3

A small sample of adolescent girls was assessed for anaemia (Haemoglobin <120 g/l) and menarchial status. Table 8.17 shows that a higher proportion of girls who have started their periods

TABLE 8.17 Presence of Anaemia in Adolescent Girls According to Menarchial Status

Menarchial status	Anaemic			
	Yes		No	
	n	%	n	%
Started periods	5	29.4 %	12	70.6 %
Not yet started	2	7.1 %	26	92.9 %

(29%) was anaemic compared with those who had not started their periods (7%). Is the relationship statistically significant? Carry out the test in three ways: using the chi-squared test without correction, with Yate's correction, and using Fisher's Exact Test.

REFERENCES

1. Values in tables adapted from: Health and Social Care Information Centre. *Health Survey for England 2015*. Physical activity in children. Health and Social Care Information Centre. London. 2016. ISBN 978-1-78386-896-4.

2. Public Health England. *The Eatwell Guide*. Public Health England. London. 2016. https://assets.publishing.service.gov.uk/government/uploads/system/uploads/attachment_data/file/551502/Eatwell_Guide_booklet.pdf

3. NHS Choices. 5 A Day Portion Sizes. https://www.nhs.uk/Livewell/5ADAY/Pages/Portionsizes.aspx

4. Campbell, I. Chi-squared and Fisher-Irwin tests of two-by-two tables with small sample recommendations. *Stat Med.* 2007; 26:3661–3675. www.iancampbell.co.uk/twobytwo/background.htm

CHAPTER 9

McNemar's Test

Learning Objectives

After studying this chapter, you should be able to:

- Identify data sets for which McNemar's test is the right test to use
- Carry out McNemar's test manually for a 2×2 table that describes change of status before and after an intervention
- Interpret SPSS output to determine the level of significance of your findings

9.1 INTRODUCTION

This chapter, I promise you, is the second shortest in the book.[1] It deals with one test: McNemar's test. Its application is limited to three circumstances:

1. Looking at change in status after an intervention, where there are only two possible states: you are in the state, or you are not in the state. 'State' might be a medical outcome (alive or dead; with a medical condition or not); or some other state (happy or sad; hungry or not hungry); or you might have a view or opinion (agree or disagree; like or dislike).

2. Relative effect of two exposures in a cross-over trial. You might compare the effect of Exposure 1 (for example, an intervention was

---

[1]The shortest chapter, Chapter 13, is really just a set of exercises on choosing statistical tests.

Statistics in Nutrition and Dietetics, First Edition. Michael Nelson.
Companion website: www.wiley.com/go/nelson/statistics

deemed satisfactory or not satisfactory) versus effect of Exposure 2. It must be a cross-over trial because the measurements have to be made in the same individuals.

3. Exposure in matched cases and controls (exposed/not exposed). The idea is that there is matching (rather than a repeat measurement) between two sets of measurements.

At first glance, a table for McNemar's test looks like a 2×2 contingency table, so you might be forgiven for thinking that a chi-squared test should be used to assess statistical significance. But the underlying purpose of the analysis is to look at status before and after an intervention or to contrast the impact of two exposures on an individual, or to contrast the impact of an exposure in matched pairs of individuals who are either cases or controls.

Statistically speaking, it is a variation on the Wilcoxon Sign Test (see Chapter 7). The reference statistic to decide whether to accept or reject the null hypothesis depends on the size of the sample. If $N > 20$, the χ^2 distribution with one degree of freedom provides a good approximation for P for the calculated test statistic. If $N \leq 20$, we refer to the binomial distribution to determine values for P.

9.2 THE BASICS

Fundamental principle

Expectation:	H_0: There is no impact of an intervention or exposure on outcome.
Decision criterion:	If there is an impact of intervention or exposure statistically significant at the 5% level, reject H_0.

Assumptions

Assumptions underpinning McNemar's test are shown in Box 9.1.

The examples below clarify how the test works for each of the three scenarios listed above.

BOX 9.1

Assumptions underpinning McNemar's test

1. Samples are random and independent
2. There is one nonnormal variable which can take one of two values (0 or 1, A or B, etc.)
3. Results are observed in one of three conditions:
   a) Status in individuals before and after an intervention
   b) Repeat observations (outcomes) within each subject on each of two treatments
   c) Exposed/not exposed status in matched cases and controls
4. Values are arranged in a table with two rows and two columns
5. The values in tables must be counts

Example 1: before and after an intervention

In my statistics classes, I had students from a range of medical sciences courses: nutrition and dietetics, medicine, nursing, and physiotherapy. To provide some observations for McNemar's test, I carried out a survey in one of my classes. At the beginning of term, I asked the students to rate their view of statistics as a discipline: 'easy', 'not too hard', 'difficult', or 'impossible'. I was surprised (and not a little shocked) to discover that no one thought statistics 'easy' or 'not too hard'. For the purposes of the survey, therefore, we agreed that everyone would rate the subject as either 'difficult' or 'impossible'. Sadly, I think this reflects their experience of statistics teaching in the past, but that is another story.

The basic question I wanted to answer (ego aside) was whether my teaching improved their view of statistics as a discipline. The best I could hope for, apparently, was that it was no longer 'impossible' and merely 'difficult'. Better than nothing, I suppose.

Fundamental principle

Expectation:	H_0: There is no impact of the course on students' view of statistics.
Decision criterion:	If the view of statistics after the course changes at the 5% level, reject H_0.

Notice that I am not saying in which *direction* I am expecting their view to change. This reflects the phrasing of the null hypothesis, that the course has no impact. If I reject the null hypothesis, it could be because the results show change in either direction.[2]

Model

The model for McNemar's test where data show the status in individuals before and after an intervention is shown in Box 9.2.

Test procedure

Arrange the data as shown in Table 9.1. The rows show the students' views before the course. The first column ('Total before') shows how many students

---

BOX 9.2

Model for **McNemar's** test: status in individuals before and after an intervention

1. Sample is random and independent
2. There is one nonnormal variable which can take one of two values: 'difficult' or 'impossible'
3. Results show status ('view of statistics') in individuals before and after an intervention (teaching on statistics)
4. Core values are arranged in a table with two rows and two columns
5. The values in tables are counts

TABLE 9.1 Number of Medical Science Students who Found Statistics 'Impossible' or 'Difficult' Before and After a Statistics Course

			After Course	
		Total Before	Impossible	Difficult
Before course	Impossible	34	a 17	b 17
	Difficult	9	c 4	d 5

put themselves into each of two response categories: 34 said statistics was 'impossible', and 9 that it was 'difficult'.

The core values are shown inside the box in the table.[3] Of the 34 students who regarded statistics as 'impossible' at the start of the course, 17 continued to find the subject 'impossible' at the end of the course, but the other 17 had shifted their position from 'impossible' to 'difficult'. 'Woohoo!' as Homer Simpson would say. Of the nine students who viewed statistics as 'difficult' at the start of the course, five continued to regard it as 'difficult', while four now saw it as 'impossible'. Not such a great outcome (ego-deflation inevitable). Not unexpected, perhaps, as some students learn about the breadth and rigours of statistical analysis and find it challenging.

At first glance, it looks like around half of each group changed their position between the start and end of the course. You might think, therefore, that the course had no impact on students' views. But let's think about this in a different way.

Those students whose view has not changed do not contribute to our understanding of the impact of the course. Thus, the number of observations in cell **a** reflect those students on whom the course has had no impact (statistics was seen as 'impossible' at the start of the course, and 'impossible' at the end). Similarly, those who found it 'difficult' at the start and at the end (**d**) have not contributed to our understanding of the impact of the course. In fact, only

---

[2]This illustrates nicely how statistical analysis can help take the ego out of scientific experimentation.

[3]Note that we have labelled the cells **a**, **b**, **c**, and **d**, as we did initially for the 2×2 contingency table.

those cells where a subject had *changed* their position (**b** and **c**) that we have useful information (statistically speaking) about the impact of the teaching on their view of statistics as a discipline.

When $\mathbf{b}+\mathbf{c} > 20$, the test statistic is T_1:

$$T_1 = \frac{(b-c)^2}{b+c} = \frac{(17-4)^2}{17+4} = \frac{13^2}{21} = \frac{169}{21} = 8.048$$

EQUATION 9.1   Formula for T_1 for McNemar's test

Please note that T_1 is not the same as the Wilcoxon T statistic

Decision and interpretation

> **Rejection rule**: If the calculated value for T_1 is *greater than* the value in the table for $\chi^2_{1,0.05}$ when $P = 0.05$, reject H_0.

To decide whether to accept or reject the null hypothesis, we refer to the χ^2 Table (Appendix A7) with one degree of freedom:

$$\chi^2_{v=1,P=0.05} = 3.841$$
$$\chi^2_{v=1,P=0.01} = 6.635$$
$$\chi^2_{v=1,P=0.001} = 10.828$$

The calculated value for T_1 (8.048) is greater than the tabulated value at $P = 0.05$ ($\chi^2 = 3.841$), so we can reject the null hypothesis at the 5% level. We then go on to find the level of confidence at which the null hypothesis can be rejected. Our calculated value is greater than the tabulated value at $P = 0.01$ ($\chi^2 = 6.635$), so we can reject the null hypothesis at the 1% level. That is as far as we can

go; the calculated value is less than the value in the table at $P = 0.001$ ($\chi^2 = 10.828$). We can therefore reject H_0 at the 1% level, $P < 0.01$.

The conclusion is that the course had a beneficial impact on the view of statistics held by members of the class. (Phew!). Sadly, there was a small group who, at the outset, thought statistics was 'difficult', but for whom learning more about statistics and statistical tests created greater confusion, not less, and it became 'impossible'. It is difficult (if not impossible) to know what to do about this group.

Example 2: repeat observations (outcomes) within each subject on each of two treatments

A study was planned to explore the risks of retinopathy during pregnancy in women with Type 2 diabetes. A pilot study was undertaken to compare retinopathy status during and after pregnancy. The results are shown in Table 9.2.

Fundamental principle

Expectation:	H_0: There is no association between pregnancy in women with Type 2 diabetes and the presence of retinopathy
Decision criterion:	If the probability of the presence of retinopathy changing after pregnancy is less than 5%, reject H_0.

Model

The model for McNemar's test where data show the status in individuals before and after an intervention is shown in Box 9.3.

TABLE 9.2   Number of Women with or without Retinopathy during and After Pregnancy

			After Pregnancy	
		Total during Pregnancy	Retinopathy	No Retinopathy
During pregnancy	Retinopathy	20	a 20	b 0
	No retinopathy	16	c 6	d 10

BOX 9.3

Model for McNemar's test: status in individuals before and after an intervention

1. Sample is random and independent
2. There is one nonnormal variable which can take one of two values: retinopathy or no retinopathy
3. Results show status in individuals during and after an intervention (pregnancy)
4. Core values are arranged in a table with two rows and two columns
5. The values in tables are counts

As in Example 1, the useful information in the table is from those individuals whose status has changed. How many of the women with retinopathy during pregnancy were without retinopathy after pregnancy? How many women without retinopathy during pregnancy had retinopathy after pregnancy? Those women whose status did not change (cells **a** and **d**) do not contribute to our understanding of the impact of the intervention (pregnancy) on the outcome (retinopathy).

If the null hypothesis were true, our expectation is that there would be changes in status (cells **b** and **c**) in equal and opposite directions: of the women whose status had changed ($n = 6$), three would have moved from Retinopathy to No Retinopathy, and three would have moved from No Retinopathy to Retinopathy. Of course, because of random sampling variation, the changes might not be equal in both cells. Perhaps **b** $= 2$ and **c** $= 4$. Or maybe **b** $= 1$ and **c** $= 5$. What seems very unlikely is that **b** $= 0$ and **c** $= 6$. The probabilities associated with each of these outcomes can be looked up in the Binomial Table (Appendix A1).

Test procedure

When **b** + **c** ≤ 20, the test statistic is T_2, the smaller of the two values **b** or **c**. We refer to the binomial table (Appendix A1) for the probabilities.

Let us label the information we have so that we can interpret the findings using the binomial table:

$$\mathbf{b} = 0$$
$$n = 6$$
$$p = 0.500^4$$

Our expectation if the null hypothesis were true is that half of the women would have changed status in each direction, that is, the proportion that would have changed position is $p = 0.500$. The value for n is the value shown in the binomial table. The value for **b** (the one to look up probabilities for) is shown in the binomial table as r. Our question is, what is the probability of observing 0 changes out of 6 when our expectation is that there would be similar changes in both directions (that is, $r = 3$, or something close to it). Find the column for $p = 0.500$. Look down the column, find the block in which $n = 6$ and $r = 0$. The associated probability (the value for P in the table) is $P = 0.0156$. Make sure you note and understand the difference between lower-case p (the proportion of observations that we expect to see in the population, $p = 0.500$, assuming the null hypothesis is true) and upper-case P (the probability of observing what we have observed).

Decision and interpretation

Rejection rule: If the value of P in **both tails** *is less than* 0.05, reject H$_0$.

We conclude that the probability of observing what we observed, assuming the null hypothesis is true, is $P = 0.0156$. At this point, you might assume that because $P < 0.05$, we can reject the null hypothesis. But we are not quite finished.

The null hypothesis made no assumptions about the *direction* in which any differences might lie. So, another possibility (with an equal probability) is that **b** $= 6$ and **c** $= 0$. This makes our test two-tailed, following the model that we have used in previous tests. The probability for observing what we observed in either direction is therefore

---
[4]Remember, this is p the proportion, not P the probability.

$P = 0.0156 \times 2 = 0.0312$.[5] Our value for P is still less than 0.05, so we can reject the null hypothesis. As this is an exact probability (there is only one set of values in the binomial table that match the assumptions underlying the null hypothesis), we do not need to look further to see if we can reject the null hypothesis with a greater degree of confidence (e.g. at the 1% or 0.1% level). Of course, there is roughly a 3 in 100 chance that we are making the wrong decision by rejecting the null hypothesis.

Example 3: exposed/not exposed status in matched cases and controls

McNemar's test can also be used to analyze the results from a case-control study. The layout is again a 2×2 table, but the thinking behind it is a little more complicated than for the previous examples. The analysis provides a quick answer to the question of whether being 'exposed' is associated with changes in the occurrence of the outcome of interest.

Iodine supplementation has been used worldwide to prevent goitre and the consequences of iodine deficiency [1]. Most countries use iodized salt as the vehicle, but New Zealand and Australia chose to use bread, in part because there were concerns about the association between salt intake and hypertension.[6] More central to the issue of iodine supplementation, there were concerns about risks of thyrotoxicosis or Graves' disease in individuals with existing hyperthyroidism. A pilot case-control study was planned to explore the risk of developing increased levels of thyroid-stimulating immunoglobulin (TSI) in subjects with existing hyperthyroidism. Elevated levels of TSI cause over-secretion

TABLE 9.3   Numbers of Case-Control Matched Pairs with or without Hyperthyroidism Disease Exposed to Bread either Iodine-Fortified or not Fortified who had Thyroid-Stimulating Antibodies Detected after Six Months

			Controls (Normal Thyroid Function)	
			Fortified Bread	Bread not Fortified
Cases (hyperthyroidism)	Fortified bread		a 4	b 11
	Bread not fortified		c 3	d 241

of thyroid hormone. Exposure in the case-control study was to either fortified or unfortified bread. The results are shown in Table 9.3.

Fundamental principle

Expectation:	H_0: There is no association between eating iodine fortified bread and risk of elevated TSI in subjects with existing hyperthyroidism
Decision criterion:	If the probability of observing TSI levels rising after eating iodine-fortified bread is less than 5%, reject H_0.

Model

The model for McNemar's test where data show the status in individuals in a matched case-control study is shown in Box 9.4.

Test procedure

There are four types of matched case-control pairs: exposed–exposed, exposed–unexposed, unexposed–exposed, and unexposed–unexposed. Analogous to the previous examples for McNemar's test, the useful information in the table is from the matched case-control pairs where the exposures are different, cells **b** and **c**. We refer to these as the discordant pairs (exposed–unexposed, unexposed–exposed). Cells **b**

---

[5]*For the nerds*: The values for the two tails are actually both given in the binomial table. The probability for $r = 0$ when $n = 6$ is, as we have seen, $P = 0.0156$. The probability for $r = 6$ when $n = 6$ is given in the table as $P = 1.000$. But that is the cumulative probability for all values up to 6. The area under the tail for values up to but not including 6 is $P = 1.000 - 0.9844 =$ (lo and behold) 0.0156. We add the values for both tails together, and we get $P = 0.0312$, same as before.
[6]They chose to add iodized salt to bread, rather than making it available to the entire population through salt purchases.

BOX 9.4

BOX 9.4

Model for McNemar's test: status in individuals in a matched case-control study

1. Sample is random and independent
2. Results show status in *matched case-control pairs* depending on whether they are exposed or not exposed
3. Core values are arranged in a table with two rows and two columns
4. The values in tables are counts of *matched pairs*

and **c** give us information about the outcome of interest where there are differences in exposure between cases and controls. The concordant pairs (both exposed or both unexposed) do not give us any information about the likely impact of exposure on outcome. This same arrangement can be used for crossover trials (see Exercises at the end of the chapter).

If the Null Hypothesis were true, we would expect to see equal numbers of the two types of discordant pairs. As **b** + **c** = 14, we would expect to see seven of each type of discordant pair. As in the previous example, when **b** + **c** ≤20, the test statistic is T_2. We have also seen that T_2 can be taken as equal to the smaller of the two values **b** or **c** (because we are going to make this a two-tailed test, not predicting in which direction we might expect to see discordance). We refer to the binomial table (Appendix A1) for the probabilities. Look down the column headed $p = 0.500$ (the proportion in the population expected in each group of discordant pairs if the null hypothesis is true) and find the block where $n = 14$ (because **b** + **c** = 14). Find the probability for getting 3 or fewer exposed–unexposed discordant pairs out of 14: $P = 0.0287$. Multiply the probability times 2 for a two-tailed test, so we say that the two-tailed probability $P = 0.0574$.

Decision and interpretation

Rejection rule: If the value of *P* **in both tails** is *less than* 0.05, reject H_0.

As $P > 0.05$, we accept the null hypothesis, that is, there is no increased likelihood of having elevated TSI in hyperthyroidism as a result of eating iodine-fortified bread. The scheme for fortifying bread went ahead. Unfortunately, after the trial, there was some evidence of a rise in hyperthyroidism in at-risk individuals [2].

9.3 SPSS

SPSS offers two ways of accessing McNemar's test. The first uses what are called 'legacy dialogs'[7] (easier to set up but less comprehensive analyses). The second uses the main menus. It takes a little longer to set up but gives a better overall analysis. Let us look at both.

9.3.1 Legacy Dialogue

Enter the data for Example 1 such that each line (case) shows status Before in the first column and After in the second column. There are four possible entries for a case: 'Impossible', 'Impossible', and 'Difficult, Difficult' (for the concordant pairs), and 'Impossible', 'Difficult', and 'Difficult, Impossible' (for the discordant pairs). The start of the data file in SPSS is shown in Figure 9.1. Enter the data for all 43 pairs of observations (43 rows).

Click on Analyze>Nonparametric Tests>Legacy dialogs>Two Related Samples. Click Before_stats and then the curved arrow to enter it as the first variable in Pair 1, and After_stats to be entered as the second variable. In the Test Type rectangle, untick Wilcoxon, and tick McNemar. Click Options, and tick Descriptive. Click Continue, then Paste to copy the syntax to the syntax file, or OK to run the test.

The output is shown in Figure 9.2.

The table generated by Descriptive is the same as the core values in Table 9.1 (inside the box). The Test Statistics are based on McNemar's test, and $P = 0.007$ is based on the binomial distribution. SPSS can use the

---

[7] Or 'dialogues,' as we spell it in traditional English and American English.

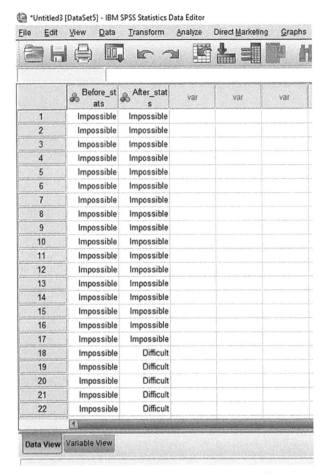

FIGURE 9.1   SPSS data layout for McNemar's test relating to impact of statistics course on students' views of statistics for use with 'Legacy Dialogs'. *Source*: Reproduced with permission of International Business Machines Corporation.

binomial distribution rather than chi-squared (which is what we did earlier) because it has a bigger table to refer to (Appendix A1 only goes up to $n = 20$).[8] This finding for $P = 0.007$ accords with what we found earlier using the chi-squared distribution and test statistic as an approximation for the binomial distribution: $0.001 < P < 0.01$.

---
[8]You may remember from Chapter 8 that we said for $N > 20$, the chi-squared distribution provides a good approximation of the binomial distribution. Yates' Correction for Continuity addresses the issue because when $N \leq 20$ the chi-squared distribution provides a less good approximation for the binomial distribution.

McNemar test

Crosstabs

Before_stats and After_stats

Before_stats	After_stats	
	Impossible	Difficult
Impossible	17	17
Difficult	4	5

Test statistics[a]

	Before_stats and After_stats
N	43
Exact sig. (2-tailed)	0.007[b]

[a]McNemar test.
[b]Binomial distribution used.

FIGURE 9.2   SPSS output for McNemar's test relating to impact of statistics course on students' views of statistics. *Source*: Reproduced with permission of International Business Machines Corporation.

9.3.2 New Commands

Let's use the same data ('views on statistics') arranged for analysis with the new commands. This analyzes the aggregated data rather than the case-by-case data, as shown in Figure 9.3.[9]

Before you run McNemar's test with the new commands you need to weight the data. This means that when you run McNemar's test, SPSS will see how many discordant pairs to use for the analysis. Click on: Data>Weight Cases, then click on 'Weight Cases by' and select Frequency for the weights. Click

---
[9]The image is from the 'Data View' screen in a .sav file. Data show the Value Labels for the variables. Variable Labels, and Value labels are easily added in the 'Variable view' screen in the data set. In the Data View screen, if you click on View in the command bar at the top of the screen, you can toggle back and forth between the numerical data entered and labels by clicking on the Value Labels tick box.

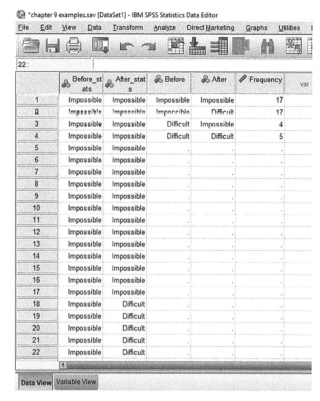

FIGURE 9.3 Aggregated data for use with SPSS new commands for McNemar's test relating to impact of statistics course on students' views. *Source*: Reproduced with permission of International Business Machines Corporation.

on OK or Paste (to copy to syntax file – you then need to run the procedure from the syntax file).

Now click on: Analyze>Nonparametric Tests> Related Samples, click on Fields, and select 'Before' and 'After' (the aggregated data). Click on Settings, Customize tests, and select 'McNemar's test (2 samples).' If you click on Test Options, you can change the level for rejecting the null hypothesis, which by default is set at 0.05 (5% level). Now click OK or Paste (to run from the syntax file). The output is shown in Figure 9.4.

This is like previous outputs in which SPSS provides not only an exact *P* value but also tells you whether to accept or reject the null hypothesis. (You may see a Warning about missing values for this data setup, but you can ignore it – it relates to

Hypothesis test summary

	Null hypothesis	Test	Sig.	Decision
1	The distributions of different values across Before and After are equally likely.	Related-samples McNemar test	0.007[a]	Reject the null hypothesis.

Asymptotic significances are displayed. The significance level is 0.05.
[a]Exact significance is displayed for this test.

FIGURE 9.4 SPSS output for McNemar's test relating to impact of statistics course on students' views using new commands. *Source*: Reproduced with permission of International Business Machines Corporation.

the missing values shown as full stops in the data.) Unsurprisingly, the results are exactly as before.

9.4 EXERCISES

9.4.1

Patients' walking ability was assessed in two categories before and after surgery. The results are shown in Table 9.4. Was there a significant change in walking ability as a result of surgery?

TABLE 9.4 Number of Patients Classified by Walking Status ('Moderate to no Restriction' or 'Unable to Walk or Severe Restriction') Before and After Surgery

		After Surgery	
Before surgery	Total Before	Moderate to No Restriction	Unable to Walk or Severe Restriction
Moderate to no restriction	18	17	1
Unable to walk or severe restriction	8	3	5

9.4.2

In a clinical trial of two drugs (A and B) for gastro-oesophageal reflux disease (GORD), patients were given each drug in a randomized crossover study and asked whether they were 'satisfied' or 'not satisfied' with the drug. 150 patients were 'satisfied' on both A and B, and 50 were 'not satisfied' on either. However, 30 were 'satisfied' on A but were 'not satisfied' on B, and 20 were 'satisfied' on B but not on A. Set up a 2×2 table which shows the concordant and discordant pairs appropriate for a McNemar analysis. Carry out the test and say whether there was a statistically significant difference in the level of satisfaction derived from A and B.

9.4.3

Prior to a public debate on salt and hypertension, 100 members of the public were asked their opinion on the hypothesis that salt is a causative factor in hypertension. Sixteen people favoured the hypothesis, and 84 were in some doubt. Following the debate, the same 100 people were again asked their opinion. Exactly one fourth of each group changed their minds.

Determine if there has been a statistically significant change in opinion following the debate.

REFERENCES

1. Iodine Global Network. http://www.ign.org/ Accessed 13.06.18
2. Adams DD, Kennedy TH, Stewart JC, Utiger RD, Vidor GI. Hyperthyroidism in Tasmania following iodide supplementation: measurements of thyroid-stimulating autoantibodies and thyrotropin. *J Clin Endocrinol Metab.* 1975 Aug;41(2):221–228.

CHAPTER 10

Association: Correlation and Regression

Learning Objectives

After studying this chapter, you should be able to:

- Understand what is meant by correlation and regression, and the difference between them
- Know when to use correlation and regression, and their purposes and limitations
- Carry out the calculations for correlation and regression manually
- Interpret SPSS output to determine the level of significance of your findings

10.1 INTRODUCTION

With the widespread use of statins to control serum cholesterol levels, previous concerns about dietary cholesterol consumption may no longer seem relevant [1]. Indeed, an acquaintance of mine was worried that his diet might be problematic. 'In what way?' I asked. 'Well', he said, 'I usually have two eggs for breakfast every morning. I am also very fond of shrimp and lobster'. He knew that there might be a problem with his cholesterol consumption, given the levels of cholesterol in eggs and shellfish. He was taking statins, he said. Was there still a cause for concern? Did he need to change his diet?

One way to address this would be to look at the association between dietary cholesterol intake and fasting levels of serum total cholesterol. I would need to have measurements of both variables at the same time point in a group of men of similar age and weight and statin dosage as my acquaintance. I could then draw a scattergram of serum total cholesterol versus dietary cholesterol intake for this group of men and see if there was an association.

Figure 10.1 shows six possible associations between paired variables (x,y). The measure of association between the two variables is the correlation coefficient, denoted by lower

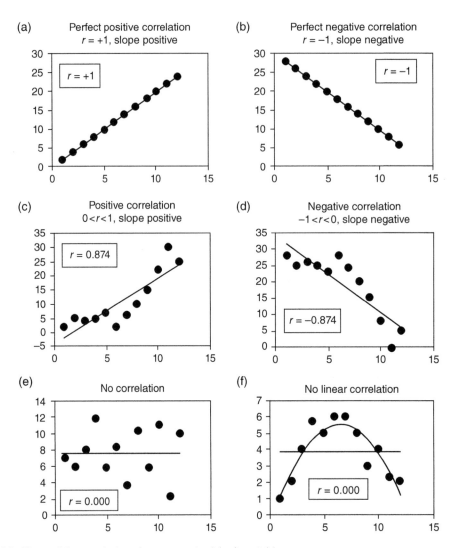

FIGURE 10.1   (a)–(f) Possible associations between paired (x,y) variables.

case 'r'.[1] Figure 10.1a shows a 'perfect' positive correlation. For every increment in variable x, there is an exact corresponding increment in variable y. If two subjects differ in their cholesterol consumption

---

[1]Yes, I know, I have used r before: when I was presenting the notion of 'n choose r' in the binomial coefficient; with a subscript (r_1) to denote the total number of observations in the first row of a contingency table; and now as the symbol for a correlation coefficient. You need to be alert to the fact that (i) there is a limited number of letters in the alphabet to denote all these different concepts; and (ii) the context in which the letter is being used will always alert you to its meaning.

by a known amount, I could tell you by exactly how much their serum total cholesterol values would differ. All of the pairs of values (x,y) fall on a straight line with a positive slope. The correlation coefficient $r = 1.0$. In Figure 10.1b, there is also a perfect correlation, but this time it is negative; $r = -1.0$. For a given increase in x, there is an exact corresponding *decrease* in y. The results fall on a straight line, as before, but this time the slope of the line is negative.

The maximum and minimum values for r are $+1.0$ and -1.0, respectively. Anything outside this range, you have made a mistake in your calculations.

In Figure 10.1c, the points do not fall on the line, but values for y typically increase as values for x increase (but not always). The correlation coefficient r will be greater than zero but less than 1.0. The closer the points are to the line, the closer to 1.0 the value for r will be. For the scatter of points in Figure 10.1c, where the points are near the line, $r = 0.874$. If, on average, y decreased as x increased (Figure 10.1d), the correlation coefficient would be negative, but this time $0 > r > -1.0$ (in this case, $r = -0.874$).

Figures 10.1e and 10.1f show situations in which there is no association between x and y, and $r = 0.0$. In Figure 10.1e, there is a cloud of points around the line, and no obvious relationship between x and y. In Figure 10.1f, there is a relationship, but it is not linear. The correlation coefficient that we are considering at the moment measures the *linear* association between two sets of observations.

Regression, on the other hand, tells us by *how much*, on average, y changes as x changes. Again (for the moment) we assume that the relationship between the two variables is linear. The concepts of correlation and regression are closely interlinked both conceptually and mathematically, as we shall see in this chapter.

Just before we get on to the subject matter at hand, please remember: **Association does not imply causation**. Keep muttering this to yourself as you read the chapter and later, when you are conducting statistical analyses of correlation and regression.

Let's start by looking at the correlation coefficient.

10.2 THE CORRELATION COEFFICIENT

Correlation measures the strength of association between paired variables (x,y). It also tells us whether the association is positive or negative.

We have already considered one example: whether serum total cholesterol is associated with dietary cholesterol intake. Here are other examples:

1. *Height and weight.* The taller you are, the heavier you are likely to be. The association is positive.

2. *Class attendance and exam results.* The more classes you miss, the poorer your exam results are likely to be. The association is negative.

3. *Body Mass Index and percentage body fat.* The higher your BMI, the higher your percentage body fat is likely to be.

4. *Eye colour and intelligence.* There is no convincing evidence that eye colour and intelligence are associated.

Of course, there will be many factors that have an impact on these associations. This explains why most correlations are not 'perfect' but have an element of variability so that not all pairs of observations fall on a straight line. In the serum total cholesterol example, dietary factors other than cholesterol intake, medication with statins, and genetic characteristics will have an impact. People of the same height will differ in weight because of the amount of food they eat and how much exercise they take. A student who misses lots of classes might spend the time learning the lecture material by reading textbooks instead, and so do well in their exams. Some individuals can have a high BMI but a low percentage body fat and a high percentage lean tissue because they take a lot of exercise or are into body-building. Eye colour and intelligence do not appear to be associated.[2]

Let's look in detail at the concept and interpretation of correlation, and the parameters that define it. There are two types of correlation coefficients that we are going to consider in detail: the Pearson product-moment correlation coefficient, and the Spearman rank correlation coefficient.

10.2.1 The Pearson Product-Moment Correlation Coefficient

For each element in our sample, we need to have paired observations for two variables: x and y. By convention, observations for the first element in the sample would be denoted as (x_1, y_1), the next element (x_2, y_2), and so on up to (x_n, y_n), where there are n

---

[2] Lots of people have looked, but no one has yet come up with any convincing evidence.

pairs of observations in the sample. Variables should be interval or ratio and follow a normal distribution. The calculations will work for both discrete and continuous variables, provided the discrete variables follow a normal distribution. If one or both variables does not follow a normal distribution, you can try using transformations (see Chapter 4).[3] The association between the variables should be linear. Again, by convention, the y variable is designated as the dependent or response variable, and the x variable as the independent or explanatory variable. This does not imply causality, of course – we are looking simply at whether the two variables are associated.

Fundamental principle

Expectation:	H_0: There is no association between x and y
Decision criterion:	If the probability of observing the measured association (the Pearson correlation coefficient r) is less than 5%, reject H_0.

Assumptions

The assumptions underpinning the Pearson product-moment correlation coefficient r are shown in Box 10.1.

Here is an example. Death rates from cirrhosis and alcoholism per 100 000 population/year and levels of alcohol consumption (litres per year per person aged 14+) were tabulated for 15 high income countries (Table 10.1). A scattergram of the data is shown in Figure 10.2. It looks on the face of it that as alcohol consumption per head increases, the risk of dying of cirrhosis or alcoholism also increases. France seems well ahead of the crowd. Let's find the Pearson product-moment correlation, r, to see how strong the association is mathematically.

---

[3] We will discover that there is a lot of rule breaking when correlation coefficients are calculated: it is possible to carry out the calculations even when the data do not conform to this underlying model. This is often done to give a sense of how variables are associated, but caution in interpretation is then needed. I will say more later.

BOX 10.1

Assumptions underpinning the Pearson product-moment correlation coefficient r

1. Observations for two variables have been collected in pairs (x,y) for every element of the sample
2. The variables are continuous or discrete, interval or ratio
3. The variables are normally distributed
4. The association between the variables is linear

TABLE 10.1 Death Rate from Cirrhosis and Alcoholism (per 100 000 Population) versus Alcohol Consumption (Litres per Year per Person Aged 14+) in 15 High-Income Countries

Country	(x) Alcohol Consumption (litres/annum/person age 14+)	(y) Death Rate (/100 000 population)
France	24.7	46.1
Italy	15.2	23.6
W. Germany	12.3	23.6
Australia	10.9	7.0
Belgium	10.9	12.3
USA	9.9	14.2
Canada	8.3	7.4
England and Wales	7.2	3.0
Sweden	6.6	7.2
Japan	5.8	10.6
Holland	5.8	3.7
Ireland	5.6	3.4
Norway	4.2	4.3
Finland	3.9	3.6
Israel	3.1	5.4

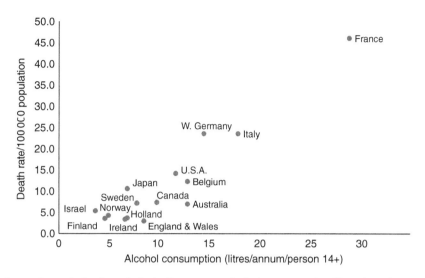

FIGURE 10.2 Death rate from cirrhosis and alcoholism versus alcohol consumption (litres/year/person aged 14+) in 15 high-income countries.

Model

The model for the Pearson product-moment correlation coefficient r is shown in Box 10.2.

Test procedure

The calculation and test procedure for the Pearson product-moment correlation coefficient r are shown in Box 10.3.

1. *Find the sum of x, the sum of x^2, the sum of y, and sum of y^2, that is* (to use our shorthand from Chapter 2): Σx, Σx^2, Σy, and Σy^2

2. *Multiply the values of each x,y pair together and find the sum of the products.* The shorthand for this is Σxy, the sum of the products of each *x,y* pair. This is the key piece of information that allows us to see how x and y are related.

3. *Calculate the sum of squares in x, the sum of squares in y, and the sum of squares in xy,* as follows:

$$S_{xx} = \Sigma x^2 - \frac{\left(\Sigma x\right)^2}{n}$$

BOX 10.2

The model for the Pearson product-moment correlation coefficient r

1. Observations for two variables (death rates from cirrhosis and alcoholism [y] and average alcohol consumption [x]) have been collected in pairs (x,y) for 15 countries
2. The variables are continuous and ratio
3. The variables are normally distributed
4. The association between the variables is linear

$$S_{yy} = \Sigma y^2 - \frac{\left(\Sigma y\right)^2}{n}$$

$$S_{xy} = \Sigma xy - \frac{\Sigma x \Sigma y}{n}$$

EQUATION 10.1 Equations for the sum of squares in x, y, and xy

I have used upper case S to denote the sum of squares. The value for n is the number of *pairs* of observations in the sample.

BOX 10.3

Calculation and test procedure for the Pearson product-moment correlation coefficient r

1. Find the sum of x, the sum of x^2, the sum of y, and sum of y^2
2. Multiply the values of each x,y pair together and find the sum of the products
3. Calculate the sum of squares in x, the sum of squares in y, and the sum of squares in xy
4. Find the value for the Pearson correlation coefficient r
5. Calculate the test statistic t and compare with the tabulated value in Appendix A3 for given values of ν and P

The first two formulae should look familiar as the numerators in the Standard Deviation calculations.[4] Look closely at the third formula, the one for S_{xy}. This is called 'the sum of squares in xy'. You will see it is to similar the previous two. The difference is that instead of multiplying x by itself or y by itself and finding the sum (that is $\sum x^2$ and $\sum y^2$), we multiply x times y and find the sum of those products $\sum xy$. Similarly, in the second term in the third equation, instead of multiplying $\sum x$ by $\sum x$ to yield $(\sum x)^2$ ('sum of x **all** squared') and $\sum y$ by $\sum y$ to yield $(\sum y)^2$ ('sum of y **all** squared'), we multiply $\sum x$ by $\sum y$ to yield $\sum x \sum y$.

If you recall, the Sum of Squares in x and the Sum of Squares in y tell you about the amount of variation of the values for x and y around their respective means. By analogy, the third formula above tells you about the way in which x and y vary around each other's means.

4. Find the value for the Pearson correlation coefficient r using the following formula:

---

[4] You might want to refer back to Chapter 2 to refresh your memory about the sum of squares.

$$r = \frac{S_{xy}}{\sqrt{S_{xx}S_{yy}}}$$

EQUATION 10.2   Formula for the Pearson product-moment correlation coefficient r

Once we have the values for the sums of squares, we simply plug them into the equation. For the sake of clarity, I have extended Table 10.1 to demonstrate how the values are determined (Table 10.2).

Let's plug the values into the equations for the sums of squares:

$$S_{xx} = \sum x^2 - \frac{(\sum x)^2}{n} = 1633.44 - \frac{18063.36}{15} = 429.216$$

$$S_{yy} = \sum y^2 - \frac{(\sum y)^2}{n} = 3954.88 - \frac{30765.16}{15} = 1903.869$$

$$S_{xy} = \sum xy - \frac{\sum x \sum y}{n} = 2419.98 - \frac{134.40 \times 175.40}{15}$$
$$= 848.396$$

Plug these values into our equation for r, and we get:

$$r = \frac{S_{xy}}{\sqrt{S_{xx}S_{yy}}} = \frac{848.396}{\sqrt{429.216 \times 1903.869}} = 0.9385$$

This looks like a 'strong' correlation. It is not 'perfect' ($r < 1.0$), but it suggests that if you live in a country in which the average *per capita* alcohol consumption is high, you are more likely to die of cirrhosis or alcoholism. This may not come as a big surprise, but it is always comforting to have evidence to support one's prejudices.

Now, just as you were beginning to feel cocky and confident, I have to ask an awkward question. Could this apparent association have arisen by chance? Might it be that there really is no association between alcohol consumption and risk of cirrhosis and alcoholism, that the null hypothesis is true, and

TABLE 10.2 Death Rate from Cirrhosis and Alcoholism (per 100 000 Population) versus Alcohol Consumption (Litres per Year per Person Aged 14+) in 15 High-Income Countries, Showing Sums and Sums of Squares Needed to Calculate the Pearson Product-Moment Correlation Coefficient r

	x	y	x²	y²	xy
	Alcohol Consumption (litres/annum/person age 14+)	Death Rate (/100 000 population)			
Country					
France	24.7	46.1	610.09	2 125.21	1 138.67
Italy	15.2	23.6	231.04	556.96	358.72
W. Germany	12.3	23.6	151.29	556.96	290.28
Australia	10.9	7.0	118.81	49.00	76.30
Belgium	10.9	12.3	118.81	151.29	134.07
USA	9.9	14.2	98.01	201.64	140.58
Canada	8.3	7.4	68.89	54.76	61.42
England and Wales	7.2	3.0	51.84	9.00	21.60
Sweden	6.6	7.2	43.56	51.84	47.52
Japan	5.8	10.6	33.64	112.36	61.48
Holland	5.8	3.7	33.64	13.69	21.46
Ireland	5.6	3.4	31.36	11.56	19.04
Norway	4.2	4.3	17.64	18.49	18.06
Finland	3.9	3.6	15.21	12.96	14.04
Israel	3.1	5.4	9.61	29.16	16.74
	$\sum x = 134.40$	$\sum y = 175.40$	$\sum x^2 = 1\,633.44$	$\sum y^2 = 3\,954.88$	$\sum xy = 2\,419.98$
	$(\sum x)^2 = 18\,063.36$	$(\sum y)^2 = 30\,765.16$			

that what we have observed is due to random sampling variation? And now, what do I hear? It is the t statistic thundering to the rescue!

Decision and interpretation

Ah, t! Using the values for r and n, we can estimate a value for t and look up that value in Appendix A3 (with given degrees of freedom). The t statistic will tell us the probability of observing what we have observed if the null hypothesis is true. Very simple and straightforward.

$$t = r\sqrt{\frac{n-2}{1-r^2}}$$

EQUATION 10.3 Formula for t relating to the Pearson product-moment correlation coefficient

We need to know r, of course. We also need a value for ν, degrees of freedom. You might think that ν would be equal to $n-1$, as it was for the t test. But we need to apply the same principal that told us that degrees of freedom for the t-test had to allow for the freedom to choose values for our variables to reach $\sum x$ and $\sum x^2$, and in the chi-squared test had to allow for the sums in the rows (r_i) and the sums in the columns (c_j). We need to allow one degree of freedom for *each* of our two variables (that is, allow one degree of freedom for $\sum x$ and one for $\sum y$). For the purposes of determining t in relation to the correlation coefficient, ν will be equal to $n - 2$. This explains the numerator in the formula for t.

The denominator also has a logical explanation. As the value for r gets bigger, the denominator will get smaller, the value for t will get larger, corresponding values for P will be smaller, and there will be an increased probability that we can reject the null hypothesis. Bigger correlation coefficients are therefore more likely to be statistically significant than small correlation coefficients. If we had a perfect correlation, for which $r = 1.0$, the denominator would be $1 - 1^2 = 0$. The calculated value for t would be equal to infinity, however many observations (degrees of freedom) we had. If t were infinity, the probability of this observation occurring is essentially zero if the null hypothesis were true, so we would reject the null hypothesis. This is all nicely consistent.

If we think further, however, we realize two things. First, we must have at least three pairs of observations to make sense of a correlation coefficient. We cannot base a correlation on two observations. Two points would (of course) be connected by a straight line, there would be $n - 2 = 0$ degrees of freedom (so we could not look up the value in the t table), the correlation would be 1, and t would be equal to 0/0, which is meaningless.[5] Second, having very few observations increases the risk of incorrectly rejecting a true null hypothesis. Is there a minimum 'safe' number of observations when calculating a correlation coefficient? The answer turns out to be more complicated than just a 'rule of thumb' guide. We will come back to this question when we look at Power in Chapter 12.

We can think logically about the whole expression for t.

- As the number of observations increases, the value for the numerator, $n - 2$, will get bigger, and the value for t will get larger. So large samples are more likely to give us a higher value for t, and we will be more likely to be able to reject the null hypothesis (if that is the right thing to do).
- The larger the value for r (i.e. the stronger the correlation), the smaller the value for the denominator ($1 - r^2$), and the larger the value for t. For a given number of observations, bigger correlation coefficients are more likely to yield values for t for which $P < 0.05$.

I hope these thoughts are comforting and help to clarify our understanding of the way in which our ability to test for the significance of a correlation coefficient accords with common sense.

Let us get back to our example, calculate t, and look up the value in Appendix A3.

$$t = r\sqrt{\frac{n-2}{1-r^2}} = 0.9385\sqrt{\frac{15-2}{1-0.9385^2}}$$

$$= 0.9385\sqrt{\frac{13}{1-0.8808}} = 0.9385\sqrt{\frac{13}{0.1192}} = 9.802$$

If we look in Appendix A3 for $\nu = n - 2 = 15 - 2 = 13$ when $P = 0.05$, the value for $t = 2.160$. Our calculated value for $t = 9.802$ is greater than the tabulated value, so we can reject the null hypothesis at the 5% level.

Conclusion

We can conclude that there is a statistically significant association between national alcohol consumption levels and death rates from cirrhosis and alcoholism. We can go further and find the level of confidence at which to reject the null hypothesis. When $\nu = 13$ and $P = 0.001$, $t = 4.221$. Our calculated value for $t = 9.802$ is greater than the tabulated value,

---

[5]Unless you are Eugenia Cheng, in which case it can mean lots of things – see her books on infinity, which are good fun, well-written, and intriguing [3].

so we can reject the null hypothesis at the 0.1% level. There is less than one in a thousand chance that we are making a mistake (a Type I error) by rejecting the null hypothesis that there is no association between national alcohol consumption levels and death rates from cirrhosis and alcoholism.

There is another very important concept in the values that we have been looking at: r^2, the square of the correlation coefficient. r^2 tells us how much of the variation[6] in y is explained by the variation in x. If the correlation was perfect ($r = 1$), r^2 would be equal to 1.0. We would say that all of the variation in y is explained by the variation in x. In our present example, $r^2 = 0.8808$. If we express $r^2 = 0.8808$ as a percentage, we can say that 88.08% of the variation in y (deaths from cirrhosis and alcoholism in these 15 countries) is explained by the variation in x (the variation in alcohol consumption). That's a lot. Only 12% of the variation in deaths between countries is explained by other factors. From a public health perspective, if we wanted to tackle the problem of deaths from cirrhosis and alcoholism, it would be difficult to find a more effective intervention than to try and get people to drink less. Of course, this does not take into account variations in consumption *within* populations – some people will drink much more heavily than others and are likely to be at greater risk. This highlights one of the weaknesses of correlation when using population level data.[7]

What other issues do we need to consider? First, there is one data point (France) that appears to lie a long way from the others. To what extent is this one point influencing the apparent strength of the correlation? If we ignored France and looked at the remaining countries, the correlation would clearly not be as strong. We know, however, (don't we) that

it is wrong to omit data that look a bit odd (the outliers) unless we have an *a priori* reason for doing so. In which case, why did we include them in the sample? We need to accept that the strength of the correlation, determined in part by France's position in relation to the other 14 countries, is a good reflection of the relationship being investigated across all 15 countries. Even within the 14 countries not including France, there is clearly an increase in risk of death from cirrhosis and alcoholism as average alcohol consumption increases.

Second, we can say (as we did for the *t*-test) that the Pearson product-moment correlation coefficient is 'robust'. This means that it provides a good estimate of the strength of the correlation between two sets of observations even if the distributions differ somewhat from normal. There is no formal measurement to say when the Pearson correlation coefficient is no longer a good estimate of the strength of association.[8] As you become more familiar with statistical testing, you will get a sense of when a finding is robust and when it is not, over and above what the P value tells you.

Finally, there is a vocabulary in the scientific literature used to describe the strength of a correlation coefficient. Terms include words like 'strong', 'good', 'moderate', and 'weak'. My (wholly unofficial) interpretation is shown in Table 10.3.

Here is another one from the internet [2]:

- 0.00–0.19 'very weak'
- 0.20–0.39 'weak'
- 0.40–0.59 'moderate'
- 0.60–0.79 'strong'
- 0.80–1.0 'very strong'

Take your pick. Anything less than 0.1 is, in my book, less than 'weak': it is so close to zero as to be unimportant. Think about r^2. If $r = 0.1$, $r^2 = 0.01$, which means only 1% of the variation in y is

---

[6]Strictly speaking, in statistical terms, we are talking about the variance (remember s^2?) rather than 'variation'. For the sake of clarity, authors talk about this concept using the word 'variation', but the concept here is the same. Should authors be purists? Answers on a postcard, please...

[7]It also raises questions about the most effective public health interventions. Target the high-risk group, or have a campaign to change drinking culture generally? Or both? But that is a discussion for public health nutrition.

[8]We looked at the Kolmogorov–Smirnov one-sample test in Chapter 6 and will use it again in Chapter 11 to decide if a set of sample observations is likely to have been derived from a population which is normal in character.

TABLE 10.3 Unofficial Vocabulary for Describing the Strength of a Correlation Coefficient

Description of Strength of Correlation	Likely Range
Strong	1.0–0.8
Good	<0.8–0.6
Moderate (or modest)	<0.6–0.3
Weak	<0.3–0.1

explained by the variation in x, and 99% of the variation in y is explained by other factors.

Another confusion arises when authors talk about a 'significant' correlation. A weak correlation, for example $r = 0.2$, may also be highly statistically significant at the 0.1% level if there are enough observations in the sample (calculate t using Equation 10.3 when $r = 0.2$ and $n = 300$ and find the value for P in Appendix A3). Some authors will, wrongly in my view, describe this as a 'highly significant' correlation. What they mean, of course, is that it is a 'weak but highly statistically significant' correlation. The calculated correlation probably reflects the truth (the probability of making a Type I error being only 0.1%, or 1 in 1000). But if $r = 0.2$, $r^2 = 0.04$, which means that only 4% of the variation in y is explained by the variation in x; 96% of the variation in y is explained by other factors. What they do *not* mean, but which the word 'significant' may imply, is that the correlation is 'important'.[9] It is *not* important in terms of any hypothesis which sets out to explain the way in which measurements on the y axis vary from one observation to the next in terms of the explanatory variable on the x axis.

10.2.2 The Spearman Rank Correlation Coefficient

If we are concerned about the influence of France as an outlier, there is an alternate statistical strategy that would still give us a measure of correlation. It does not rely on the absolute measures but on the rank positions of the pairs of observations. It allows us to find a correlation coefficient that does not depend on variables having a normal distribution.

The Spearman rank correlation coefficient is denoted by the symbol 'ρ', (lower-case Greek letter 'rho') or by r_S. It makes no assumption about the underlying distribution of the variables. It is the nonparametric version of the correlation coefficient. It can also be used to overcome the problem highlighted above about France being an outlier. It is perfectly legitimate to transform ratio or interval data into ordinal data to overcome concerns about the data not fitting the statistical model on which the test is based. (Of course, by carrying out such a transformation, we are throwing away some useful information.) In fact, the Spearman rank correlation coefficient does not make assumptions about linearity. Because it uses ranks, it can provide a useful measure of association for any *monotonic* relationship. A monotonic relationship is one in which values for y typically either increase or decrease over the whole of the range of x, whether in a linear fashion (Figure 10.3a) or nonlinear fashion (Figure 10.3b). The Spearman rank correlation coefficient cannot, however, cope with relationships which are non-monotonic, in which (for example) y increases over part of the range for x and then decreases over another part of the range (Figure 10.3c).[10]

Fundamental principle

Expectation:	H_0: There is no association at country level between death rates from cirrhosis and alcoholism and average alcohol consumption
Decision criterion:	If the probability of observing the measured association (the Spearman rank correlation coefficient ρ) is less than 5%, reject H_0.

---

[9]The first word listed in the Thesaurus when you look up 'significant' in Word using 'shift-F7'.

[10]For those, you might have to consider higher-order equations (above quadratic), but that is beyond the scope of this textbook.

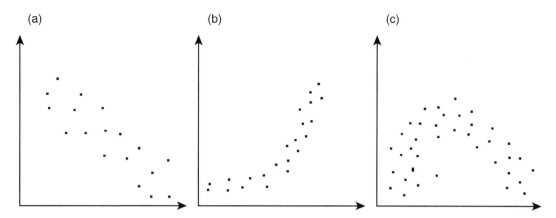

(a)   (b)   (c)

FIGURE 10.3   Examples of monotonic and nonmonotonic relationships. (a) Linear; (b) nonlinear; (c) nonmonotic.
Source: Adapted from https://statistics.laerd.com/statistical-guides/spearmans-rank-order-correlation-statistical-guide.php (accessed 22 June 2018)

Assumptions

The assumptions underpinning the Spearman correlation coefficient ρ or r_s are shown in Box 10.4

Model

The model for the Spearman correlation coefficient ρ or r_s is shown in Box 10.5.

The data fit the model.

Table 10.4 shows, in the first two columns, the data on deaths from cirrhosis and alcoholism versus alcohol consumption from 15 countries. This time, however, we will not use the original observations, but instead consider their ranks in relation to one another. The observations in the table are ordered according to the average alcohol consumption in each country. The country with the highest consumption is assigned a rank of 1, that with the lowest consumption a rank of 15. We deal with ties as we have previously for nonparametric statistical tests, assigning to the tied values the average of the ranks that would have been assigned if the values had not been tied. The next column shows the corresponding rank of death rate (y). The death rates are also ranked from 1 to 15 from the highest value to the lowest. Ties are dealt with in the same way as for x.

> **BOX 10.4**
>
> Assumptions underpinning the Spearman correlation coefficient ρ or r_s
>
> 1. Observations for two variables have been collected in pairs (x,y) for every element of the sample
> 2. The variables may be continuous or discrete, ordinal, interval or ratio, but the observations for the test must be expressed in terms of ranks
> 3. The variables may have a parametric or nonparametric distribution
> 4. The relationship must be monotonic

> **BOX 10.5**
>
> The model for the Spearman correlation coefficient ρ or r_s
>
> 1. Observations for two variables (death rates from cirrhosis and alcoholism (y) and average alcohol consumption (x)) have been collected in pairs (x,y) for 15 countries
> 2. The variables are continuous and ratio
> 3. The observations for the variables are expressed in ranks
> 4. The association between the variables is monotonic

TABLE 10.4   Death Rate from Cirrhosis and Alcoholism (per 100 000 Population) versus Alcohol Consumption (Litres per Year per Person Aged 14+) in 15 High-Income Countries, Showing the Rankings, the Difference in Rank Within Pairs (d), and the Square of the Differences Needed to Compute the Spearman Rank Correlation Coefficient ρ, or r_s

	x	y	Rank of x	Rank of y	d	d²
	Alcohol Consumption (litres/annum/person age 14+)	Death Rate (/100 000 population)				
Country						
France	24.7	46.1	1	1	0	0
Italy	15.2	23.6	2	2.5	−0.5	0.25
W. Germany	12.3	23.6	3	2.5	0.5	0.25
Australia	10.9	7.0	4.5	9	−4.5	20.25
Belgium	10.9	12.3	4.5	5	−0.5	0.25
USA	9.9	14.2	6	4	2	4
Canada	8.3	7.4	7	7	0	0
England and Wales	7.2	3.0	8	15	−7	49
Sweden	6.6	7.2	9	8	1	1
Japan	5.8	10.6	10.5	6	4.5	20.25
Holland	5.8	3.7	10.5	12	−1.5	2.25
Ireland	5.6	3.4	12	14	−2	4
Norway	4.2	4.3	13	11	2	4
Finland	3.9	3.6	14	13	1	1
Israel	3.1	5.4	15	10	5	25
						$\sum d^2 = 131.5$

Test procedure

The test procedure for the Spearman correlation coefficient ρ or r_s is shown in Box 10.6.

We notice a couple of things. First, the maths is much easier for finding the Spearman rank correlation coefficient than the Pearson product-moment correlation coefficient. This is partly because we have reduced the amount of information that we are using about each pair of observations to find the correlation. Rather than interval or ratio, we have limited ourselves to ordinal data.

Second, if we think through the formula for ρ (as we did for the Pearson correlation coefficient, r), we can work out which elements of the formula would have an impact on the size of the calculated value for ρ. If the ranks for both sets of observations were the same, there would be a perfect, positive correlation, the difference d would be zero for every pair of observations, the denominator $6\sum d^2$ would also be zero, and $1 - 0 = 1.0$. So, the largest value the correlation coefficient could take would be 1.0. We could also show that if the ranks were perfectly paired in opposite directions, the value for the

BOX 10.6

Test procedure for the Spearman correlation coefficient ρ or r_s

1. Rank the values for each variable separately
2. Find the difference (d) between the ranks for each x,y pair
3. Square the difference (d^2) to get rid of the sign
4. Find the sum of the squares of the differences $\sum d^2 = 131.5$
5. Find ρ using the formula:

$$\rho = 1 - \frac{6\sum d^2}{n^3 - n} = 1 - \frac{6 \times 131.5}{15^3 - 15} = 0.765$$

second term in the formula for ρ would be 2, and $\rho = -1$. The limits of the Spearman rank correlation coefficient, therefore, are the same as the Pearson product-moment correlation coefficient: +1 and −1. If there is no association between the two sets of observations, we would discover that the second term in the formula would be equal to 1.0, and ρ would equal 0, again mimicking the Pearson correlation coefficient. Finally, it is worth noting that the more pairs of observations in the sample, n, the larger the denominator will be. But don't be tempted to think this might have an impact on the size of the correlation coefficient. The sum of d^2 ($\sum d^2$) is partly dependent on the number of pairs of observations in the sample. $\sum d^2$ has the capacity to increase as n increases. There is no suggestion that a larger sample size will automatically generate a larger correlation coefficient.

Finally, it is worth noting that the value for the Spearman correlation coefficient, calculated as we have done, is the same as the Pearson correlation coefficient based on the ranks. We have found the value for ρ more efficiently using the method set out above.

Decision and interpretation

We are now faced with the same question as before. We have a rank correlation coefficient, $\rho = 0.765$. Although less than the Pearson correlation coefficient (I will say more about that shortly), it is not far from 1.0. This suggests (as common sense would tell us looking at the scattergram) that there is an association between alcohol consumption and death from cirrhosis and alcoholism. But as before, we must ask ourselves if the result is statistically significant (i.e. unlikely to have arisen just by chance due to random sampling variation).

For values of $n \leq 50$, the t distribution does not provide an accurate estimate of the probability of observing what we observed for ρ assuming the null hypothesis is true. We therefore refer to a table of probabilities (Appendix A8) that relate probabilities to statistically significant values for ρ. The layout shows the values for n down the left-hand side, and values for P across the top. The values in the body of the table are values for ρ. Findings are statistically significant if the calculated value for ρ is equal to or above the value given in the table.

In the present example, $n = 15$ and $\rho = 0.765$. In Appendix A8, we use n rather than $n - 2$. Find the row where $n = 15$. Which column do we look in? We will follow previous examples in the book, and assume that the null hypothesis is true, and that $\rho = 0$. The question then is, how far away from zero does our value for ρ need to be before we think it unlikely to have arisen just by chance due to random sampling variation? We do not make an assumption about the direction in which ρ differs from zero – it could be greater than zero, or less than zero. This matches the criterion for a two-tailed test. Statistically (as we shall see shortly), this is the more conservative test, i.e. we are less likely to make a Type I error.

> **Rejection rule:** If the calculated value is *equal to or greater than* the tabulated value at *P (two-tailed)* = 0.05, reject the null hypothesis at the 5% level.

Find the column in the row 'P, two-tailed' that is headed 0.05. The intersection of this column with the row headed $n = 15$ gives us the minimum value for ρ that is statistically significant at the 5% level. In this example, *if the calculated value is* **equal to or greater than** *the tabulated value*, 0.521, we can reject the null hypothesis at the 5% level. Our calculated value for $\rho = 0.765$, so we can reject the null hypothesis at the 5% level. We can look further along the row to find the level of significance at which the null hypothesis can be rejected. At $P = 0.01$, $\rho = 0.604$. At $P = 0.002$, $\rho = 0.750$. So, we can reject the null hypothesis at the 0.2% level. When $P = 0.001$, $\rho = 0.779$. This is greater than the calculated value, so we are not able to reject the null hypothesis at the 0.1% level.[11]

For the sake of comparison, let's look at the value for ρ using the values for P in the row headed 'P, one-tailed'. This is the row we would use if we thought that there was only one direction in which the findings could be associated if the null hypothesis were not true. We find that the value for ρ for the one-tailed test at $P = 0.001$ is the same as the value for ρ for the two-tailed test when $P = 0.002$, $\rho = 0.750$. If we had used the one-tailed test, we would have rejected the null hypothesis at the 0.1% level, whereas using the two-tailed test, we were able to reject the null hypothesis only at the 0.2% level. The result would appear to be more highly statistically significant using the one-tailed test compared with the two-tailed test. Some students will say to themselves, 'Oh, my result appears to be more statistically significant if I use the one-tailed test, so I'll use that one!' That, of course, is not the way to think. It is best practice to be statistically conservative, err on the side of caution, and use the highest (not the lowest) value for P when reporting the significance of statistical tests. That way you will be lest likely to make a Type I error.[12]

[11]Remember, of course, that this does not mean we accept the null hypothesis at the 0.1% level. Once we have rejected the null hypothesis at the 5% level, it is gone, finished, kaput.
[12]I will repeat the phrase 'Less likely to make a Type I error' until it is a mantra in your head. It will guide the appropriate choice of statistical tests and stop you from going 'fishing' for the most statistically significant result to report, **which is the wrong thing to do**, however tempting.

You will also have noted that ρ is less than r. Statistically speaking, ρ is more conservative than r, as ordinal data inherently contain less information than interval or ratio data. By using the ordinal rather than the interval or ratio data, you are less likely to make a Type I error and incorrectly reject the null hypothesis. If you have doubts (for example, about outliers), then it is safer to take the more conservative approach. Of course, you should always use the test that best fits the data. We will explore this in more detail in Chapter 13.

Appendix A8 provides values for ρ up to $n = 50$. For values of $n > 50$, you can use the following formula for u, the standard normal deviate, and refer to the values in the normal distribution in Appendix A2 to find values for $\frac{1}{2}P$. For example, if $\rho = 0.280$ for a sample in which there were 60 pairs of observations ($n = 60$), would you be able to reject the null hypothesis? Use the formula:

$$u = \rho\sqrt{n-1}$$

EQUATION 10.4 Formula for u (the standard normal deviate) for estimating $\frac{1}{2}P$ to test the statistical significance of the Spearman correlation coefficient when $n > 50$

In the present example, $u = \rho\sqrt{n-1} = 0.280\sqrt{60-1} = 0.280\sqrt{59} = 0.280 \times 7.681 = 2.151$. When you look up 2.151 in Appendix A2, you see that the value for $\frac{1}{2}P$ lies one tenth of the way between the value for $\frac{1}{2}P$ when $u = 2.15$ (0.015 78) and the value for $\frac{1}{2}P$ when $u = 2.16$ (0.015 39). By interpolating within the table, we can say that the value for $\frac{1}{2}P$ when $u = 2.151$ is: $\frac{1}{2}P = 0.015\ 78 - (0.015\ 78 - 0.015 39) \times 0.1 = 0.015\ 741$. We then need to double this (because we want the test to be two-tailed), so $P = 2 \times \frac{1}{2}P = 0.0315$. As $P < 0.05$, we can reject the null hypothesis at the 5% level.

10.2.3 Kendall's Tau

Kendall's tau (τ) is another commonly used correlation coefficient. Its computation is based on concordant and discordant pairs, which in turn is based on the relative ranks of observations. Like Pearson and Spearman correlation coefficients, its value ranges from −1.0 to +1.0, with zero implying no association between the variables. It has some merits over the Spearman correlation coefficient, in that it may be less sensitive to the impact of extreme values. It is also better for looking at associations between observations that are in categories (a seven-point Likert scale on food preferences, for example) versus an outcome in categories (weight status rated in four categories). Kendall's tau-b makes adjustment for ties. For the purposes of this book, it is much more complicated to compute, so I will not go into detail here. Your friend and mine, SPSS, will compute both without fuss, but a word with your friendly statistician will help you to decide which correlation coefficient is best suited to your data.

We will now move from correlation to regression, its close cousin.

10.3 REGRESSION

When I was nine years old, I learned how to draw a straight line through a set of points in a scattergram, working out on average how much y changed for a given change in x. It was all estimates and fillings-in on graph paper, but I was very proud of myself. My teacher gave me a big green tick and a 'Well done!' at the top of my homework. Imagine my delight (go on, imagine it!) as a precocious 13-year-old when I discovered that the line could be drawn with mathematical precision. Not only could I discover the slope of the line that best fit the data, I could also pinpoint the intercept.[13] Heaven! I had been introduced to *linear regression*.

Regression measures the direction of association between two variables. *Simple linear regression* assumes that the association is linear (i.e. a straight line)[14] and that we are dealing with only two

variables, x and y.[15] It is also referred to as *least squares regression*, or the 'line of best fit'. (I will come back to these concepts shortly.) The calculations enable you to find the equation for a straight line, $Y = a + bx$, where Y is the *predicted* value of y at a given value of x (based on the regression line equation), a is the intercept (the point at which the line crosses the y-axis), and b is the slope (or gradient) that tells you, for a given unit change in x, the corresponding average change in y. Most values for Y will be different from the observed values of y for a given value of x, although if there is a pair of observations (x_i, y_i) that falls on the regression line, then Y_i *will* be equal to y_i.

Let's continue using our cirrhosis/alcohol example.

Fundamental principle

Expectation:	H_0: There is no change in death rates from cirrhosis and alcoholism at country level as average alcohol consumption changes.
Decision criterion:	If the probability of observing the measured change (slope = b) is less than 5%, reject H_0.

Assumptions

The assumptions underpinning regression analysis are shown in Box 10.7.

---

[13]The value at which the line crossed the y-axis.

[14]Other types of regression exist for associations that are non-linear: quadratic, logarithmic, harmonic – and the regression equations reflect these more complex relationships. We will stick with linear regression for the time being.

[15]There is also *multiple regression*, in which the influence of more than one independent variable on the dependent variable can be considered at the same time. The assumptions underpinning multiple regression include multivariate normality, no or little multicollinearity, no auto-correlation and homoscedasticity. If these terms frighten you, they are not meant to. They simply illustrate that a thorough analysis of the data is needed before a robust multiple regression analysis is carried out, and that a statistician's input is crucial at this juncture. Do not be lured into undertaking complex analyses in SPSS because of the simplicity of the dropdown menus when clarity and insight are needed.

BOX 10.7

Assumptions underpinning regression analysis

1. Observations for two variables have been collected in pairs (x,y) for every element of the sample
2. The variables are continuous or discrete, interval or ratio
3. The variables are normally distributed
4. The association between the variables is linear

Depending on who you talk to, some statisticians will argue that you shouldn't carry out a linear regression on fewer than 20 pairs of observations. Not everyone is in agreement, and it can be a very useful way of exploring relationships between variables. This is, perhaps, another example of why the rules governing statistics are not hard and fast (as you might once have thought) and that good guidance is essential if you 'want sense' (as the Dodecahedron would say).

$$Y = a + bx$$

Test procedure

Regression relies on the same sums of squares that we calculated for correlation, so it is a small step, mathematically speaking, to find the slope and intercept of the regression line. Correlation looked at the way in which x and y varied in relation to each other using Equation 10.2:

$$r = \frac{S_{xy}}{\sqrt{S_{xx}S_{yy}}}$$

The formula to find the slope for the best-fit linear regression line looks similar, but omits the sum of squares in y. The formula for the slope,

designated by the letter b, tells us how y varies as x varies:

$$b = \frac{S_{xy}}{S_{xx}}$$

EQUATION 10.5 Formula to find the slope, b, of the linear regression line

The formula for a straight line is $y = a + bx$. Once we know b, we can find a, the intercept, by solving the following equation:

$$a = \overline{y} - b\overline{x}$$

EQUATION 10.6 Formula to find the intercept, a, of the linear regression line

We know this is right, because simple maths will show that the regression line passes through the point $(\overline{x}, \overline{y})$.

If we plug in our values for the sum of squares in x,y and the sum of squares in x, we find:

$$b = \frac{S_{xy}}{S_{xx}} = \frac{848.396}{429.216} = 1.9766$$

And

$$a = \overline{y} - b\overline{x} = 11.693 - 1.9766 \times 8.96 = -6.0172$$

So,

$$Y = -6.0172 + 1.9766x$$

If we plot this on our graph showing the relationship between alcohol consumption and death rates, we get Figure 10.4.

One more thought. If the null hypothesis were true, there would be no relationship between x and y. So, on average, y would not change as x changed, and the slope of the line would be zero (it would be flat, parallel with the x-axis). We need to make sure that the value for b did not arise by chance through random sampling variation. We will use the t distribution, as we did before for r, to see if the value for the slope is statistically significantly different from zero.

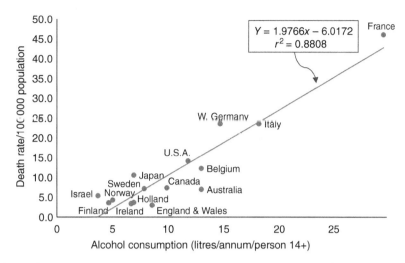

FIGURE 10.4 Death rate from cirrhosis and alcoholism versus alcohol consumption (litres/year/person aged 14+) in 15 high-income countries, with regression line.

We say that $t = b/\text{SE}(b)$. The standard error of b, $\text{SE}(b) = \sqrt{s^2/S_{xx}}$, where s^2, the variance of b, is given by the formula $s^2 = (S_{yy} - b^2 S_{xx})/(n-2) = (1903.869 - (1.9766)^2 \times 429.216)/(15-2) = 17.455$. So, $\text{SE}(b) = \sqrt{s^2/S_{xx}} = \sqrt{17.455/429.216} = 0.2017$ and $t = b/\text{SE}(b) = 1.9766/0.2017 = 9.802$.

This, you will notice, is exactly the same value for t that we found when we calculated the value of t for r, the correlation coefficient. (Ta Da!) Thus, we can say that the value for the slope can be regarded as highly statistically significantly different from zero $(P < 0.001)$.

In the long run, it is easier to calculate the value for t using the correlation coefficient, $t = r\sqrt{(n-2)/(1-r^2)}$, rather than finding the standard error for b and using the alternative formula for t. If the values are not the same using both formulae, you've made a mistake in your calculations.

Why is the line that we have calculated called the 'least squares' regression line? For each value x_i, the *predicted value* of y (denoted by the symbol Y_i) is the value of y at the point where x_i intersects the regression line. The *observed* value for y for each value x_i is, of course, the value for y_i in the (x_i, y_i) pair. We seek to find the minimum value for the sum of the *squares* of the *differences* between the *predicted* and the *observed* values for y for each value of x, that

is, the line for which $\sum(y_i - Y_i)^2$ is a minimum. The $y_i - Y_i$ differences are referred to as the 'residuals'. They are shown in Figure 10.5. Why square the values to find the minimum? Because (as with the standard deviation) some of the residuals are positive and some are negative. If you simply add the residuals together, you can easily show that the sum is zero: $\sum(y_i - Y_i) = 0$.

Decision and interpretation

We know from t that the slope of the line is statistically significantly different from zero at $P < 0.001$. This implies that at country level there are changes in mortality of a given size associated with corresponding changes in alcohol consumption.

The value for $b = 1.9766$. What does this mean? If we go back to basic principles regarding the slope of a line, we can say that for every unit change in x, there is a corresponding change in y equal to the value of the slope. For our current example, we can say that across the 15 countries in the sample, for every additional litre of alcohol consumed over one year in the population aged 14 and older, there will be roughly two additional deaths from cirrhosis and alcoholism per 100 000 population. That may not sound like very much. But if we start multiplying

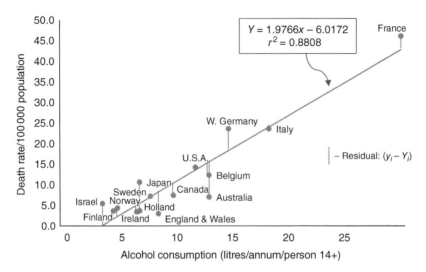

FIGURE 10.5   Death rate from cirrhosis and alcoholism versus alcohol consumption (litres/year/person aged 14+) in 15 high-income countries, with regression line, showing the residuals $(y_i - Y_i)$ for each value x_i.

up, we begin to see its public health implication: 20 additional deaths per million. 1000 additional deaths in a country with a population of 50 million. As an example, look at the difference between Norway and Italy where the average consumption levels are 4.2 and 15.21 per year, respectively. In theory, if Italy consumed alcohol at the level consumed in Norway, there would be roughly 13 000 fewer deaths per year from cirrhosis and alcoholism in Italy (1.9766 deaths per 100 000 per litre change in alcohol consumption times $15.2 - 4.2 = 11$ l difference times 60 million [the population of Italy] $= 13 046$). It becomes clear that there is potentially a major health issue that could be addressed by reducing the level of alcohol consumption in Italy.

What about the intercept, $a = -6.0172$? How do we interpret this? If alcohol consumption in a country were zero, does it mean that, on average, 6 people come back from the dead having not died of cirrhosis or alcoholism per 100 000 population? The answer, of course, is 'Don't be ridiculous'. It shows, however, that to create a meaningful estimate of the way in which two variables are related, we need to use a mathematical model that may not wholly reflect reality. If we had more data from other countries, including those where levels of alcohol

consumption are low or close to zero and there were, nevertheless, deaths from cirrhosis from other causes, we would gain further insight into how these two variables are related. But that discussion is for a different book.

Conclusion

We have shown that the value for b is statistically significantly different from zero. We have also calculated a standard error for b. This means we can calculate a confidence interval around the regression line itself. Effectively, that is asking, 'What is the 95% confidence interval for each value of Y_i?' This is best seen graphically.

The formula for finding the confidence interval around the regression line is not simple but is worth considering in detail. (Get a damp towel and wrap it round your head.) It takes into account the errors that arise when finding Y (the predicted value of y for a given value of x). Stop and think for a moment. As you get further and further from $(\bar{x}, \bar{y})$, you have less information on which to base the estimate of error. This means that the errors for Y_i are going to be greater at the ends of the line than in the centre. You will be right in saying that 95% of the time, the

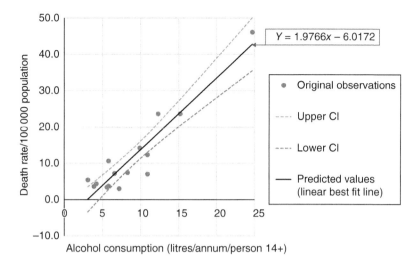

FIGURE 10.6 Death rate versus alcohol consumption in 15 countries, with regression line and confidence intervals.

value for Y_i will lie within the interval $Y_i \pm \Delta Y_{CI, i}$, where the error term for the predicted value of Y_i is:

$$\Delta Y_{CI,i} = t_{\nu,P} \times SE_Y \times \sqrt{\frac{1}{n} + \frac{\left(x_i - \bar{x}\right)^2}{S_{xx}}}$$

$t_{\nu, P}$ is the value for t for when $P = 0.05$, and ν is our old friend, degrees of freedom.[16] SE_Y is the standard error for the predicted values of Y: $SE_Y = \sqrt{\Sigma\left(y_i - Y_i\right)^2 / \left(n - 2\right)}$, where $y_i - Y_i$ are the residuals for all the values of x. The symbol Δ (upper-case Greek letter 'delta') stands for 'difference' or 'change'. In this instance, $n = 15$, $\nu = n - 2 = 13$, $t_{\nu = 13, P = 0.05} = 2.160$ (from Appendix A3), and S_{xx} is (of course) the sum of squares in x, equal to 429.216. If we find values for the confidence interval around each value of Y_i and plot them around the regression line, we obtain Figure 10.6.

As we get further from the centre of the distribution, the lines for the confidence interval get wider and wider, as predicted. This estimate of the error associated with regression helps us not to become overconfident about the importance of the predicted values based on regression lines, and to recognize that any time we are dealing with sample data, we risk misinterpretation if we do not take random sampling errors into account.

10.4 SPSS

SPSS is a wonderful tool for undertaking correlation and regression analyses. Let's use the alcohol and mortality data again.

Open 'ch10d01.sav'. This has the country, alcohol, and death rate data entered.

For correlation and regression, it is sensible to start by creating a graph. It is simplest to use Graphs>Legacy Dialogs>Scatter/Dot, choose Simple Scatter, put Alcohol on the x-axis and Death rate on the y-axis, and click OK or Paste.

For a graph that labels the points with the names of the countries, you need to click on Graphs>Chart Builder. Click on the Gallery tab, select Scatter/dot. Drag the death rate variable to the y-axis box, and alcohol to the x-axis box. Click on Groups/Point ID,

---

[16]Earlier in the chapter we said that we were allowing one degree of freedom for each of our variables, x and y, so $\nu = n - 2$, where n was the number of (x, y) pairs. For the regression equation, we can argue that we are allowing one degree of freedom for each of the two defined variables in our function, the intercept and the slope. Again, it means that $\nu = n - 2$, where n is the number of (x, y) pairs whose values are used to define the regression line.

Correlations

		Alcohol	Death_rate
Alcohol	Pearson correlation	1	0.939**
	Sig. (2-tailed)		0.000
	N	15	15
Death_rate	Pearson correlation	0.939**	1
	Sig. (2-tailed)	0.000	
	N	15	15

**Correlation is significant at the 0.01 level (2-tailed).

```
NONPAR CORR
   /VARIABLES=Alcohol Death_rate
   /PRINT=SPEARMAN TWOTAIL NOSIG
   /MISSING=PAIRWISE.
```

Nonparametric correlations

Correlations

			Alcohol	Death_rate
Spearman's rho	Alcohol	Correlation coefficient	1.000	0.765**
		Sig. (2-tailed)		0.001
		N	15	15
	Death_rate	Correlation coefficient	0.765**	1.000
		Sig. (2-tailed)	0.001	
		N	15	15

**Correlation is significant at the 0.01 level (2-tailed).

FIGURE 10.7   SPSS output for correlation analysis of death rate versus alcohol consumption in 15 countries. *Source*: Reproduced with permission of International Business Machines Corporation.

and click on Point ID Label. A new box appears on the graph template. Drag Country to the box labelled Point ID. Click Paste. The syntax for the Chart Builder is much more complex than for the Legacy Graph command. Make sure you click on all the commands to create the graph from the pasted syntax, starting with GGRAPH and ending with END GPL. You can add the regression line to both graphs by double-clicking the figure and selecting the linear regression line from the symbols *immediately* above the scatter-plot ('Add Fit Line at Total' appears when you hover over the right symbol). The regression line, the regression equation and the value for r^2 (R^2) appear on the graph. In the graph made with Chart Builder, I have added not only the regression line but also the confidence intervals for the mean (in the Properties box that appears when you double click the figure,

click the Fit Line tab, and under Confidence Intervals, choose Mean, then click on Apply). This will create the same lines as in Figure 10.6.

When you have created the graph and have a sense of the relationship (if it is monotonic, for example),[17] compute the correlation coefficient. Click on Analyze>Correlate>Bivariate. Highlight both variables and select with the curved blue arrow so they appear in the Variables box. Tick both Pearson and Spearman. Click on OK or Paste. You are done. The output is shown in Figure 10.7.

Because SPSS makes no assumptions about which variable is dependent and which one is

---

[17]You can explore other types of relationships by choosing different options in the Fit Method section of the Fit Line tab in the Properties box.

Coefficients[a]

Model		Unstandardized coefficients B	Std. error	Standardized coefficients Beta	t	Sig.	95.0% confidence interval for B Lower bound	Upper bound
1	(Constant)	−6.017	2.104		−2.859	0.013	−10.563	−1.471
	Alcohol	1.977	0.202	0.939	9.802	0.000	1.541	2.412

[a]Dependent varibale: Death_rate

FIGURE 10.8 SPSS output for linear regression analysis of death rate versus alcohol consumption in 15 countries. *Source*: Reproduced with permission of International Business Machines Corporation.

independent, it presents the values for the correlation coefficients and *P* values twice for each analysis. The correlation coefficients in the output match the values computed manually (as one would hope). The *P* values are not exactly the same, because SPSS has used slightly different methods for finding *P*. The conclusion cited in the footnote in both tables ('Correlation is significant at the 0.01 level (2-tailed))' is more conservative than the *P* values cited in the tables.

The nonparametric correlation in SPSS also gives the same value that we calculated manually, with a *P* value slightly less than that which we determined from Appendix A8 because SPSS uses a different algorithm for estimating *P*.

For the regression analysis, click on Analyze> Regression>Linear... Choose Death_rate as the dependent variable and Alcohol as the independent variable. Click on Statistics and choose Confidence Intervals and Descriptives. This will give you a full range of outputs, the last of which is shown in Figure 10.8. You see not only the regression coefficient and intercept but also whether or not they are statistically significantly different from zero (the null hypothesis).

10.5 EXERCISES

10.5.1

The data in Table 10.5 show the relationship between age (*x*) and typical dietitian salaries in the NHS (*y*). Plot the data. Assuming that the distribution of the

data is normal for both variables, carry out manual calculations to find the Pearson product-moment correlation coefficient and the equation for the regression line. Calculate: the significance level of the correlation coefficient; the slope of the regression line; and the intercept. Plot the regression line using Excel and the 95% confidence lines for the mean using SPSS.

TABLE 10.5 Typical Dietitian Salaries in the NHS in England, by Age (from Dietetic Support Workers to Senior and Specialist Dietitians)

Age (years)	Salary (1000 £/year)
19	15
21	18
23	20
24	22
26	24
29	24
30	25
32	27
33	27
35	28
44	30
45	31
48	35
51	36

TABLE 10.6   Glucocorticoid Therapy (Months) and Bone-Density (*T*-Score) in 14 Women Treated for Inflammatory Bowel Disease (IBD)

GC Therapy (Months)	T-score
20	0.15
23	−1.55
24	−0.25
27	−0.3
29	−0.6
32	−1.8
33	−1.4
36	−1.5
38	−1.65
40	−2.85
42	−2.25
44	−2.35
47	−1
48	−2.55

10.5.2

The data in Table 10.6 show the relationship between the duration of glucocorticoid therapy (months) and bone-density (*T*-score) in 14 women treated for inflammatory bowel disease (IBD). Plot the data. Without making any assumptions about the nature of the distribution of the variables, manually calculate the Spearman correlation coefficient ρ.

REFERENCES

1. Spence JD, Jenkins DJA, Davignon J. Dietary cholesterol and egg yolks: Not for patients at risk of vascular disease. *Can J Cardiol.* 2010 November; 26(9): e336–e339.

2. http://www.statstutor.ac.uk/resources/uploaded/spearmans.doc (accessed 13 February 2019).

3. Eugenia Cheng. *Beyond Infinity: An Expedition to the Outer Limits of Mathematics.* Basic Books. New York. 2017.

CHAPTER 11

Analysis of Variance

Learning Objectives

After studying this chapter, you should be able to:

- Understand what is meant by analysis of variance (ANOVA)
- Know when to use one-way analysis of variance, and its purposes and limitations
- Understand the concepts of two-way and n-way analysis of variance
- Know when to use the nonparametric equivalents for one-way and two-way analysis of variance (Kruskal–Wallis and Friedman tests)
- Carry out the calculations for one-way analysis of variance manually
- Interpret SPSS output for ANOVA to determine the level of significance of your findings

11.1 INTRODUCTION

One-way analysis of variance will be the pinnacle in this textbook of your experience in practical statistical testing. To be honest, we have reached only the foothills of statistical exploration. There are many peaks beyond this, where the air gets thinner and thinner and your brain has to work harder and harder to make sense of what is going on. But don't panic. At the higher altitudes, you will find the help of many Sherpa statisticians who will guide you and keep your statistical analyses fully oxygenated. Equally, by the time you finish this chapter, I hope you will have amazed yourself at the level of understanding that you have achieved since the start of this book.

It is important to note that analysis of variance is primarily the work of R.A. Fisher, who 'almost single-handedly created the foundations for modern statistical science' [1]. He introduced the term *variance*. He helped to regularize the notion that if the

Statistics in Nutrition and Dietetics, First Edition. Michael Nelson.
© 2020 John Wiley & Sons Ltd. Published 2020 by John Wiley & Sons Ltd.
Companion website: www.wiley.com/go/nelson/statistics

chance of observing a result was less than 1 in 20 (i.e. $P < 0.05$), it was reasonable to reject the null hypothesis. He was also a geneticist, which provided both the impetus and the opportunity to explore his mathematical ideas.[1] Joan Fisher Box, his daughter, wrote the definitive biography [2].

More extraordinary still, he laid these foundations less than a century ago [3]. Before then, the basic principles which we have been exploring in this book were known but not systematized and therefore less consistently applied. Be grateful that you live in a world where statistical inference has removed a vast amount of the guesswork and conjecture about the meaning of scientific findings and helped us put evidence on a firmer footing.

Enough adulation. On to the basics.

11.2 ONE-WAY ANALYSIS OF VARIANCE

Analysis of variance, or ANOVA for short, is a generalization of the t-test.[2] For practical purposes, we will start by exploring one-way analysis of variance for unmatched samples. This is equivalent to the unpaired t-test for more than two groups.[3] The paradox in nomenclature is explained by the method of analysis: it is based on sums of squares and variances (think back to Chapter 2).

The basic assumption is that the observations in each group are drawn from the same population. The expectation, therefore, is that there are no differences between the group means. Here are a few examples:

1. Analysis of growth in four groups of rats fed diets with 0%, 0.5%, 1% or 2% linoleic acid (natural order).
2. Comparison of haemoglobin levels in mothers from three different villages (no natural order).
3. Days of hospitalization for young children with three different feeding regimens following laparoscopic gastrostomy placement (natural order not established).

The aim in each case is to test for evidence of real differences between group means as opposed to differences which may have arisen by chance due to sampling error. As in previous chapters, we need to clarify our assumptions and delineate a model which will enable us to undertake the test.

Assumptions

The assumptions underpinning one-way analysis of variance are shown in Box 11.1.

As for previous statistical tests, we are going to need to introduce some new symbols. This new shorthand encapsulates ideas that we have developed in earlier chapters; the symbols just make it easier to manipulate the formulae for analysis of variance.

For one-way analysis of variance, the new symbols are set out in Table 11.1.

---

[1] He also had some misplaced ideas about race and eugenics, but they did not undermine his mathematical genius. For more information, see: https://en.wikipedia.org/wiki/Ronald_Fisher#cite_note-Hald98-4

[2] Or we could say, the unpaired t-test is a specific instance of one-way analysis of variance. The t-test came first, of course, but not by much (1908 for the t-test, 1925 for analysis of variance).

[3] If you carried out an analysis of variance for only two groups, you would discover that it is identical to the unpaired t-test. Although in practice it uses a different approach, the underlying statistics are the same.

BOX 11.1

Assumptions underpinning one-way analysis of variance

1. There are three or more groups of observations drawn from the same population
2. The distribution of the variable is normal
3. The samples are random and independent
4. There is no matching between samples
5. The variances of the samples are the same

For clarity, I have described the formulae for the new symbols in detail below (*An explication*). If they make sense already, just skip the explication and go on to '**The fundamentals**'. All the new symbols equate to our old symbols but make it easier to set out the formulae for calculating the F statistic. The F statistic is the equivalent of the t statistic when we want to compare more than two groups. (And 'yes', F is for Fisher.)

An explication of the new symbols in Table 11.1

We have k groups, numbered from 1 through i to k. In previous chapters, we used the subscript i to indicate a particular value for x in a set of n observations from 1 to n ($x_1, x_2, \ldots x_i, \ldots x_n$). Here, we are using the subscript i to indicate a particular group in a set of k groups labelled from 1 to k. The number of observations in each group is given by n_1, n_2 through n_i up to n_k. The grand total of the number of observations N is given by the formula:

$$N = \sum_{i=1}^{k} n_i$$

I have included the full version of the formula with upper case sigma (meaning, of course, 'the sum of') and the subscript and superscript to indicate that we are taking the sum of the numbers of observations from group 1 through group k.

I have used upper-case T with a subscript (T_1 through T_k) to indicate the sum of x in each of the groups. In previous chapters, we said simply that the sum of x was represented by $\sum x$. Now we have introduced a subscript, so our previous formula now reads $T_1 = \sum_1 x$, indicating that the sum is for a particular group. In keeping with our 'lazy' ethos, it easier to write T_1 than $\sum_1 x$, which is why we have introduced a new symbol. And I am sure you would agree that T (the sum of observations across all groups) is easier to write than:

$$T = \sum_{i=1}^{k} \sum_i x$$

Similarly, S_1 is easier to write than $\sum_1 x^2$ (the sum of the squares of the values for x [x^2] for all the observations in group 1), and S is easier to write than:

$$S = \sum_{i=1}^{k} \sum_i x^2$$

TABLE 11.1 Symbols Used for Calculation of F Statistic in One-Way Analysis of Variance

Group	1	2	...i...	k	All Groups Combined
Number of observations	n_1	n_2	$...n_i...$	n_k	$N = \sum_{i=1}^{k} n_i$
Sum of x	T_1	T_2	$...T_i...$	T_k	$T = \sum_{i=1}^{k} T_i$
Sum of x^2	S_1	S_2	$...S_i...$	S_k	$S = \sum_{i=1}^{k} S_i$
Mean of x	$\bar{x}_1$	$\bar{x}_2$	$...\bar{x}_i...$	$\bar{x}_k$	$\bar{x} = \dfrac{T}{N}$

(the sum of the values for x^2 for all the observations in groups 1 through k).

In the final row, $\bar{x}_i$ indicates the mean of the values for x for each group ($\bar{x}_1$ through $\bar{x}_k$), and $\bar{x}$ indicates the mean of all values of x across all the groups, that is $\bar{x} = \sum x / \sum n_i = \sum x / N = T / N$. It should be noted that $\bar{x}$ is the weighted average of the means of the groups, that is $\bar{x} = \sum n_i \bar{x}_i / \sum n_i$.

I hope that helps. If it is not clear, it is worth your while going back and re-reading the explication.

The fundamentals

Having established a new vocabulary of symbols, we need to understand exactly how analysis of variance works. Here is our new vocabulary: N, T, and S are sums. $\bar{x}$ is the average across all observations in all the groups, equivalent to the *weighted* mean of the averages of each sample. We need to introduce one new term. Denote the jth observation in group i as x_{ij}.

Way back in Chapter 2, we introduced the concept of *variance* (equal to the standard deviation before taking the square root). We come back to this concept when trying see if the group means differ statistically from one another. Start by determining how much each observation differs from the grand mean. This can be written as: $x_{ij} - \bar{x}$.

Now it gets really clever. The deviation of any observation from the grand mean, $x_{ij} - \bar{x}$, can be rewritten as $(x_{ij} - \bar{x}_i) + (\bar{x}_i - \bar{x})$. The first term is the deviation of each observation from the group mean; the second term is the deviation of the group mean from the grand mean. More formally, we can say:

$$x_{ij} - \bar{x} = (x_{ij} - \bar{x}_i) + (\bar{x}_i - \bar{x})$$

EQUATION 11.1   Splitting the difference of each observation from the grand mean into two components

Fisher established that when the terms are squared and summed, the same relationship holds true,[4] that is

$$\sum \left(x_{ij} - \bar{x} \right)^2 = \sum \left(x_{ij} - \bar{x}_i \right)^2 + \sum \left(\bar{x}_i - \bar{x} \right)^2$$

EQUATION 11.2   Splitting the difference of the total sum of squares

In Chapter 2, we defined the expression $\sum (x - \bar{x})^2$ as 'the sum of squares'.[5] We can talk, therefore, about the total sum of squares (the first term in Equation 11.2 that relates each observation to the mean of all the observations), the within-group sum of squares (the second term, that relates each observation within a group to the group mean), and the between group sum of squares (the third term, that relates the group means to the grand mean) (Box 11.2).

Now we can make the great leap that Fisher made. We say that we *partition* the sum of squares into two parts. This is blindingly obvious if you are a genius like Fisher, or mind-bogglingly clever if you're not. What can we now do with this information? Let's think logically about this.

Our succinct terminology, introduced in Table 11.1, now allows us to produce some brilliantly condensed formulae for the calculations that we need to make:

$$\text{Total SSq} = S - \frac{T^2}{N}$$

$$\text{Within group SSq} = S - \sum \frac{T_i^2}{n_i}$$

$$\text{Between group SSq} = \sum \frac{T_i^2}{n_i} - \frac{T^2}{N}$$

EQUATION 11.3   Formulae for the sums of squares needed for analysis of variance

There are two things to note. First, the *Total sum of squares* (*Total SSq*) is exactly the same as the sum of squares for a sample that we described in Chapter 2: $\sum x^2 - (\sum x)^2$ (the crude sum of squares

---

[4]I won't go into the proof for this. It is not complicated, but (let's face it) probably beyond the interest of most students reading this book.

[5]This is shorthand for: 'the sum of the squares of the differences between each observation and the mean'.

BOX 11.2

Fundamental equation for one-way analysis of variance

**The total SSq =
Within groups SSq + Between groups SSq**

minus the correction for the mean). Total SSq is therefore the sum of squares for all the observations in all our samples (the crude sum of squares, S, minus the correction for the mean, T^2/N). Second, the *Between group SSq* is independent of S, that is, it is all to do with the corrections for the mean.

Now, how do we go about testing for evidence of the statistical significance of the differences between the group means? We need to think through how we can use the information that we have about the variations in our observations between groups and within groups.

Let's start by assuming that there are no differences between the group means and that the standard deviation, σ, is the same for all groups. Moreover, if we think of the way in which random sampling works, the differences between the *group means* should also reflect the variance of the population.

Say we have three samples. If the null hypothesis is true, the three samples are from the same (or identical) populations in which $\mu_1 = \mu_2 = \mu_3$ and $\sigma_1 = \sigma_2 = \sigma_3$. We can say, therefore, $\sigma_1 = \sigma_2 = \sigma_3 = \sigma$. In theory, therefore, the variances of our three samples, s_1, s_2, and s_3, are equally good estimators of σ. They differ only because of random sampling variation. Now we can use all the information that we have about the way in which observations vary around the mean and find a way to use s_1, s_2, and s_3 in our calculations.

We have three ways of estimating s^2, our best estimate of the population variance, σ^2:

1. From the Total SSq:

$$s_T^2 = \frac{\text{Total SSq}}{N-1} = \frac{S-(T^2/N)}{N-1}$$

This estimate of the population variance is based on all the observations collected. The

number of degrees of freedom (the divisor) is equal to the total number of observations (N) minus 1.[6]

2. From the within group SSq:

$$s_W^2 = \frac{\text{Within group SSq}}{N-k} = \frac{S-\sum\left(T_i^2/n_i\right)}{N-k}$$

This estimate of σ^2 is based on the variation in observations within the groups *independent of* the variation in observations between the groups. It is analogous to the pooled estimate of variance in the unpaired t-test. There, the number of degrees of freedom was $n-2$. Here, there are $N-k$ degrees of freedom: the total number of observations minus one degree of freedom for each group.[7] This is called the *Within Group Mean Square (Within group MSq)*.

3. Since s_W^2 and s_T^2 are (in theory) both unbiased estimators of σ^2, then the expected value of the between group SSq is $\sigma^2 \times (N-1) - \sigma^2 \times (N-k) = \sigma^2 \times (k-1)$. So

$$s_B^2 = \frac{\sum\left(T_i^2/n_i\right)-\left(T^2/N\right)}{k-1}$$

s_B^2 is the *Between Group Mean Square (Between group MSq)*

Now, suppose that all the group means are not equal. s_W^2 is still an *unbiased* estimator of σ^2, since it is based purely on variation within the groups. But s_B^2 will increase as the differences between the group means increase. An appropriate test of the null hypothesis can then be based on the ratio of the between group mean square divided by the within group mean square: s_B^2/s_W^2. The distribution of this ratio, which is tabulated according to the number of

---

[6]This is exactly equivalent to what we did in Chapter 2 to find the best estimate of the population variance based on sample observations: $s^2 = (\sum x^2 - (\sum x)^2/n)/(n-1)$.
[7]You can now begin to see why the unpaired t-test is like an analysis of variance where there are only two groups.

(a)   No statistically significant differences:

- S_B^2 and S_W^2 (the widths of the ovals) are similar
- F ratio is small (for given ν_1 and ν_2)
- The sample means are close together

(b)   Statistically significant differences:

- The width of the S_B^2 oval is greater than that of the S_W^2 ovals
- F ratio is large (for given ν_1 and ν_2)
- The sample means are far apart

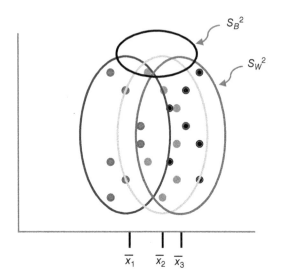
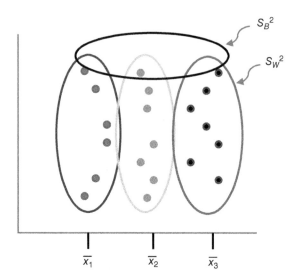

FIGURE 11.1   Schematic representation of analysis of variance when (a) the F ratio is close to 1.0 and (b) the F ratio is substantially larger than 1.0. Variances are indicated by the width of the ovals.

degrees of freedom in the numerator and denominator, follows the F distribution. We can write: $F = s_B^2 / s_W^2$. Hence, we have an 'analysis of variance' (now you know where the term comes from).

If the underling distribution of the variable is normal,[8] then s_B^2 and s_W^2 should behave like two *independent* estimates of σ^2 with $k - 1$ and $N - k$ degrees of freedom.[9] If the null hypothesis is true, we expect our two estimators of σ^2 (s_B^2 and s_W^2) to be equal. F would be equal to 1.0. If we allow for random sampling variation, the F ratio might be greater than or less than 1.0. If the differences between the group means are large in comparison to the variation in observations within the groups, and s_B^2 / s_W^2 is substantially greater than 1.0, it may be that the samples have not all have been drawn from the same or identical populations. In that case, we could reject the null hypothesis. Exactly what we mean by 'substantially greater' is the ultimate focus of analysis of variance.

The impact on F of the differences in the sizes of our two estimators of variance, s_B^2 and s_W^2, are illustrated in Figure 11.1. In Figure 11.1a, there is a lot of overlap between three sets of observations and little difference between the means. s_B^2 and s_W^2 (illustrated by the widths of the ovals) are likely to be similar. The F ratio would be close to 1.0. In Figure 11.1b, there is little overlap between the three sets of observations and marked differences between the means.

---

[8]Unlike the *t*-test, analysis of variance is not robust, in the sense that it does not give reliable values for P if the distribution of the variable of interest deviates very far from normal. The test will give a result, of course. It is a matter of deciding if the probability of the outcome justifies rejection of the null hypothesis. We saw in Chapter 6 how normality can easily be assessed in SPSS, and we looked in Chapter 4 at transformations in case we needed a better fit of our data to the normal distribution.

[9]If $k = 2$, then the situation is exactly that described for the unpaired *t*-test.

s_B^2 will be greater than s_W^2, and the F ratio large enough to warrant rejection of the null hypothesis. Now let's look at an example and see how this works in practice.

An example

In a study of postoperative feeding regimens after laparoscopic gastrostomy placement in children, hospital length of stay (time to discharge) was the outcome variable of interest. The day of initiation of postoperative feeding via gastric tube was the independent variable. Results for 17 patients in 3 groups are shown in Table 11.2. While there is clearly a degree of overlap in length of hospital stay between the three groups, the mean values suggest that earlier introduction of the feeding regimen is associated with a shorter stay in hospital. If we assume that the length of stay follows a normal distribution,[10] we can use analysis of variance to test for statistically significant differences between the three groups.

Fundamental principle

Expectation:	H_0: There is no difference in mean length of hospital stay in relation to day of initiation of feeding following laparoscopic gastrostomy placement in children.
Decision criterion:	If there is a statistically significantly difference between group means at the 5% level, we can reject H_0.

The model

The model for one-way analysis of variance is shown in Box 11.3.

If we look at Box 11.3, it appears that data fit the model and the criteria are met.[11]

TABLE 11.2   Length of Hospital Stay versus Day of Initiation of Feeding Following Laparoscopic Gastrostomy Placement in Children

	Postoperative Days (Initial Day of Feeding)			
	0	1	2+	All Children
n	6	5	6	17
Hospital length of stay	2	3	3	
	3	4	5	
	2	2	6	
	4	3	3	
	2	5	4	
	2		4	
Mean	2.6	3.0	4.2	3.4
sd	0.8367	1.1402	1.1690	1.2217

BOX 11.3

Model for one-way analysis of variance

1. k groups, where $k > 2$. There are three groups.
2. n_i observations in each group; n_i may differ between groups.
3. The observations in each group are randomly drawn from normally distributed values in the parent population.
4. The observations in the different groups are independent, i.e. no pairing or matching between groups.
5. The variances of the groups are the same.

---

[10] We will test for this later in the chapter.

[11] We will test for normality and equal variances a bit later. I would be perverse indeed if I had chosen a data set in which the underlying assumptions for normality and homogeneity of variance did not fit the model, so rest assured that all is well.

TABLE 11.3   Length of Hospital Stay versus Day of Initiation of Feeding Following Laparoscopic Gastrostomy Placement in Children

| | Postoperative Days (Initial Day of Feeding) | | | |
	0	1	2+	All Children
n	6	5	6	17
Hospital length of stay	2	3	3	
	3	4	5	
	2	2	6	
	4	3	3	
	2	5	4	
	2		4	
Mean	2.6	3.0	4.2	3.4
sd	0.8367	1.1402	1.1690	1.2217
T	15	17	25	57
S	41	63	111	215
T_i^2/n_i	37.50	57.80	104.17	191.12

Test procedure

First, we need to find the values for our sums and squares. Let's expand Table 11.2 to include the additional information for T, S, and T_i^2/n_i (Table 11.3). We now have the values that we need to compute the total, between group, and within group sums of squares, and the between group and within group mean squares.

$$s_W^2 = \frac{\text{Within group SSq}}{N-k} = \frac{S - \sum\left(T_i^2/n_i\right)}{N-k}$$

$$= \frac{215 - 199.467}{17 - 3} = \frac{15.533}{14} = 1.1095$$

$$s_B^2 = \frac{\text{Between group SSq}}{k-1} = \frac{\sum\left(T_i^2/n_i\right) - \left(T^2/N\right)}{k-1}$$

$$= \frac{199.467 - 191.118}{3-1} = \frac{8.349}{2} = 4.175$$

We can now put together the analysis of variance table (Table 11.4). This is the standard layout

TABLE 11.4   Analysis of Variance Table for Data Comparing Length of Hospital Stay in Three Groups of Children Differing in Day of Initiation of Feeding Following Laparoscopic Gastrostomy Placement (see Table 11.3)

Source of Variation	SSq	df	MSq	F
Between group	8.349	2	4.175	3.762
Within group	15.533	14	1.110	
Total	23.882	16		

for an analysis of variance. The first column shows the source of the variance, then the sums of squares using the formulae above. Note that the between group sum of squares and within group sum of squares add up to the total sum of squares, as we expected. The next column shows the degrees of freedom: $k-1$ (3 – 1 = 2) and $N-k$ (17 – 3 = 14) for the between group and within group mean squares, respectively. The total degrees of freedom is (of course) $N-1 = 17 - 1 = 16 = 2 + 14$. The next column shows the mean squares (SSq divided by degrees of freedom, df).[12]

The two values for mean square are, in theory, equally good estimates of the variance of the observations in the population. If the null hypothesis were true, we would expect them to be similar, and the ratio of the variances, F, would be close to 1.0. The value for F for the present data is

$$F = \frac{s_B^2}{s_W^2} = \frac{\text{Between group mean square}}{\text{Within group mean square}} = \frac{4.175}{1.110} = 3.762$$

Decision and interpretation

Now we can consult Appendix A9 for areas in the tail of the F distribution and find out the probability of observing what we observed (the F ratio) if we assume that the null hypothesis is true. If $P < 0.05$, we can reject the null hypothesis.

Rejection rule: If the calculated value of F is *greater than* the tabulated value of F for ν_1 and ν_2 when $P = 0.05$, reject H_0.

In Appendix A9, look in the first row of values at the top of the table for degrees of freedom (ν_1) for the numerator (the between group mean square). $\nu_1 = k - 1 = 3 - 1 = 2$ degrees of freedom for the between group mean square, so find the column headed '2'. In the left-hand column of the table, find the row for the number of degrees of freedom (ν_2) for the denominator (within group mean square): $\nu_2 = N - k = 17 - 3 = 14$. The block of values in the second column shows four values for P: 0.05, 0.02, 0.01, and 0.005. The block of four values at the intersection of $\nu_1 = 2$ and $\nu_2 = 14$ show the cut-off values for F at each level of probability. If the calculated value for F is *greater than* the tabulated value at a given level of P, we can reject the null hypothesis at that level. (Note that the values for F increase as the value for P decreases. In terms of the little diagram at the top of the table, this makes sense: the larger the value for F, the smaller the area under the curve

in the tail to the right, P.) In the current example, the calculated value for F is 3.762. This is greater than the tabulated value for F when $P = 0.05$, 3.74. We can therefore reject the null hypothesis at the 5% level. If the calculated value for F had been greater than 5.24, we would have been able to reject the null hypothesis at the 2% level, and so on.

We can conclude that there is a statistically significant difference between the mean number of days stay in hospital and the initiation of the feeding regimen. The mean value is lowest for those children whose feeding regimen started on the day of the operation (2.6 days), in the middle for those who started feeding the day after the operation (3.0), and highest for those whose feeding regimen started 2 or more days after the operation (4.2 days).

11.3 SPSS

When we use SPSS to carry out the test, we get Table 11.5.

The only difference between this table and Table 11.4 is the inclusion of the column labelled 'Sig.' (what we have been calling 'P'). As we have seen in previous SPSS output, instead of giving values for P in bands with cut-off points (as the tables in the Appendices generally do), SPSS computes and displays an exact value for P. In the present analysis, SPSS says Sig. $= 0.49$.[13] So, we are in agreement: using the cut-off value in Appendix A9, we said

---

[12] SPSS and other software uses df rather than ν in their output tables, so I am following that convention here.

[13] This corresponds (roughly) to what we would find if we interpolated P within the F table in Appendix A9: if $\nu_1 = 2$ and $\nu_2 = 14$, $F = 3.74$ when $P = 0.05$, and $F = 5.24$ when $P = 0.02$. Our calculated value for F is 3.762. The maths is simple: the value for P is the same distance between 0.05 and 0.02 as 3.762 is between 3.74 and 5.24. That is:

$$P = 0.05 - \frac{3.762 - 3.74}{5.24 - 3.74} \times (0.05 - 0.02) = 0.04956$$

Our interpolated value is slightly larger than the value produced by SPSS because we have carried out a linear interpolation for simplicity, whereas the relationship between P and F is not exactly linear (see the curve in the graph in the upper left-hand corner of at the top of the table in Appendix A9).

TABLE 11.5   SPSS Output for One-Way Analysis of Variance Based on Laparoscopic Gastrostomy Data

| ANOVA | | | | | |
Days	Sum of Squares	df	Mean Square	F	Sig.
Between groups	8.349	2	4.175	3.762	0.049
Within groups	15.533	14	1.110		
Total	23.882	16			

Source: Reproduced with permission of International Business Machines Corporation.

$P < 0.05$. We come to the same conclusion: reject H_0. Now, there is one final issue to address.

Comparing groups

When we carried out the unpaired t-test, it was simply a matter of saying if there was a statistically significant difference between two group means. But now there are three groups. Does the statistical significance of the difference apply to all three groups (are groups 1, 2, and 3 all different from each other)? Or is it that group 1 is different from group 3, but not from group 2? Is group 2 different from group 3?

Having established through analysis of variance that there is a statistically significant difference between groups (that is, all three groups were NOT drawn from the same or identical populations), you might think that the simplest approach to find out which groups differ from which other groups would be to undertake a series of t-tests for every pair of comparisons that we could make. This is not the best approach for two reasons, however. First, it does not take into account that we have data from three groups when we make our comparisons. The error mean square (within group mean square) is our best unbiased estimate of the population variance (σ^2), so we should use it, rather than relying on variances based on only two sets of observations if we were to compare two samples at a time. Second, the more comparisons we undertake, the more likely it is that (just by chance) one of them will be statistically significant (see Box 11.4).

SPSS uses *post hoc* tests to compare groups without asking you to make assumptions about the ways in which you think the groups are likely to differ from one another before you begin the research.[14] You should look at the *post hoc* tests *if and only if* your analysis of variance has yielded a statistically significant F value, with $P < 0.05$.

There is a vast literature about the strengths and weaknesses of the different *post hoc* tests available in SPSS. The tests vary in their application according to the size of the sample, the number of groups, whether observations are matched between groups, and whether there is a control group for comparison. They also differ in how liberal or conservative they are.[15]

With the equal variances assumption, two of the most commonly used *post hoc* tests are LSD (Least Significant Difference) and Tukey's HSD (Honest Significant Difference). LSD is generally regarded as too liberal – you are likely to think there are statistically significant differences between two groups when in fact there are none.[16] HSD gives a more conservative view which is widely accepted. Generally

---

[14] If you think you know in advance how groups are likely to differ, you can carry out *a priori* tests. The approach to *a priori* testing is different from that for *post hoc* testing. We will not discuss this here. Consult your friendly statistician for advice if you are convinced that you know beforehand how your groups will differ. Some *post hoc* tests allow you to compare intervention groups specifically with control groups, but that is different from *a priori* testing.

[15] 'Liberal' tests are more likely to suggest that there are statistically significant differences between groups. 'Conservative' tests are less likely to suggest that there are statistically significant differences between groups. Generally speaking (from a statistical perspective, you understand), it is better to be conservative, i.e. to accept the null hypothesis rather than to risk rejecting it in error.

[16] A Type I error: incorrect rejection of a true null hypothesis.

BOX 11.4

Why making multiple comparisons between groups can be problematic

Making multiple comparisons

Once we have established (through analysis of variance) that there is a statistically significant difference between a set of groups (i.e. they do not all come from the same or identical populations), we can use LSD (Least Significant Difference) to make pairwise comparisons between every possible pair of groups, like a series of t-tests (paired or unpaired according to whether or not the data between groups are matched). LSD does use the error mean square (based on all the information available from the entire sample). The problem is, the more groups there are, the more comparisons you can make. For example, if you have four groups, you can make six comparisons (group 1 with groups 2, 3, and 4; group 2 with groups 3 and 4; and group 3 with group 4). If there are five groups, you can make 10 comparisons, six groups allow 15 comparisons, and seven groups allow 21 comparisons. The problem? If your comparisons are all at the 5% level of significance ($P = 0.05$), and you use the value for t for the given number of degrees of freedom, every 20th comparison risks generating a Type I error. LSD does not make any correction for the number of groups being compared. If there are seven groups being compared, one of the comparisons (just by chance) is likely to be statistically significant at the 5% level. Bonferroni is like LSD with a correction for the number of comparisons, but it is seen as a bit heavy handed (overly conservative). Tukey's HSD (Honest Significant Difference) takes into account the number of groups being compared while at the same time ensuring that there is only a 5% chance of a Type I error if the assumption is that $P = 0.05$.

speaking, HSD is the best *post hoc* test to opt for with the equal variances assumption. If variances are heterogeneous ('not equal'), Dunnett's T3 is good for small samples and Dunnett's C for large samples. If you are in any doubt, consult your friendly statistician.

Let's look at some output from SPSS for comparisons between pairs of groups. Put the data from Table 11.2 into the correct format for analysis of variance in SPSS: the observations for number of days in hospital are all in one column ('days'), and the group number for each observation in the second column ('group') (see online file ch11d01. sav). Click on Analyze/Compare Means/One-way ANOVA, then select Dependent List ('days', the variable of interest) and Factor ('group', the variable that identifies which group each observation belongs to). Click PostHoc. You are then presented with a list of 14 *post hoc* tests to use when making the equal variances assumption, and another four if equal variances are not assumed. In the present example, tick the box labelled 'Tukey'. In addition to the analysis of variance output that we saw in Table 11.5, you will generate two further tables.

An exploration of Table 11.6 will help you discover which groups differ from one another at the 5% level. The first two columns show which group (column 1) is being compared with which other groups (column 2). The third column shows the mean difference between the two groups being compared. There is some repetition in the values in the table, some positive and some negative, according the direction in which the difference between the group means is being taken (I – J in column three of the table).

If the null hypothesis were true, we would expect the values for the differences to be equal to zero. Because of random sampling variation, however, we know that they will not be exactly zero. We know also from the result of our analysis of variance that at least one of these differences will be statistically significantly different from zero (although we do not yet know which one). The next column is labelled 'Sig.' (SPSS for P). If $P < 0.05$, we can say that the group means differ significantly from zero at the 5% level. There are two values in the column where $P = 0.04$. We can say, therefore, that these

TABLE 11.6 SPSS Output for Multiple Comparisons Based on Tukey (HSD) *post hoc* Analysis

		Multiple Comparisons				
		Dependent Variable: days				
		Tukey HSD				
(I) Group	**(J) Group**	**Mean Difference (I − J)**	**Std. Error**	**Sig.**	**95% Confidence Interval**	
					Lower Bound	**Upper Bound**
1.00	2.00	−0.90000	0.63783	0.362	−2.5694	0.7694
	3.00	−1.66667[a]	0.60815	0.040	−3.2584	−0.0750
2.00	1.00	0.90000	0.63783	0.362	−0.7694	2.5694
	3.00	−0.76667	0.63783	0.471	−2.4360	0.9027
3.00	1.00	1.66667[a]	0.60815	0.040	0.0750	3.2584
	2.00	0.76667	0.63783	0.471	−0.9027	2.4360

Source: Reproduced with permission of International Business Machines Corporation.
[a]The mean difference is significant at the 0.05 level.

group means differ significantly from one another. When we look further, we see that they are, in fact, the same comparison: Group 1 versus Group 3, with the difference taken comparing Group 1 versus Group 3 in the first comparison, and Group 3 versus Group 1 in the second comparison. The mean difference (I − J) is the same magnitude for both comparisons, but with opposite signs. Finally, look at the bounds for the 95% confidence interval. Where the bounds include zero, the value for the difference is not statistically significant from zero ($P > 0.05$). Where the bounds do not include zero (for Group 1 versus Group 3, for example, the lower bound is −3.2584 and the upper bound is −0.0750, and $P = 0.04$). It ties together very satisfactorily.

The next table in the SPSS output for the Tukey *post hoc* analysis is for Homogenous subsets (Table 11.7). This is a very neat way of showing which groups are likely to be from the same population (are homogeneous). There are two subsets of groups which are homogeneous at alpha (P) = 0.05, that is, groups which are likely to have come from the same population. The two subsets, however, represent different populations. The first subset contains Groups 1 and 2 and the second subset contains Groups 2 and 3. Group 2, it appears,

TABLE 11.7 SPSS Output for Homogeneous Subsets Based on Tukey (HSD) *post hoc* Analysis

		Days		
	Group	**N**	**Subset for alpha = 0.05**	
			1	**2**
Tukey HSD[a,b]	1.00	6	2.5000	
	2.00	5	3.4000	3.4000
	3.00	6		4.1667
	Sig.		0.352	0.461

Source: Reproduced with permission of International Business Machines Corporation.
Means for groups in homogeneous subsets are displayed.
[a]Uses Harmonic Mean Sample Size = 5.625.
[b]The group sizes are unequal. The harmonic mean of the group sizes is used. Type I error levels are not guaranteed.

could have come from either population. Group 1 and Group 3 appear to come from different populations. Again, we have a story consistent with the results in Table 11.6. The value for Sig. at the bottom of the table shows the probability that the two groups for Subset 1 and for Subset 2 came from the same population. In both cases, $P > 0.05$, and we accept the null hypothesis that both groups in each subset come from the same population.

How can Group 2 come from both populations? This may at first seem inconsistent. The answer is, random sampling variation in both populations produced values for Group 2 that made it not statistically different from Group 1 and also not statistically different from Group 3. This may test your logical thinking. Are you thinking: if a = b and b = c, then a = c. But the equal sign is another way of saying 'identical to', which the groups clearly are not. They are merely similar. Statistics offers a joyous resolution for this apparent inconsistency because it deals with errors and confidence limits, which help us to understand when we can regarding things (samples, groups) as identical and when they are statistically indistinguishable but at the same time different. What fun!

Normality and equal variances

In Section 11.2, Box 11.1, we made two key assumptions about conditions that need to be met before carrying out an analysis of variance. First, we assumed that the variable was normally distributed in the parent population from which our samples were drawn. Second, we said that the variances of the groups had to be equal (or more specifically, not statistically different from one another). I promised earlier in the chapter that we would come back to tests that we can use to ensure that these assumptions are met.

Again, I am going to turn to SPSS. It isn't that we couldn't do the necessary tests manually. But for the purposes of your understanding relating to analysis of variance, a couple of computer-based shortcuts seem in order. It is also worth pointing out that you would normally test for normality and equality of variances *before* you carried out the analysis of variance (otherwise you might be wasting your time). I have presented the results in this chapter in the order that I have (interesting bits about ANOVA first, less interesting but essential bits about normality and equal variances second) knowing at the outset that the data fulfilled the assumptions. But we need to fill in the gap.

Testing for normality

There are many tests for normality.[17] SPSS relies primarily on two tests: Kolmogorov–Smirnov and Shapiro–Wilk.[18] Select Analyze/Descriptive Statistics/ Explore, choose 'days', click 'Plots', then tick the box for 'Normality plots with tests'. One of the elements of output you generate will look like Table 11.8.

Both tests determine the probability that the given observations were drawn from a normally distributed parent population. The null hypothesis is that our observations came from a normally distributed population. In the current example, both tests give a value for Sig. (P) greater than 0.05, so we can accept the null hypothesis and assume that the underlying distribution for our variable is normally distributed. One of the issues here is that our sample size is small, which is potentially a problem of sensitivity with both tests. If the value for $P < 0.05$, you can reject the null hypothesis and assume that the observations did *not* come from a normally distributed parent population.[19]

TABLE 11.8 SPSS Output for Tests of Normality Using the Present Data set

	Tests of Normality					
	Kolmogorov–Smirnov[a]			Shapiro–Wilk		
	Statistic	df	Sig.	Statistic	df	Sig.
Days	0.202	17	0.064	0.892	17	0.051

Source: Reproduced with permission of International Business Machines Corporation.
[a]Lilliefors Significance Correction.

[17] The entry in Wikipedia provides a useful summary and lists more than 10 approaches. Even this is not exhaustive: https://en.wikipedia.org/wiki/Normality_test
[18] The tests differ in terms of how they deal with outliers, skewness, and kurtosis.
[19] The options then are to transform the data to see if you can generate a distribution that is normal in character or use nonparametric statistics to carry out the analysis of variance. We will look at the latter option a bit later in the chapter.

Testing for equal variances

Again, SPSS comes to the rescue. Select Analyze/ Compare Means/One-way ANOVA, then select your Dependent List ('days') and Factor ('group'), click Options, tick the box for 'Homogeneity of variance test', and run, and you will generate a table for Levene's Statistic (Table 11.9).

The null hypothesis for the Levene Statistic is that the variances for the groups do not differ (statistically speaking), that is, they are all derived from the same parent population. (Have a look at Table 11.3 and see if that is consistent with your expectation.[20]) If the value for *Sig.* is greater than or equal to 0.05, accept the null hypothesis. In this case, Sig. = 0.742, so you can accept the null hypothesis and make the 'equal variances' assumption. If Sig. < 0.05, you will need to use a different approach to your analyses that does not make the equal variances assumption (see the options in SPPS, and consult your tame statistician).

11.4 TWO-WAY ANALYSIS OF VARIANCE

You are now virtuosi[21] of one-way analysis of variance. But Statistics never sleeps. What happens, for example, if there are two independent variables? What if we had wanted to compare outcomes for our data not just between feeding regimens but also between boys and girls? Could we explore the impact on days in hospital of the day on which the feeding regimen was started and the gender of the child at the same time? The answer, of course, is 'Yes'.

I am going to turn to a larger data set to explore two-way analysis of variance. We will look at the impact of two influences, gender and diet, on weight loss, and see which factors (if either) are important, statistically speaking.

The mean values for weight loss for the three different diets are shown separately for men and women in Table 11.10.[22]

If we look in the last column ('Total'), it appears that average weight loss was greatest on diet 3 (5.1481 kg after 10 weeks). Diets 1 and 2 look like they were less effective (3.3 kg and 3.268 kg, respectively). But if we look at the differences between the diets by gender, the impact in men is not all that different, whereas the impact in women is clearly greater for Diet 3.

I could, of course, simply analyze the impact of the diets separately for men and women. But statistically speaking, it is preferable to use all the information available in a single analysis. We can then discover not only if there is a difference in impact between diets, but also if the observed differences between men and women are statistically significant (or if they arose by chance). We couldn't do that if we looked at the impact of the diet on weight loss in two separate analyses.

Assumptions

The assumptions for two-way analysis of variance are the same as for one-way analysis of variance: three or more groups of observations drawn from the same population, a normally distributed variable, random, and independent samples, no matching

TABLE 11.9   SPSS Output for Leven's Statistic for Homogeneity of Variances

Test of Homogeneity of Variances			
Days			
Levene Statistic	df1	df2	Sig.
0.304	2	14	0.742

Source: Reproduced with permission of International Business Machines Corporation.

---

[20]If you had one.

[21]Here are the Word Thesaurus synonyms for 'virtuosi': 1. Wunderkinds (n.) genii, geniuses, wizards, prodigies, aces, mavens; 2. Prodigies (n.) experts, genii, performers, maestros, artistes, artists. Take your pick – you have earned the accolade.

[22]I have used the SPSS 'Descriptives' function to generate this output:

Analyze>Descriptive Statistics>Descriptives

TABLE 11.10   Average Weight Loss after 10 Weeks in Men and Women on Three Different Diets

Diet		Female	Male	Total
		Descriptive Statistics		
		Dependent Variable: Weight Lost (kg)		
		Gender		
1	Mean	3.0500	3.6500	3.3000
	Std. deviation	2.065 00	2.536 07	2.240 15
	N	14	10	24
2	Mean	2.6071	4.1091	3.2680
	Std. deviation	2.288 92	2.525 25	2.464 54
	N	14	11	25
3	Mean	5.8800	4.2333	5.1481
	Std. deviation	1.889 52	2.716 06	2.395 57
	N	15	12	27
Total	Mean	3.8930	4.0152	3.9461
	Std. deviation	2.515 89	2.529 84	2.505 80
	N	43	33	76

Source: Reproduced with permission of International Business Machines Corporation.

between samples, and equal variances between subgroups. The added assumption is that there is a second categorical variable for which we want to assess the statistical significance of any observed differences.

As before, we test for normality. The result is shown in Table 11.11. Both Kolmogorov–Smirnov and Shapiro–Wilk show $P > 0.05$. The null hypothesis is that the data are drawn from a population in which the underlying distribution of the observations is normal. So, we accept the null hypothesis, and proceed with the two-way analysis of variance.[23]

---

[23]The second test, for homogeneity of variances, will be generated when we undertake the two-way analysis of variance itself, so we don't need to look at it right now. Don't worry, all will be well. But you need to consider the outcome of the test to make sure you use the right set of statistical analyses.

Test procedure

Effectively, we are going to partition the sources of variance as we did in the one-way analysis of variance. I am not going to set out the mathematics of this procedure, as they are far more complicated than for the one-way analysis of variance. But you understand the principle: there are elements of variation in the observations that can be attributed to within group variation, and elements that can be attributed to between group variation. The difference with two-way analysis of variance is that we now have two sources of between group variation (diet and gender) rather than just one.

To save you lots of heartache and head scratching, I am going to look at the menus and output from SPSS. The starting point in SPSS is Analyze>General Linear Model>Univariate. This takes you to the menu shown in Figure 11.2.

TABLE 11.11   Analysis of Weight Loss Data for Normality

	Tests of Normality					
	Kolmogorov–Smirnov[a]			Shapiro–Wilk		
	Statistic	df	Sig.	Statistic	df	Sig.
Weight lost (kg)	0.062	76	0.200*	0.990	76	0.790

Source: Reproduced with permission of International Business Machines Corporation.
[a]Lilliefors Significance Correction.
*This is a lower bound of the true significance.

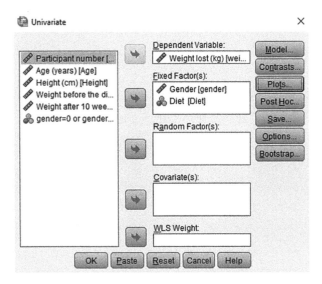

FIGURE 11.2   Introductory screen in SPSS for Analyze>General Linear Model>Univariate. *Source:* Reproduced with permission of International Business Machines Corporation.

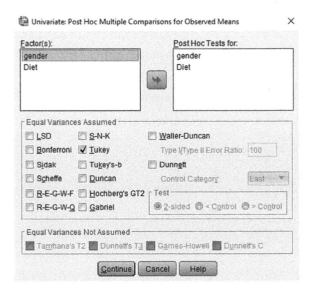

FIGURE 11.3   'Post hoc' menu for Analyze>General Linear Model>Univariate. *Source:* Reproduced with permission of International Business Machines Corporation.

The variables in the data set are listed in the box on the left-hand side.[24] The dependent variable is Weight Lost, and the two 'Factors' (the categorical variables whose impact we wish to explore) are Gender and Diet.

If we click on Post *Hoc*, we see the menu in Figure 11.3. Select Gender and Diet, and click on Tukey for the *post hoc* test. Click Continue.

Finally, from the starting Univariate menu, click on Options to generate the menu in Figure 11.4. Because we are interested not just in the differences between men and women and between diets but also in the interaction between diet and gender, select 'gender*Diet' for the 'Display means for': box. Tick 'Descriptive

---

[24]Data set 'Diet' used with permission, University of Sheffield. See ch11d02.sav in the online resources for Chapter 11. The link to the original data set is here: https://maths.shu.ac.uk/mathshelp/StatsTests/ANOVA.html

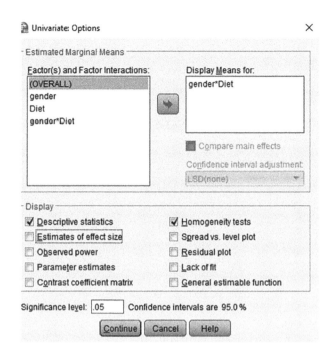

FIGURE 11.4 'Options' menu for Analyze>General Linear Model>Univariate. *Source:* Reproduced with permission of International Business Machines Corporation.

statistics' and 'Homogeneity tests' and click 'Continue'. Then click 'OK' or 'Paste'.[25]

The output that you generate will include several tables. I am not going to look at all of them, just the key ones that are similar to those that we looked at for one-way analysis of variance.

First, you will see a **Warning**. This says: 'Post hoc tests are not performed for Gender because there are fewer than three groups'. Fair enough. The *post hoc* tests (which groups means into subsets) can work only if you have three or more groups to

TABLE 11.12 Levene's Test of Equality of Error Variances

Levene's Test of Equality of Error Variances[a]			
Dependent Variable: Weight Lost (kg)			
F	df1	df2	Sig.
0.382	5	70	0.860

Source: Reproduced with permission of International Business Machines Corporation.
Tests the null hypothesis that the error variance of the dependent variable is equal across groups.
[a]Design: Intercept + gender + Diet + gender * Diet

compare. The second part of the output shows the results we saw in Table 11.10. Third, you will see the results for 'Levene's test of Equality of Error Variances' (Table 11.12). The model (as indicated in the footnote) includes both sets of categorical variable – gender and diet – as well as the interaction between them. As Sig.(P) = 0.860, we accept the null hypothesis that the variances of the groups are equal.

Finally, we see the analysis of variance table (Table 11.13). Do not blench.

Many elements in the table are similar to those for the one-way analysis of variance. The Source of the variance is shown in the first column. The sums of squares add up to the Total. The Mean Square values are the sums of squares divided by the number of degrees of freedom. The F value is the quotient of the mean square for each element of the Source (of the variance) divided by Error Mean Square (the unbiased estimate of variance independent of all the other sources of variation). This generates five values for F, each of which has a level of significance associated with the value and the numbers of degrees of freedom in the numerator and denominator.

The first two lines show F values for the 'Corrected model' and 'Intercept'. They are statistically significant (*Sig.* equals 0.007 and 0.000,[26]

---

[25]Because I am 'old-school', I like to have a copy of the syntax that I generate to run the analyses that I carry out. So, I click 'Paste' rather than 'OK'. This copies the syntax to an SPSS syntax file. This has two advantages. (i) You run the procedure from the syntax file. As you gain experience with SPSS, you get to learn what SPSS syntax looks like. With enough experience, you can begin to write your own. (ii) If you need to run the procedure again, you don't need to go back and click through the menus. If you want to make a minor adjustment to the syntax, you can just copy the block of syntax in the .sps file, make the change, and run it again.

[26]When SPSS says 'Sig. = 0.000,' it doesn't mean the probability of that outcome is equal to zero. It means, rather, that $P<0.0005$. If you round a value that is less than 0.0005 to three decimal places, you get 0.000.

TABLE 11.13   Two-Way Analysis of Variance Table Showing the Impact of Gender, Diet, and The Interaction Between Gender and Diet on Weight Lost

| | Tests of Between-Subjects Effects | | | | | |
| | Dependent Variable: Weight Lost (kg) | | | | | |
Source	Type III Sum of Squares	df	Mean Square	F	Sig.	Partial Eta Squared
Corrected model	94.600[a]	5	18.920	3.519	0.007	0.201
Intercept	1144.438	1	1144.438	212.874	0.000	0.753
Gender	0.428	1	0.428	0.080	0.779	0.001
Diet	49.679	2	24.840	4.620	0.013	0.117
Gender * Diet	33.904	2	16.952	3.153	0.049	0.083
Error	376.329	70	5.376			
Total	1654.350	76				
Corrected total	470.929	75				

Source: Reproduced with permission of International Business Machines Corporation.
[a]R squared = 0.201 (adjusted R squared = 0.144).

respectively) in the overall analysis. The 'Corrected model', (as we talked about in Chapter 4) takes into account the total sum of squares corrected for the means of the groups. This is the overall F test of whether there are differences between the groups and whether the intercept of the model is statistically significantly different from zero.[27] When we

look up the value for F (3.519) in Appendix A9 for df_1 (numerator) = 5 and df_2 (denominator) = 60 (we do not have a block in the Appendix for $df_2 = 75$, so I am using the nearest **lower** value in order to be statistically conservative, as the F values are larger), we see that the computed value for F is greater than the tabulated value for F when $P_{5,60,0.01} = 3.34$ and less than the value when $P_{5,60,0.005} = 3.76$. So, $0.005 < P < 0.01$, exactly what SPSS tells us ($P = 0.007$). On the basis of this test, we can reject the null hypothesis and accept the hypothesis at the 0.7% level and say that there are statistically significant differences between groups (gender and/or diet) and (possibly) in the interaction between gender and diet.

The next four rows will help us understand which groups are different from which other groups. The sources of variance are gender and diet; the interaction term (Gender * Diet) tells us if the impact of diet on weight loss is the same or different in men and women; and the error term is the best unbiased estimate of the variance for the sample as a whole. These rows are treated as they were for the one-way analysis of variance, that is, the mean squares of the sources of variance that we are interested in (gender, diet, and their interaction) are divided by the error

[27]The IBM SPSS support desk puts it like this: 'The Total Sums of Squares are sums of squares around 0, i.e. if you simply squared each value of the dependent variable and summed these squares, you would get the Total SS. The corrected Sums of Squares are the sums of squares around the grand mean of the dependent variable. If you subtracted the grand mean from each observation of the dependent variable and squared that deviation, the sum of these squared deviations would be the Corrected Total SS. It is 'corrected' for the grand mean. The Corrected model SS are sums of squares that can be attributed to the set of all the between-subjects effects, excluding the intercept, i.e. all the fixed and random factors and covariates and their interactions that are listed on the Between-Subjects table. These are sums of squares around the grand mean as well, and therefore the 'corrected model' SS. The F-test for the corrected model is a test of whether the model as a whole accounts for any variance in the dependent variable'.
Source: https://www.ibm.com/support/pages/corrected-model-sums-squares-unianova-and-glm-multivariate

mean square[28] to yield three F values of interest. These in turn are assessed for the probability of their occurrence if the null hypothesis is true (no differences between genders, no differences between diets, no interaction between gender and diet).

We can conclude that there are no differences between men and women in the impact of diet on weight loss (Sig. = 0.779); that there *are* differences between diets in their impact on weight loss (Sig. = 0.013); and that there is a borderline interaction between gender and diet (Sig. = 0.049), that is, the diets have a different impact in men compared with women. These statistical findings confirm the impression that we had from the mean values presented in Table 11.10. There are no overall differences in outcome between men and women, but there are differences between diets, which are different for men and women.

Lastly, we can identify the homogeneous subgroups for the dietary impact, as we did in the one-way analysis of variance (Table 11.14). There are two subgroups, with diets 2 and 1 in one group, and diet 3 in the other group. The Sig. = 0.999 for subset 1 tells us that impact of diets 2 and 1 is essentially the same – this is what we would expect to see if the null hypothesis were true.

To put a bit of icing on the cake, here is the graph that makes clear why the interaction gender*diet is statistically significant (even if it is of borderline significance, $P = 0.49$) (Figure 11.5):

In footnote '27', the description of the model mentions 'covariates'. We did not add any to the model, but in an experiment of this kind, we could have included age as a covariate, for example, or weight or BMI at the start of the study. This would have produced a more complex version of Table 11.13, with additional rows for the covariates and any interactions that were specified, but the same principles would have applied: you can discover the impact of

TABLE 11.14 Homogeneous Subsets Based on Tukey Analysis of the Impact of Diet, Taking Gender into Account

Weight lost (kg)			
Tukey HSD[a,b,c]			
Diet	N	Subset	
		1	2
2	25	3.2680	
1	24	3.3000	
3	27		5.1481
Sig.		0.999	1.000

Source: Reproduced with permission of International Business Machines Corporation.
Means for groups in homogeneous subsets are displayed.
Based on observed means.
The error term is Mean Square (Error) = 5.376.
[a]Uses Harmonic Mean Sample Size 25.273.
[b]The group sizes are unequal. The harmonic mean of the group sizes is used. Type I error levels are not guaranteed.
[c]Alpha = 0.05.

the covariates in relation to the outcome by finding values for F (covariate Mean Square divided by Error Mean Square) and the corresponding values for P.

11.5 N-WAY ANALYSIS OF VARIANCE AND BEYOND

There is not much to say here, except that we are now getting above our pay grade. Understand that we have been looking at relatively simple experimental models. There are many others

A warning!

If you spend time splashing around in SPSS trying to find your own way, it is likely you will quickly get out of your depth and drown. Be humble. You are not stupid, just unknowing. Let someone who has spent their entire career grappling with the complexities of statistical analysis guide you.

---

[28]The 'error mean square' is the equivalent to the Within Group mean square in the one-way analysis of variance. It is the best unbiased estimate of the variance of the population from which the observations were drawn (s^2) once the differences between the groups have been taken into account.

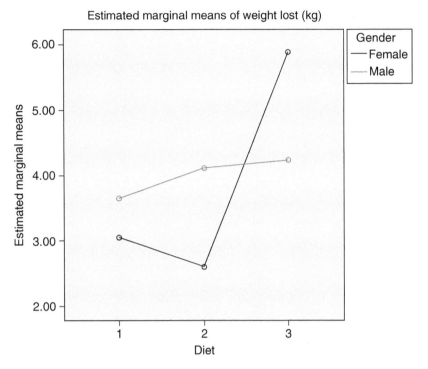

FIGURE 11.5   Mean weight loss by diet and gender. *Source:* Reproduced with permission of International Business Machines Corporation.

(repeat measures, mixed methods analysis of variance, etc.). It is beyond the scope of this text even to begin to describe the levels of complexity involved.

11.6 NONPARAMETRIC ANALYSIS OF VARIANCE

There will be times, of course, when the requirement to have a normally distributed variable for analysis of variance cannot be met: no amount of data transformation helps you to achieve the goal of generating a normally distributed variable. The fallback, therefore, is a nonparametric analysis of variance.

As we saw when we contrasted the *t*-test with its nonparametric equivalents (Mann–Whitney and Wilcoxon), the nonparametric tests are more conservative, that is, if you carry out a nonparametric analysis on a borderline *t*-test for which *P* is, say 0.049, there is a good possibility that the nonparametric test will lead you to accept the null hypothesis when

the *t*-test would have you reject it. This is because (as we have discussed in Chapter 7), ordinal data contain less information than scale (interval or ratio) data.

There are two options available for nonparametric analysis of variance: the Kruskal–Wallis test for unmatched (independent) sample data; and the Friedman test for matched (related) sample data. These are the extension of the Mann–Whitney test and the Wilcoxon test, respectively, when you have more than two groups. Kruskal–Wallis compares medians, while Friedman's compares distributions (the shapes of the histograms, if you like, and their position on the scale of the outcome variable).

You now understand the principles that govern comparisons of more than two groups: you use all the information from the observations across all the samples (whether related or independent) to decide if it is likely that the samples were drawn from the same or identical populations. I am not going to take you through the manual calculations of

Hypothesis test summary

	Null Hypothesis	Test	Sig.	Decision
1	The distribution of days is the same across categories of group	Independent-samples Kruskal–Wallis test	0.052	Retain the null hypothesis

Asymptotic significances are displayed. The significance level is 0.05

FIGURE 11.6 SPSS output for Kruskal–Wallis analysis. *Source:* Reproduced with permission of International Business Machines Corporation.

Kruskal–Wallis or Friedman, as their basis is similar to that for the Mann–Whitney and Wilcoxon tests. Moreover, SPSS provides a direct analysis of your raw data. You do not have to transform your observations to ordinal data if they are scale measurements, as SPSS does the transformation behind the scenes. The sequence for selection is Analyze>Nonparametric Tests>Independent Samples (for Kruskal–Wallis) or Analyze>Nonparametric Tests>Related Samples (for Friedman's). In the more recent versions of SPSS (v.24 onwards), when you select nonparametric tests for more than two groups, SPSS looks at the data to decide which test is the best fit for the data. You simply specify whether your samples are independent (for the Kruskal–Wallis test) or related (for Friedman's test).

The SPSS output for the nonparametric tests is very simple compared with that for one-way and two-way analysis of variance. **For illustrative purposes only**, I have analyzed the laparoscopic gastroscopy data using the Kruskal–Wallis test.[29] The results are shown in Figure 11.6.

[29]As I said earlier, you should **NEVER** 'shop around' for significant *P* values using different tests. You should always use only one test for your statistical analysis, the test that best fits the data. If you start shopping around for the test that gives you the *P* value that you want to see (usually one that shows statistical significance), you will get into serious trouble with the God of Statistics. We will discuss this in Chapter 13. When I say, 'For illustrative purposes only', I mean I am analyzing a data set with which you are familiar (but for which we demonstrated normality) simply to show you what the nonparametric analysis of variance looks like. **We know** that the data meet the assumptions for one-way analysis of variance (data in the parent population from which the sample is drawn are normally distributed) so that is the test we **should** (rightly) be using.

You can now see two things. The first part of the Kruskal–Wallis output (Figure 11.6) suggests that you should accept the null hypothesis, whereas the one-way analysis of variance suggested the null hypothesis should be rejected (in Table 11.15, Sig. = 0.049). This illustrates what I was saying above about the nonparametric test being more conservative than the parametric test. If you apply both tests to the same data, you are more likely to accept the null hypothesis using the nonparametric test.[30]

Second, if you want clarity regarding the interpretation of the analysis, the subsidiary output from SPSS[31] (Figure 11.7) shows a graph which plots the medians and the limits of the range (box-and-whisker plot), and a table showing the test statistic *H*, which follows the chi-squared distribution with two degrees of freedom (because we have three groups, so $\nu = k - 1 = 3 - 1 = 2$).

The SPSS output from the Friedman's test is very similar to that from Kruskal–Wallis. As we have not explored analysis of variance for matched data, I will not illustrate it here. Given the aims of this book, suffice it to say that you are entering the realms of analysis where you should be consulting a statistician for advice.

11.7 EXERCISES

Given that there is perfectly good software to undertake one-way and two-way analysis of variance, it

[30]Now re-read footnote 29.
[31]In the SPSS output file, double-click on the first part of the output (as illustrated in Figure 11.6) to see the subsidiary output (as illustrated in Figure 11.7).

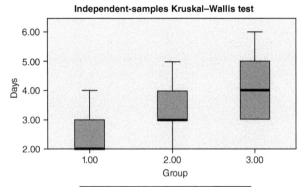

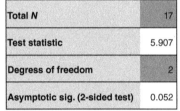

Total N	17
Test statistic	5.907
Degress of freedom	2
Asymptotic sig. (2-sided test)	0.052

1. The test statistic is adjusted for ties.
2. Multiple comparisons are not performed because the overall test does not show significant differences across samples.

FIGURE 11.7   Subsidiary SPSS output for Kruskal–Wallis analysis. *Source:* Reproduced with permission of International Business Machines Corporation.

would be cruel and unnatural to ask you to do the calculations for ANOVA by hand. For the exercises for this chapter, use SPSS with the data set for this exercise (ch11e01.sav).

11.7.1

Four groups of amateur cyclists were arguing about the impact of carbohydrate intake on their performance. The levels of performance were different for each group, '1' indicating the lowest level and '4' the

TABLE 11.15   Carbohydrate Intake (g/d) in Four Groups of Cyclists

Group	Carbohydrate intake (g/d)			
	1	2	3	4
	279	378	172	381
	338	275	335	346
	334	412	335	340
	198	265	282	471
	303	286	250	318

highest. The club nutritionist measured their diet using a food frequency questionnaire and obtained the results shown in Table 11.15.

Set out the data for analysis in SPSS using Analyze>Compare Means>Oneway ANOVA.

1. Show the mean, standard deviation, and other relevant statistics for each group.
2. Are there statistically significant differences between the groups?
3. Should you carry out *post hoc* tests?

REFERENCES

1. Hald, Anders. *A History of Mathematical Statistics.* Wiley. New York. 1998. ISBN 0-471-17912-4.
2. Box, Joan Fisher. *R. A. Fisher: The Life of a Scientist.* Wiley. 1978. ISBN 0-471-09300-9.
3. Fisher, Ronald. *Statistical Methods for Research Workers.* Oliver and Boyd. Edinburgh. p. 47. 1925. ISBN 0-05-002170-2.

PART 3

DOING RESEARCH

Introduction

Part 3 deals with the design and presentation of research.

Chapter 12 adds to the design ideas presented in Part 1, particularly randomization of procedures to complement the randomization of sampling that we discussed in Chapter 2. We also look at how to determine the size of sample that will give you the best chances of finding a statistically significant result, if one exists (that is, you are doing the right thing in rejecting the null hypothesis).

Chapter 13 is quite short, essentially a series of exercises in which you are given a brief description of a study and asked to choose which is the right statistical test to use, with the help of a useful flow chart.

In Chapter 14, you are invited to design a research protocol. The chapter is set out as an extended tutorial (for indeed, that is what it was). You are asked to design a student-sized research project (i.e. not too ambitious) and to reflect on your work with a tutor or mentor. The work should be both challenging and fun. If you complete all of the stages, you will have a viable working proposal. The work will draw upon all of the preceding chapters, helping to ensure that you don't miss out any critical component and that your protocol is comprehensive, thorough, and robust.

The last chapter (Chapter 15) explores ideas for presenting your results to a variety of audiences. This is just toe-in-the-water stuff, with a number of examples from both raw data and published papers. There is much more to presenting than we have space to deal with, but there is plenty of guidance out there about how to make your presentation or report writing engaging, clear, and truthful.

By the time you have completed this section, you should feel confident about using the language of statistics and the principles of design to help you engage in real-time research. You should also recognize that there is no shame in not knowing exactly what you should do before you have had experience. Research is very much a learning process. It should always be a collaborative effort, working with people whose skills and experience can you help you achieve the best outcomes.

Statistics in Nutrition and Dietetics, First Edition. Michael Nelson.
© 2020 John Wiley & Sons Ltd. Published 2020 by John Wiley & Sons Ltd.
Companion website: www.wiley.com/go/nelson/statistics

CHAPTER 12

Design, Sample Size, and Power

Learning Objectives

After studying this chapter, you should be able to:

- Know when to use Randomized Block, Latin Square, and Factorial designs
- Understand how to calculate sample size for different experimental settings
- Understand the concept of Power
- Know how to calculate Power and sample size for different experimental designs and analysis

12.1 RANDOMIZATION OF PROCEDURES

Sampling randomizes the choice of subjects to generate a sample which is representative of the population (i.e. random and independent). There is,

however, another side to randomization. It is also necessary to randomize procedures to obtain results that are:

1. free from experimental bias which may be, for example, related to the order of treatment, or the time of day at which treatments are given
2. representative of all possible experimental results which could be obtained under similar experimental conditions.

The purpose of randomization of procedures is to obtain results which take into account factors that may influence the measured outcome but are not of primary interest. In statistical terms, we are talking about sources of error (variance) that can be identified and separated out in statistical analyses. We shall look at some examples below.

There are many established approaches to the process of randomization of procedure. A few of the more common examples are shown in Table 12.1.

Statistics in Nutrition and Dietetics, First Edition. Michael Nelson.
© 2020 John Wiley & Sons Ltd. Published 2020 by John Wiley & Sons Ltd.
Companion website: www.wiley.com/go/nelson/statistics

251

TABLE 12.1   Types of Randomization of Procedure

Design	Test
Randomized block	Two-way ANOVA
Latin square	Modified two-way ANOVA
Factorial	Complex analysis
Systematic square	**DO NOT USE!!**

12.1.1 Randomized Block Design

Farmers have always wanted to know if one variety of a crop can produce higher yields than another. Say I have a field where I want to carry out an experiment with two varieties of seeds, A and B, to see which has a higher yield. A picture of my field is shown in Figure 12.1.

I sow my two crops, as shown in Figure 12.2. I harvest the crop, get a higher yield for B, and conclude that B is the better crop.

Is this a valid finding? What if (without my being aware) there was a patch of more fertile ground in my field (Figure 12.3)? One possibility is that B outperformed A on its own merits. The other explanation is that a higher proportion of B than A was on fertile ground. As an experimental design, it is a failure. What should I have done?

First, I could have divided the field into six blocks. I could then have sown half of each block with seed A and half with seed B. Just to be on the safe side, I could have sown A on the left-hand side in alternating blocks, and B on the left-hand side in the remaining blocks (Figure 12.4). This addresses the possibility that there is another strip of fertility running from top to bottom on one side of the field.

This is a much more robust experimental design. It addresses the possibility that an unwanted ('nuisance') factor might undermine my conclusions. Other potential nuisance factors (hours of sunshine, centimetres of rainfall) are likely to be the same for the entire field, so I don't need to take these into account.

In terms of statistical analysis, I would use a two-way analysis of variance. The outcome is yield

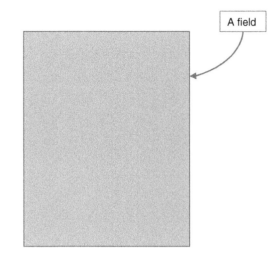

FIGURE 12.1   A field.

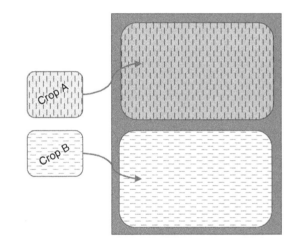

FIGURE 12.2   A field sown with two crops.

(kg/hectare). The two factors are variety (A or B) and block (1–6). Even if there were differences in yield between blocks (there could well be), any statistically significant differences in observed yield between varieties would be independent of the impact of the block. That's what I am after, statistically speaking.

Similar requirements arise in many nutritional experiments. Gender is often an important factor. In the example in Chapter 11 looking at the impact of diet on weight loss (Table 11.10), if I had studied men only I would have concluded that there was no difference between the impact of the diets, whereas

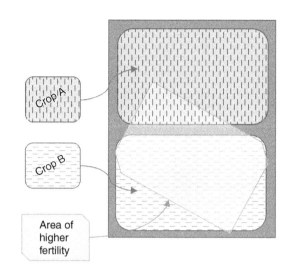

FIGURE 12.3 A field with an unknown fertile patch sown with two crops.

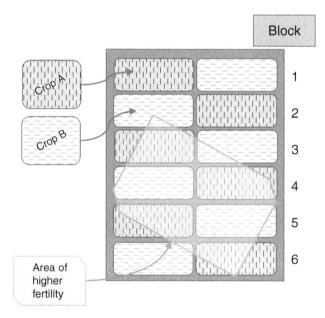

FIGURE 12.4 A field with an unknown fertile patch sown with two crops in a randomized block design.

if I had studied women only I would have concluded Diet 3 was more effective than Diet 1 and Diet 2.

Disease status can also constitute a series of blocks. Different stages of cancer, different levels of heart disease, different diagnostic categories, all represent 'blocks'. For example, the impact of the administration of different levels of anti-oxidant

TABLE 12.2 Number of Subjects in Each Block of Administration of Three Levels of Anti-oxidant Vitamins in Patients with PAD

Diabetic Status	Level of Supplement		
	Low	Medium	High
Nondiabetic	6	6	6
Prediabetic	6	6	6
Type 2 diabetes	6	6	6

vitamins on lower limb blood flow in men with peripheral arterial disease diagnosed by ankle brachial index assessment may differ according to diabetic status. Subjects with Type 2 diabetes may respond differently from subjects who are prediabetic or nondiabetic. The model therefore has three blocks (diabetic status) and three treatments (level of supplement) (Table 12.2). In this particular study, my aim is to have six patients in each group.[1]

Again, two-way analysis of variance will help us discover if and how the impact of the intervention is related to the type of intervention and the status of the subjects. Other factors that might have an influence on the outcome, such as age, weight, BMI, smoking habits, etc. can be added into the model as covariates, as they may have in influence on the outcome but will not necessarily be evenly distributed across all the groups.

12.1.2 Latin Square Design

This is often used in agricultural experiments where the number of animals and the number of treatments is equal. It can also be used in human nutrition. For example, suppose we have six members of an expert taste panel testing six varieties of a product (labelled A–F). We need to randomize the order of tasting across the members of the panel so that any potential interactions associated with tasting one specific sample (say sample D) after another specific

---

[1]The sample size will depend on how much variation I expect to see in each group. We will address this later in the chapter when we look at Power and sample size.

TABLE 12.3   Latin Square Design for Six Taste Panel Experts to Test Six Related Product Samples

Expert Panel Member	Product Sample					
	1	2	3	4	5	6
1	F	C	E	D	B	A
2	D	B	C	F	A	E
3	A	D	B	E	C	F
4	C	F	D	A	E	B
5	B	E	A	C	F	D
6	E	A	F	B	D	C

sample (say C) are minimized. This can be done using a Latin Square design, as shown in Table 12.3.[2]

This sequence is one of many.[3] The point is, it randomizes the sequence in such a way as to ensure that every taster gets to test every product (all rows and all columns contain the letters A–F in a 6×6 Latin Square) but the sequence is different for every taster and there is no circumstance in which the two products are tasted in the same succession for every taster.

Statistical analysis uses a modified form of a two-way analysis of variance to assess differences between products and tasters. Again, you will need to consult your friendly statistician to make sure you get the analysis right.

12.1.3 A Thing **Not** to Do

As a child, I used to generate random sequences for games that I played with friends.[4] The idea was simple: I wanted to make sure everyone got a turn at X.

---

[2]In the old days, I would have had a handy book of Latin Squares and, for a given $n \times n$ design, would have chosen one (literally) at random for my experiment. The internet, of course, provides a quick and easy way to do this. I used https://hamsterandwheel.com/grids/index2d.php for this example.

[3]I am not going to say how many. There is a debate amongst mathematicians and game players as to how to count unique Latin Squares for a given $n \times n$ design.

[4]Sad, I know, but I was a nerdy kid and wanted to be 'fair'. You can also imagine there were lots of arguments about who went first at what.

TABLE 12.4   A Systematic Square for Four Friends and Four Games

Friend	Game			
	1	2	3	4
1	A	B	C	D
2	B	C	D	A
3	C	D	A	B
4	D	A	B	C

If there were four of us playing, and there were four games, my square might look like Table 12.4.

While this may have worked well for a bunch of 9-year-olds, it makes for a lousy experimental design. The problem is that although everyone gets to do everything, if you perform better at D having done C, friend four is at a disadvantage. More to the point, if this is a design for a 4×4 tasting panel, and the taste of D is influenced by having eaten C, the taste of D would not be independently assessed, and taster 4 may come up with a different result for D compared with the others, whose observations could not be regarded as independent.

The design in Table 12.4 is a *systematic square*. It is one of the 4×4 Latin Squares, but one to avoid because of the potential repetition of interactions. When using Latin Squares in your design protocol, make sure that you avoid using systematic squares.

12.1.4 Factorial Design

This allows for testing combinations of treatments to see if the outcome is superior to treatments given individually. It is commonly used in drug trials.

Suppose I have two treatments: A and B. A factorial design would require four groups of patients for treatment:

- Active A, Active B
- Active A, Placebo B
- Placebo A, Active B
- Placebo A, Placebo B

This would allow me to explore the relative impact of A and B separately and in combination against a control group (placebo A, placebo B). Again, you should seek a statistician's help to undertake the analysis.

12.2 SAMPLE SIZE

It is vital at the planning stage to know how many observations will be needed to detect a statistically significant result at a given level of significance. There are effectively three conditions which one may wish to satisfy. The first two relate to observations within samples. The third relates sample observations to population values and is the one most commonly used.

12.2.1 Obtain a Standard Error of a Given Size

This is the simplest condition and is used when the aim is to relate a sample mean to some fixed standard or reference.

The standard error of the mean, $SE = \sigma / \sqrt{n}$. Solve for n:

$$n = \frac{\sigma^2}{SE^2}$$

EQUATION 12.1 Formula for sample size if you know the standard deviation of the population, σ, and the size of the difference between a sample mean and a reference value that you want to be statistically significant at a given level, in terms of number of standard errors

If the aim is to obtain a value for SE less than a given value (the *error term*, e), then Equation 12.1 can be re-written using e, and my sample size n needs to be:

$$n > \frac{\sigma^2}{e^2}$$

For example, suppose that you want to know if the mean intake of calcium for a group of women is significantly below 700 mg/d (the reference value, R). Assume (from the literature on calcium intake in women) that the value for $\sigma = 300$ mg/d. If the predicted mean intake for the group of women is about 600 mg/d, then the size of the difference between the reference measure and the actual intake is 100 mg/d. For this to be statistically significant at the 5% level, the difference needs to be at least 1.96 SE, that is, the mean for the measured intake should have a confidence interval (based on the population standard deviation) which *does not* include the reference value.

The formula for the 95% confidence interval around the population mean μ is:

$$95\% CI(\mu) = \bar{x} \pm 1.96 \times SE$$

We can use 1.96 because we know the value for σ, the true population standard deviation. If the difference between $\bar{x}$ and the reference value is to exceed 1.96 SE, then the value for e in the formula above needs to be no greater than the difference between $\bar{x}$ and the reference value (R) divided by 1.96, that is $e \leq |\bar{x} - R|/1.96$. The vertical bars indicate modulus or absolute value (i.e. ignore the sign of the difference). Using the data above, $e \leq |\bar{x} - R|/1.96 = |600 - 700|/1.96 = 100/1.96 = 51.02$.

So

$$n > \sigma^2 / e^2 = 300^2 / 51.02^2 = 90\,000 / 2\,603.04 = 34.57.$$

The sample therefore needs to contain at least 35 subjects (we need to round up to the nearest integer) if we want to be able to demonstrate that a sample mean of 600 mg/d is statistically significantly different from the reference value, 700 mg/d. If we follow through by calculating the 95% CI for μ around the sample mean, we find it is:

$$95\% CI(\mu) = \bar{x} \pm 1.96 \times SE = 600 \pm 1.96 \times \frac{\sigma}{\sqrt{n}}$$

$$= 600 \pm 1.96 \times \frac{300}{\sqrt{35}}$$

$$= 600 \pm 99.4 = 500.61,\ 699.4$$

The confidence interval for the sample around $\bar{x} = 600$ mg/d does not include the reference value $R = 700$ mg/d. So, we could say that for a sample size of 35, we could be confident that the mean of the sample is statistically significantly below the reference value at the 5% level of confidence. All well and good.

Last point: if the mean for the sample was greater than 600 mg/d, the value for e would be less than 51.02, the value for n would be greater than 34.57 and, accordingly, we would need more subjects to be able to demonstrate a statistically significant difference between the sample mean and the reference value.[5]

12.2.2 Given Difference Between Sample Means to be Significant

This can be used when you have two sample means which you believe will differ by a given amount. You want to make sure you have enough observations to show a statistically significant difference. We will use the calcium intake data from the previous example.

Suppose you want to be able to demonstrate that the difference between two sample means, $\bar{x}_1$ and $\bar{x}_2$, is greater than a given value, that is: $|\bar{x}_1 - \bar{x}_2| > d$. Then:

$$d > Z_{\alpha/2}\sigma\sqrt{\frac{2}{n}}$$

EQUATION 12.2   Formula to achieve the minimum value for d (the difference between two sample means) at a given level of statistical significance corresponding to $Z_{\alpha/2}$ (the standard normal deviate) if you know σ (the standard deviation of the population) and n (the minimum sample size in each group)

[5]I understand this can be a bit brain-tangling. Re-read this section until it makes sense to you, as the following sections depend on your understanding of the concepts being presented here.

If we choose $Z_{\alpha/2} = 1.96$,[6] and we know σ (the standard deviation of the population) and n (the minimum sample size in each group), we want to be able to demonstrate a statistically significant difference between sample means at the 5% level.

We solve for n:

$$n > 2\left(\frac{Z_{\alpha/2}\sigma}{d}\right)^2$$

EQUATION 12.3   Formula for sample size n (the size of the smallest group) if you know σ (the standard deviation of the population), and the size of the difference between two sample means, d, that you want to say is statistically significant at a given level

For example, if $\bar{x}_1 = 600$ mg/d and $\bar{x}_2 = 800$ mg/d, then $d = 200$ mg/d. If, as before, we say that $\sigma = 300$ mg/d and $Z_{\alpha/2} = 1.96$, then

$$n > 2\left(\frac{Z_{\alpha/2}\sigma}{d}\right)^2 = 2\times\left(\frac{1.96\times300}{200}\right)^2 = 17.29$$

The minimum number of subjects needed would be 18 *per group* to be able to demonstrate a difference between the two group means that was statistically significant at the 5% level.

If the difference were only 100 mg/d, as in Section 12.2.1, but instead of one of the values being a reference value both values are sample means, then the equation for n above would yield a value for $n = 69.15$, so the number of observations per group would need to be 70. This is equivalent to saying that we now have two 95% Confidence Intervals which must not overlap, so we need twice the number of observations compared with the previous calculation to ensure a small enough SE in each group.

[6]The value 1.96, you may recall, is the value for u (the standard normal deviate) outside of which (in both tails) 5% of observations fall in a normally distributed variable, or outside of which 5% of sample means fall. The symbol Z is also used to indicate the standard normal deviate that corresponds to $\frac{1}{2}P$. The numbers in the tables for Z and u differ only in that they reflect different parts of the area under the curve.

If you know the size of the difference between two sample means and the value for the standard error of the difference between two means, $SE_{diff} = \sigma_0 \sqrt{1/n_1 + 1/n_2}$, then using the logic above you can find the value for e by which to calculate n. If we wish to establish that a difference of 100 mg/d is statistically significant between two groups, then the minimum sample size per group must be $n > (2 \times \sigma^2)/e^2$. To achieve a statistically significance difference at the 5% level, the confidence intervals for the difference between the means should be $(\bar{x}_1 - \bar{x}_2) \pm 1.96 \times SE$, so $e < 100/1.96 = 51.02$ and $n > 2\sigma^2/e^2 = (2 \times 100^2)/51.02^2 = 69.15$. As before, we would require 70 subjects *per group* to be confident of finding a statistically significant difference between the samples whose means differed by 100 mg/d.

12.2.3 Given Power Against Specified Difference Between Population Means

I know parents aren't supposed to have a favourite child. The same is true of authors, I think. There shouldn't be one part of a book that is favoured above all others. But I have to tell you, reader, that the next section on Power really is my favourite section in the entire book. Power is so well-behaved, and so clever, and so useful (like the model child), that I can't get enough of it. I hope you enjoy it as much as I do. Read slowly and carefully, to appreciate its full character. It's all about

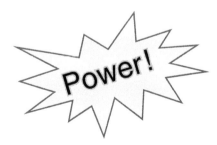

FIGURE 12.5   Power.

The example in Section 12.2.2, when estimating sample size, started with the premise that the *sample* means differ from each other. But it would be more sensible, wouldn't it (yes, it would), to be sure that the *population* means differed, not just the sample means. To undertake this calculation, we need to invoke the concept of **Power**. What is Power? Power is the chance of detecting a statistically significant result *if one exists*.

Up till now, we have been dealing with level of significance, P, which relates to our ability to reject a true null hypothesis. We know that when $P = 0.05$, at the 5% level, there is a 5% chance that we are making a mistake when we reject the null hypothesis. That is, we might reject the null hypothesis when it is in fact true. This is a Type I error. But what if the null hypothesis is false? We *would* want to reject it. But what chance is there of accepting a false null hypothesis? This is a Type II error: the incorrect *acceptance* of a false null hypothesis.

Power reflects the probability that we are making the correct decision in rejecting a false null hypothesis. By introducing Power into our deliberations, we are effectively 'hedging our bets', that is, choosing a sample size that gives us the best chance of coming up with the correct answer whether H_0 is true or H_0 is false. These ideas, and the terms used, are summarized in Table 12.5.

Table 12.5 is wildly important! It is based on two axioms. First, the null hypothesis is either true or false. It cannot be both. If that is the case, then it stands to reason that the probabilities of a Type I error and a Type II error are independent. Hence, α and β are independent. So, when we determine how big we want our sample to be, we can decide at what level we want to set the probability of both types of error. By convention, the *largest* value for P at which we reject the null hypothesis is 0.05. This means that the chance of making a Type I error is 5% or (hopefully) less. Similarly, the *largest* value (by convention) that we select for β is 0.2. This means that there is a 20% chance of the incorrect acceptance of a false null hypothesis.

We can redefine that concept as *Power*, equal to $(1 - \beta) \times 100$. If β equals 0.2, it means there is an 80% chance that you will be making a *correct* decision when you reject a false null hypothesis. You are giving yourself a four out of five chance that you will correctly reject a false null hypothesis. You can, of course, opt for higher values for Power (90% or 95%)

TABLE 12.5   The Relationships between H_0, *P* Value (also Referred to as α), Power, and Type I and Type II Errors

The True Situation	The Decision	
	Accept H_0	Reject H_0
H_0 **is true**	Correct decision: Probability = $1 - \alpha$	Type I error: Probability = α (level of significance)
H_0 **is false**	Type II error: Probability = β	Correct decision: Probability = $1 - \beta$ POWER = $(1-\beta) \times 100$

to reduce the chances of a Type II error, in the same way that you can opt for lower cut-off points for *P* (0.02, 0.01, etc.) to reduce the chances of a Type I error. The smaller the value for *P*, or the higher the Power you want to achieve, the bigger your sample will need to be.

12.2.4 Calculating Sample Size using P and Power

In Section 12.2.2, when determining the minimum sample size that we would need to assess if a statistically significant difference between two sample means exists, we took into account only the value for *P* set at 0.05 (hence we chose $Z_{\alpha/2} = 1.96$). Assume now that our aim is to detect a statistically significant difference between two population means, that is $d > \mu_1 - \mu_2$. Now we need to consider values for $Z_{\alpha/2}$ (relating to the value for *P*, which is two-tailed) *and* Z_β (relating to the value for β, which is one-tailed).[7]

The formula that relates $Z_{\alpha/2}$, Z_β, *d*, and *n* is:

$$Z_{\alpha/2} \times \sigma \sqrt{\frac{2}{n}} < d - Z_\beta \times \sigma \sqrt{\frac{2}{n}}$$

EQUATION 12.4   The relationship between $Z_{\alpha/2}$, Z_β, *d* (the difference between two population means, $\mu_1 - \mu_2$), and *n* (the minimum number of observations needed in *each* sample)

[7]I have added an annex at the end of this chapter to explain why α is two-tailed and β is one-tailed.

Note that this looks very similar to Equation 12.2, but we have added a new term to take Power into account. If we want to know sample size, we rearrange Equation 12.4 to $d > \left(Z_{\alpha/2} + Z_\beta \right) \times \sigma \sqrt{2/n}$ and then solve for *n*, the minimum sample size *per group*:

$$n > \frac{2\sigma^2 \left(Z_{\alpha/2} + Z_\beta \right)^2}{d^2}$$

EQUATION 12.5   Formula for sample size if you know σ (the standard deviation of the population), $Z_{\alpha/2}$ (level of statistical confidence to be achieved), Z_β (level of Power to be achieved), and *d* (the difference between two population means, $\mu_1 - \mu_2$)

Let's look at an example.

In assessing treatment of anaemia in rural women tea plantation workers in the Cameroon, the mean haemoglobin level was 10.0 g/dl, and the standard deviation, $\sigma = 1.5$.[8] If the women were randomly allocated to two groups, and one group was given an iron supplement, and the other group a placebo, how many subjects would be needed to show that a Hb of 11.0 g/dl in the iron supplement group was statistically significantly different from the Hb in the placebo group (assuming it stayed at 10.0 g/dl), at $P = 0.05$ and with a Power of (i) 80% or (ii) 90%?

As we established above, the number of subjects required is $n > 2\sigma^2(Z_{\alpha/2} + Z_\beta)^2/d^2$. If $P = 0.05$ then $Z_{\alpha/2} = 1.96$, and if we want to achieve a Power of 80%

[8]In most circumstances, you will need to estimate σ by looking in the literature for published values which relate to the variable you are interested in. Of course, you will not find *exact* values for σ, but you will find a range of values for standard deviation in different articles. Choose a value for σ that you think is representative. A very high value for σ will, of course, increase the value that you calculate for *n*, thereby increasing the likelihood of having a high Power to your study. But choosing the largest published value for standard deviation is not necessarily the most representative, so use common sense. In the text below is the alternative formula for circumstances when a value for σ is not available and you can only estimate the coefficient of variation (CV%).

TABLE 12.6   Values for $(Z_{\alpha/2}+Z_\beta)^2$ used in the Calculation of Sample Size According to Levels of α (Probability of Making a Type I Error) and β (Probability of Making a Type II Error) and Power $((1-\beta)\times100)$. Values for $Z_{\alpha/2}$ are two-tailed, values for Z_β are one-tailed (see Annex).

	Beta	0.2	0.1	0.05
	Power	80%	90%	95%
	Z_β	0.842	1.282	1.645
Alpha	$Z_{\alpha/2}$			
0.05	1.96	7.85	10.51	13.00
0.01	2.576	11.68	14.88	17.82
0.001	3.291	17.08	20.91	24.36

(i.e. $\beta=0.2$), and Power$=1-\beta$, then $\beta=0.2$, $Z_\beta=0.842$, and $(Z_{\alpha/2}+Z_\beta)^2=7.85$ (see Table 12.6).

So $n>(2\times1.5^2\times7.85)/1.0^2=35.3$, and at least 36 subjects *per group* would be required. If Power $=90\%$, then $(Z_{\alpha/2}+Z_\beta)^2=10.51$, and $n>47.295$, so at least 48 subjects would be required per group.

If you had the resources to study only 30 subjects, then you could solve Equation 12.4 to work out the Power (i.e. the chance of finding a statistically significant difference if one exists) by solving for Z_β.

$Z_\beta=\left(d\sqrt{n/2}/\sigma\right)-Z_{\alpha/2}=1.0\sqrt{30/2}/1.5-1.96$, and in this example $Z_\beta=0.622$. Look this up in Appendix A2 for the normal distribution (for one tail, i.e. use $\frac{1}{2}P$), and you find (with a little interpolation) that the probability of $\beta=0.2669$, so Power $=1-\beta=0.7331$, or around 73%. At this level of Power, you might decide not to do the study (you have only a three-in-four chance of detecting a statistically significant result if one exists). Alternatively, if you think you will be able to show a change in Hb of 1.5 g/dl, then $Z_\beta=1.913$, $\beta=0.0279$, and the Power will be over 97%.

If we consider the example relating to calcium from Section 12.2.2, where $\sigma=300$ mg/d and $d=100$ mg/d, then $n>(2\times300^2\times7.85)/100^2=141.3$, or 142 subjects per group. This is 72 more subjects than in the estimate we made in Section 12.2.2,

when we did not include Power in our calculation. The larger sample size will ensure that given sampling variation, if a true difference of 100 mg/d exists between sample means, we would have a four out of five (80%) chance in our study to detect it.

There are at least a zillion online routines for Power calculation. You don't need to do the calculations manually, but I have shown them in detail in this chapter to support your understanding of how Power is derived and used. Feel free to use the online calculators available – there is no need to martyr yourself on the altar of maths for maths sake. You will need two of the three elements – difference, standard deviation, number of observations per sample – to find the third. Use caution and, as usual, seek advice.

12.2.5 More Variations

Other formulae exist to determine:

- The number of sets of observations needed to establish a statistically significant correlation of a given size
- The number of subjects per group needed to establish a statistically significant difference in proportion between two groups
- The number of subjects per group needed to establish a statistically significant odds ratio in a case-control study
- The number of subjects per group needed to establish a statistically significant relative risk in a cohort study.

Table 12.7 shows the appropriate formula for use in each circumstance, with notes regarding the variables. If this is starting to feel a bit heavy weight, don't panic. It is by way of illustration, simply so that you don't try and use an inappropriate formula that you think might be a 'good enough' fit. As usual, my advice is to consult with a qualified statistician.

The formulae in Table 12.7 for the determination of n, Power and d for case-control, cohort and experimental studies correspond to the simplest study designs. Matching, in particular, introduces

TABLE 12.7 Formulae for Calculation of n, Z_β (for Power) or d, Given You Know Values for the Other Parameters in Each Case

Type of Comparison	Formula for Finding Sample Size (n per Group) for Given Values and Power. n is Minimum Sample Size	Formula for Finding Z_β (See Text on How to Calculate Power) for Given Values and n.	Formula for Finding d or r for Given n and Power. Relates to Smallest Value Likely to be Statistically Significant.	Comment
Significant difference between means	$n = \dfrac{2\sigma^2\left(Z_{\alpha/2}+Z_\beta\right)^2}{d^2}$	$Z_\beta = \dfrac{d\sqrt{n/2}}{\sigma} - Z_{\alpha/2}$	$d > \left(Z_{\alpha/2}+Z_\beta\right)\times\sigma\sqrt{\dfrac{2}{n}}$	See Table 12.6 for values for $(Z_{\alpha/2}+Z_\beta)^2$. Epidemiological studies: cross-sectional.
Statistically significant correlation	$n = \dfrac{\left(1-r^2\right)\left(Z_{\alpha/2}+Z_\beta\right)^2}{r^2} + 5$	$Z_\beta = \sqrt{\dfrac{r^2(n-5)}{1-r^2}} - Z_{\alpha/2}$	$r = \sqrt{\dfrac{\left(Z_{\alpha/2}+Z_\beta\right)^2}{\left(Z_{\alpha/2}+Z_\beta\right)^2 + n-5}}$	n is number of (x,y) pairs of observations. Epidemiological studies: ecological
Significant difference between proportions	$n = \dfrac{2\bar{p}(1-\bar{p})\left(Z_{\alpha/2}+Z_\beta\right)^2}{d^2}$	$Z_\beta = \dfrac{d\sqrt{n/2}}{\sqrt{\bar{p}(1-\bar{p})}} - Z_{\alpha/2}$	$d > \left(Z_{\alpha/2}+Z_\beta\right)\sqrt{\bar{p}(1-\bar{p})}\sqrt{\dfrac{2}{n}}$	For use with binary variables and two groups.[a] Epidemiological studies: Case-control.
Significant odds ratio	$n = \dfrac{2\bar{p}(1-\bar{p})\left(Z_{\alpha/2}+Z_\beta\right)^2}{d^2} \times \dfrac{r+1}{2r}$	$Z_\beta = \dfrac{d}{\sqrt{\bar{p}(1-\bar{p})}}\sqrt{\dfrac{nr}{r+1}} - Z_{\alpha/2}$	$d > \left(Z_{\alpha/2}+Z_\beta\right)\sqrt{\bar{p}(1-\bar{p})}\sqrt{\dfrac{r+1}{nr}}$	Formulae allow for one or more controls per case.[b] n is the number of cases. Epidemiological studies: Case-control, unmatched
Significant relative risk	$n = \dfrac{2\bar{p}(1-\bar{p})\left(Z_{\alpha/2}+Z_\beta\right)^2}{d^2} \times \dfrac{r+1}{2r}$	$Z_\beta = \dfrac{d}{\sqrt{\bar{p}(1-\bar{p})}}\sqrt{\dfrac{nr}{r+1}} - Z_{\alpha/2}$	$d > \left(Z_{\alpha/2}+Z_\beta\right)\sqrt{\bar{p}(1-\bar{p})}\sqrt{\dfrac{r+1}{nr}}$	Epidemiological studies: Cohort.[c]
Significant relative risk	$n = \dfrac{2\bar{p}(1-\bar{p})\left(Z_{\alpha/2}+Z_\beta\right)^2}{d^2}$	$Z_\beta = \dfrac{d\sqrt{n/2}}{\sqrt{\bar{p}(1-\bar{p})}} - Z_{\alpha/2}$	$d > \left(Z_{\alpha/2}+Z_\beta\right)\sqrt{\bar{p}(1-\bar{p})}\sqrt{\dfrac{2}{n}}$	Epidemiological studies: Experimental (intervention).[d]

Source: Cole [1]. Reproduced with permission of Oxford University Press.

[a] p_0 and p_1 are the proportions in the two groups. $d = p_1 - p_0$; $\bar{p} = (p_0 + p_1)/2$.

[b] p_0 and p_1 are the proportions of controls and cases exposed, respectively. Find $p_1 = (p_0 \times \text{OR})/(1 + p_0 \times (\text{OR} - 1))$, where p_0 and OR (Odds Ratio) are estimated from the literature. $d = p_1 - p_0$; $\bar{p} = (r \times p_0 + p_1)/(1 + r)$, where r is the number of controls per case. If $r = 1$, the formula is the same as that for the comparison of proportions (see Footnote a).

[c] p_0 and p_1 are the proportions of unexposed and exposed people who get the disease, respectively. $p_1 = p_0\text{RR}$, where RR is the relative risk. r = the ratio of the number of unexposed to exposed people in the population. $p_0 = \bar{p}(1 + r)/(\text{RR} + r)$. $d = p_1 - p_0$.

[d] p_0 is the proportion of placebo subjects succumbing to the disease, and $p_1 = p_0\text{RR}$, where RR is the effect of the treatment on disease rate.

further variations into the formulae (and tends to reduce the sample size needed). For further discussion on Power and sample size, see Chapter 3 (*Sampling, study size and power*) in Design Concepts in Nutritional Epidemiology [1].

There will be some circumstances in which no values for σ or decent estimates of standard deviation are published in the literature. It will then be necessary to use common sense to estimate the likely size of the difference (or other measure) in percentage terms. The value for σ can then be expressed as a CV (coefficient of variation which, of course, is the standard deviation expressed as a percentage of the mean). The formula for these alternate data is then:

$$n > \frac{2\text{CV}^2 \left(Z_{\alpha/2} + Z_{\beta} \right)^2}{\left(\%\text{difference} \right)^2}$$

EQUATION 12.5 Formula for sample size if you know CV (the coefficient of variation of the population), $Z_{\alpha/2}$ (level of statistical confidence to be achieved), Z_{β} (level of Power to be achieved), and %d (the difference between two population means, $\mu_1 - \mu_2$, expressed as a percentage)

Appropriate variations for all the formulae in Table 12.7 can be developed in a similar fashion for CV.

REFERENCE

1. Cole TJ. Sampling, study size, and power. In: Margetts BM and Nelson M. *Design Concepts in Nutritional Epidemiology*. 2nd edition. Oxford University Press. 1997.

Annex – why is β one-tailed?

P is two tailed. Throughout this book, when considering deviations in tests relating to the Normal or *t* distributions, we concluded that it is better scientifically to consider the deviation from zero in both directions rather than just in one direction. When the test statistic distribution is itself one-tailed (e.g. chi-squared, or the *F* statistic for analysis of variance), it is because we have squared values of the observations in the test procedure (for example $(O - E)^2$, $\sum \left(x_{ij} - \bar{x} \right)^2$), but we still assume that deviations that we see in the sample could be in either direction away from what we expect if the null hypothesis is true. Using a two-tailed approach is the more conservative position, statistically speaking, and the one that is safer to adopt, because it is associated with a lower risk of a Type I error. β, on the other hand, is one-tailed. Why?

If we make a Type 1 error, it is because we have decided that (for example) two group means are different when in fact they are the same (incorrect rejection of a true null hypothesis). The probabilities associated with this error are in both tails of the distribution of the values for $\bar{x}_1 - \bar{x}_2$ which we expect to centre around zero. We reject the null hypothesis if we are a long way from zero, in either direction, but there is always the chance we are making a Type I error, the probability of which we define by α. If, on the other hand, there really is a difference between the sample means, but we say there is not a difference (a Type II error, the incorrect acceptance of a false null hypothesis), the error that we have made can be in only one direction, between the value for the real difference (call it *d**) and zero, the value that we have incorrectly chosen to accept. The probability of this error, β, is therefore one-tailed.

We take our values for probabilities from the Normal distribution (Appendix A2). $Z_{\alpha/2}$ follows the distribution of *u*, the standard normal deviate. If we want to make the probability of a Type I error 0.05, then the value for α (also known as *P*) that we want is 0.05. The values tabulated in Appendix A2 are for ½P (the area in one tail of the distribution). The value in the table for *u* when ½P = 0.0250 is 1.96. So, when P = 0.05, $Z_{\alpha/2}$ = 1.96.

We want the value for Z_{β} to reflect the value for *u* in one tail of the area under the normal curve. So, if we want β = 0.2 (that is, Power = 80%), the value for *u* when the area in one tail is 0.2 is equal to 0.842.

CHAPTER 13

Describing Statistical Models and Selecting Appropriate Tests

Learning Objectives

After studying this chapter, you should be able to:

- Know how to describe statistical models
- Use the statistical flow chart to choose statistical tests appropriate for your model

13.1 DESCRIBING STATISTICAL MODELS

This is the shortest chapter in the book, but pithy and full of meaning. It is one that you will need to come back to time and again when confronted with a set of data for analysis. The chapter is in effect a short set of exercises getting you to describe data sets and choose the relevant statistical tests.

Assuming that you have all the necessary information about the study design, how the data were collected, and the hypothesis being tested, you must decide two things:

1. Which statistical model do the data best fit?
2. What can you infer about the populations from the sample data?

Each time you carry out an analysis, you must answer the questions in Box 13.1.

The answers to these questions will help you to establish how well your data fit a variety of statistical models. You must then decide what characteristics of the population you want to infer from the sample data and select the appropriate statistical tests from those which are available.

To help you with this, I have prepared a flow chart in Appendix A10 that is designed to help you select the appropriate statistical test for a given data set. The answers to the questions in Box 13.1 will

---

Statistics in Nutrition and Dietetics, First Edition. Michael Nelson.
Companion website: www.wiley.com/go/nelson/statistics

BOX 13.1

Questions about your data set
to be answered when seeking the best
statistical test

1. How many variables are there?
2. How many separate samples (groups) are there?
3. How many observations per subject have been made?
4. If there is more than one observation per subject, are the observations repeat measures or paired?
5. If there is one observation per subject in two or more samples, are the samples paired or unpaired (matched or unmatched)?
6. Are the data parametric or nonparametric?

---

lead you to the right test. For example, if you have one variable measured once in one sample, you may wish to know the central value and measure of spread (the 95% confidence interval or interquartile range, for example). First, you will need to decide if your sample is parametric or nonparametric. You can use common sense and your knowledge of the distribution of nutritional or biological variables to decide whether the data are likely to be normally or nonnormally distributed. To be on surer ground, you can plot the data and *see* whether or not they look normal. And of course, more formally, you can compare your data distribution to the binomial, Poisson, or normal distributions (using chi-squared, regression, and Kolmogorov–Smirnov one sample tests, respectively). These goodness-of-fit tests are available in SPSS. For tests of this type, SPSS does not require you to make a decision about the best test to use: if you select Analyze>Nonparametric Tests>One Sample, on the Objective tab choose *Automatically compare observed data to hypothesized*; on the Fields tab, select the data you want to test; and on the Settings tab choose *Automatically choose the tests based on the data*; then click on Paste (to save and inspect the syntax) or Run (if you are certain the parameters have been correctly selected). If you click on the Help button, you will get more information about the tests, their functionality, and

limitations. You can, if you prefer, specify which test you want.

When you have decided on the distribution characteristics of the data, you can determine the measures of central tendency and spread:

- If parametric, the mean and standard deviation (or standard error or 95% confidence interval, whichever is most helpful to the story you want to tell your audience)
- If nonparametric, the median and interquartile range, or proportion, or other relevant measure.

This systematic approach to characterizing any data set and knowing the type of test or comparison you want to undertake will allow you to determine which statistical model is appropriate.

The following pages contain brief descriptions of data sets or experiments and a question which illustrates the purpose for which the experiment was carried out. For each description, decide which statistical test or tests would be appropriate. If the description of the model seems incomplete, choose the *simplest* model that requires the fewest assumptions (e.g. if you are told that there are two samples but not whether or not they are paired, assume that they are not paired). The answers are given in Section 13.3.

Just before we start the exercise on selecting the right statistical test for your data, please read the warning about 'fishing' in Box 13.2.

13.2 CHOOSING STATISTICAL TESTS

Below are 14 descriptions of data with a question that needs to be answered. Use the flow chart in Appendix A10 to decide which statistical test you should use.[1]

---

[1] Another version of a flow chart that I like, and that links well to SPSS, can be found in Laerd Statistics (https://statistics.laerd.com/premium/sts/index.php). It is behind a paywall, but the wall is very low (£4.99 for 1 month, £8.99 for 6 months), so worth investigating. Once you get into it, the site is more friendly and explanatory than the SPSS help pages. It has lots of other good stuff about statistics generally, and tests and their limitations. See notes online relating to available software.

BOX 13.2

Do not go fishing to find statistically significant values of *P*

A stern warning

There is a strong temptation to go 'fishing' for statistically significant results. By that, I mean trying out different statistical tests until you find one that yields a *P* value less than 0.05. I described this type of danger in Box 11.4: by making lots of comparisons between pairs of means when carrying out post hoc tests in an analysis of variance, for example, you increase the risk of making a Type I error (incorrect rejection of a true null hypothesis).

There is only one model which your data fit, and only one statistical test that is relevant. If you start 'fishing', the *P* values that you determine will not necessarily reflect the true probability of observing what you have observed in relation to the null hypothesis.

However tempting, **DON'T DO IT!**

1. A group of 8 year-old children have had their height measured. What is the average height of children of this age in the population?

2. Two groups of 8 year-old children have their height measured. Is there a difference in height between the two groups?

3. Vitamin A intake was estimated by 24-hour recall in 500 middle-aged women. What was the average intake?

4. A group of children had their BMI measured at age 11 and again at age 16. How closely is BMI at age 16 associated with BMI at age 11?

5. Twelve subjects have their transit time measured before and after a 20 g/d bran supplement given over three weeks. Is there a significant change in mean transit time as a result of the supplement?

6. Eight pairs of rats are matched for sex and weight. One member of each pair is fed a low protein diet, the other a high protein diet. At the end of three months, the rats are timed as they run a maze. Most complete it in a short time, but a few take much longer. Is there a

significant effect of dietary protein on the time it takes to run the maze?

7. Three groups of subjects – thin, normal and obese – were given a standard lunch of 700 kcal, and their satiety measured two hours later on a scale from 0 (starving) to 100 (replete). Assume the satiety measure is normally distributed. Is there a significant difference in mean satiety at two hours between the groups?

8. 5000 Canadian lumberjacks categorized according to level of education – high school graduate, Bachelor's degree, or PhD – were given a questionnaire on nutritional knowledge and classified into three groups based on the results – good, average, and ignorant. Is there an association between level of education and nutritional knowledge?

9. Urinary ascorbate excretion was measured in two groups of women from different income groups. Was there a difference in median excretion between the groups?

10. Age–sex standardized mortality from cirrhosis of the liver was compared with average annual alcohol consumption in 15 countries. Is there a significant association between cirrhosis mortality and alcohol consumption?

11. 100 highly intelligent housewives were asked to say which of two brands of margarine they preferred. On average, was one brand preferred to the other?

12. 100 highly intelligent housewives were asked to say which of two brands of margarine they preferred. They were then given a Marxist tract on the value of highly poly-unsaturated vegetable oils to the development of third world economies, told which of the margarines was the approved Marxist variety, and asked to restate their preference. Did the tract alter their preference?

13. The level of fluoride present in drinking water (ppm) and the percentage of children aged 5–15 years without caries was measured in 20 towns. By how much does the percentage of children without caries vary according to the variation in fluoride levels?

14. Eighty 10-year-old children were matched for IQ in groups of four. In each group, the children were randomly assigned to one of four nutrition education programmes and assessed for changes in dietary behaviour after 6 months. Were changes in behaviour after 6 months different on the different programmes? Was IQ an important factor in response to the programmes?

13.3 SOLUTIONS

1. Mean and 95% CI
2. Unpaired t-test
3. Median and inter-quartile range
4. Pearson r
5. Paired t-test
6. Wilcoxon signed-rank test
7. One-way analysis of variance
8. Chi-squared test
9. Mann–Whitney test
10. Spearman ρ (rho)
11. Wilcoxon sign test
12. McNemar's test
13. Linear regression
14. Two-way analysis of variance

CHAPTER 14

Designing a Research Protocol

Learning Objectives

After studying this chapter, you should be able to:

- Design and set out a research protocol
- Understand and justify each element of the protocol
- Know how to tailor a protocol to the time and resources available
- Avoid being overambitious

14.1 INTRODUCTION

The notes in this chapter were prepared for students undertaking research suitable for undergraduate and MSc courses in nutrition and dietetics at King's College London. The purpose of this phase of the course was to develop a viable protocol for a research project that could be undertaken by the student. The timelines and details set out here provide a useful template for protocol development.

At PhD level, of course, you would go into much more detail and spend far more time than this chapter recommends.

14.2 THE RESEARCH PROTOCOL

There is no standard outline for a research protocol, but most protocols contain most of the following:

- A **TITLE** which makes clear the main area of research and study design
- The **BACKGROUND** to a topic that informs the reader about what has been done to date and describes a key bit of information missing that your research will address
- The **HYPOTHESIS** that is to be tested
- The **RATIONALE**, a concise paragraph about why the proposed research needs to be undertaken
- **STUDY DESIGN**. This describes the experimental approach you plan to use to test your hypothesis. It could be cross-sectional, or longitudinal, or compare two or more groups, or

Statistics in Nutrition and Dietetics, First Edition. Michael Nelson.
© 2020 John Wiley & Sons Ltd. Published 2020 by John Wiley & Sons Ltd.
Companion website: www.wiley.com/go/nelson/statistics

require an intervention and control group. It should be informed by previous research (as set out in the background) and explain how the research validates the rationale and is the right approach for testing the hypothesis.

- **AIMS and OBJECTIVES**. The **Aim** provides a clear, simple, one sentence statement of your overall purpose. If you can't put your Aim into a single sentence, or at most two, you might need to think again about what you hope to show or achieve. The **Objectives** set out a series of strategic targets or milestones that you hope to achieve.
- The **METHODS** which are to be used, justifying their choice where necessary and referencing previous work done in the field of your research. Methods typically include sampling frame and procedures, the methods of measurement and data collection and how they will be administered or applied, and (always) a section on statistical analysis of the data, including Power calculations. They need to be detailed enough so someone else could replicate your research and test your findings.
- **ETHICAL APPROVAL**. Most studies need research ethics approval. This applies to both human and animal studies.
- **PROJECTED OUTCOMES**. These are clear statements of what you hope to demonstrate and include speculation on how the conclusions from your research will facilitate further research or be of benefit generally.
- **REFERENCES**. Your Background will be underpinned by good academic research and citations. The references to your Methods need to refer to published descriptions of the methods you plan to use, including validation studies.
- **APPENDICES**. This is where you put documents showing ethical approval, study information sheets, questionnaires, data collection and recording forms, equipment specifications, etc. All of these are important to include in a protocol or written thesis but should not be part of the body of the text unless your research is specifically to explore the develop-

ment of a new questionnaire or laboratory technique, for example.

In a 'real' protocol (where you were bidding for funds to carry out your research), you would also need to set out your **COSTS**. These typically set out the costs for staff salaries, equipment, running costs (including chemicals, stationery, telephone, postage, travel, etc.), and any overheads (e.g. costs for office space, lighting, heating, etc.). *For student research projects, you do not normally need to estimate costs. You do need to be aware of resource implications, however, and discuss these with your tutor. An undergraduate or MSc research project will usually have limited resources available (time, technical expertise and support, access to equipment, money to pay for consumables, travel costs, incentive payments, etc.). You may be asked to elucidate costs as an exercise in your protocol development.*

14.3 STAGES OF DEVELOPMENT

Three stages of development are outlined for this exercise:

Stage 1.   Initiation (2 days)
- Title, background (cited research), rationale, hypothesis, study design, aims and objectives

Stage 2.   Development (1 week)
- Review of Stage 1
- Sampling and methods

Stage 3.   Full protocol (2 weeks)
- Review of Stages 1 and 2
- Finalize protocol for submission

The timings suggested above reflect the times within which I expected students to complete each stage. The timings for Stages 2 and 3 included date deadlines for submission but allowed time for discussion and reflection with tutors and other members of staff. For undergraduate students, we allowed two or three days per week for each stage (given that they had other activities such as lectures to attend and coursework to complete). For MSc students, the work was undertaken mainly after exams were completed, so essentially full-time.

The evaluation scheme given at the end of these notes (Section 14.9) is based on a marking scheme for submitted protocols. They highlight the extent to which students were successful in developing the elements of the protocol and responding to criticisms as it developed.

In the course which led to the development of this textbook, the protocol development began in the lecture. We discussed these notes on the development of the protocols. After a *brief* discussion, students were asked to go to the library (preferably in pairs) and undertake research over a few hours, bounce research ideas off one another, and decide (tentatively) on a research topic. Further discussion with a classmate[1] or a tutor (especially the tutor whose area of research you are interested in) and conversations with oneself[2] help to develop the basis for a viable hypothesis.

14.4 STAGE 1: INITIATION[3]

Read through the whole of Stage 1 BEFORE TAKING ANY ACTION. Then complete the four Actions set out in Stage 1.

The aim of Stage 1 is to begin preparation of a protocol for a research project that could be carried out by an undergraduate or MSc student. You will not necessarily carry out the research (although some of you may), but we can look at the stages involved in preparing a research protocol.

The work for Stage 1 is submitted *two days* after the class discussion.

The reason for giving students so little time for Stage 1 is set out in Box 14.1.

---

[1]Most libraries have discussion areas or bookable work rooms so you can carry out your discussions without disturbing others.

[2]I have the annoying habit of talking out loud to myself when I am writing syntax for SPSS or working through a problem. I try to do these things in private so as not to disturb others in the room.

[3]Throughout the rest of the chapter, the text is addressed directly to the student.

> **BOX 14.1**
>
> Less haste, more speed
>
> **Why are students given so little time to develop Stage 1?**
>
> This question arises every year. The reason is simple. While some students will succeed in identifying a research idea suitable for an undergraduate or MSc project, many will present either an over-ambitious project or one in which the hypothesis is flawed. In either event, considerable re-thinking is required. There is therefore little to be gained by spending too long on this first stage. When the initial idea has been reviewed and clarified with your tutor, it is then worth putting in more time and effort to the development of a protocol to test your hypothesis.

14.4.1 Choosing a Research Topic

This is an opportunity for you to follow some of your own interests. They might range from aspects of biochemistry through energy or nutrient metabolism to the effects of social factors on diet and health. It might involve use of animals or human subjects. It could include the validation of measurement techniques or an investigation of factors that influence clinical outcomes or recovery. The research should involve some practical element of investigation and not be wholly library or computer based.

14.4.2 Limitations to the Research

1. For both undergraduate and MSc projects, there is a limited amount of time that you will be able to devote to your research. For undergraduates, assume that you will have two days per week in the first term (10 weeks) in which to plan and collect your observations and two days per week in the second term (10 weeks) in which to analyze your data and write up your report. Assume also that you will have a supervisor who will help you obtain samples, animals, chemicals for

analysis, etc., and technical help in the lab, where needed. MSc students have longer, from the completion of exams in April to the first week in August (typically around three months) from inception to submission. Some preparation can be done in February and March, provided it doesn't interfere with other work and revision for exams.

2. The research must be possible with the resources that are available in the Department. Assume that biochemical analyses of most nutrients, nutrient markers, DNA profiles, etc., are possible; that a limited number of animals (say 40 rats or mice) could be available for an animal experiment; that you have access to the human metabolic rooms for up to 48 hours at a time for measurements of energy expenditure; that any specialized equipment that is used in the nutrition practicals (e.g. skinfold callipers, equipment for collection and analysis of respired air, etc.) will be available; and that you can obtain venous blood samples, urine samples, and records of diet. If in doubt, check with your departmental technicians concerning availability of equipment and technical procedures. If the study is field based, ensure that you have enough time to identify your sample (through a GP surgery, for example, or a school or community centre) and that you have the necessary permissions to approach your subjects and obtain consent. You will need to have approval from the relevant research ethics committee.

Assume that you will **NOT** have access to doubly labelled water, computer-assisted tomography (e.g. CAT scans), nuclear magnetic resonance, mass spectrometry, etc., unless your proposed research is part of a larger ongoing research project into which your proposed research could be integrated (evidence of such on-going work in the department would be required).

3. If you plan to sample a specific section of the population (e.g. pregnant women, school children, people with diabetes or raised cholesterol levels, etc.), make sure that they are reasonably available in the locale where you are studying (i.e. do not choose Peruvian llama herders[4] or people who weigh over 45 stone as your sample).

Action 1. Go to the library and find between 6 and 10 recent articles which relate to the area of research that you are interested in, and which together suggest a hypothesis that needs testing. These articles will form the core of the Background that you will be writing and will need clear citations[5] to be included in the References. Write a short paragraph about previous research, and a short Rationale that justifies why your chosen research topic is worth investigating.

As you develop the protocol, the rationale will grow to be a short paragraph which justifies both the need to test the hypothesis and the choice of methods (the choice of a particular method for measuring your main variable(s) may need to form a part of the background). It should state clearly *why* the research needs to be undertaken, *why* the methods are the right ones to use, and *how* the conclusions will be of benefit.

14.4.3 Developing a Hypothesis

A good hypothesis addresses a new, important and interesting research question. It may break new ground, or it may help to confirm or shed light on existing research. It should not, therefore, simply be a repeat test of someone else's hypothesis, but should address some flaw or omission in previous research or propose a new idea which has not been tested before.

---

[4]Unless, perhaps, you live in the Andes, but even then, you might want to think about the generalizability of your findings to other populations.

[5]The method of citation may be Harvard (citing the author(s) in the text, with a date of publication; the full citations appear in the References section at the end of the document alphabetically by first author); or Vancouver (references are numbered in the order in which they appear in the text [in brackets, or superscript], and the full citations are listed in the References section in numerical order). Follow the method advocated by your institution or tutor.

It should be *specific*, e.g. 'Coarse oat-bran is more effective at reducing glycemic response than fine oat-bran' rather than general e.g. 'Oat bran affects glycemic response'.

A good hypothesis must be *testable*. This means that within the resources that are available (personnel, time, equipment, money) you will be able to make the necessary and relevant measurements in the sample so you can test your hypothesis. For example, for the purposes of this exercise, there is no point in putting forward a proposal to test a hypothesis which will require an intervention with baseline and follow-up observations made 12 weeks apart, when you have only 5–10 weeks in which to collect your data. Your hypothesis may need to be modified when you consider more closely the methods that you propose to use. Also, you will need to consider Power (the likelihood of being able to detect a statistically significant outcome if one exists – see Chapter 12), which depends, in part, on the number of observations that you make. This will help you to decide if it will be worthwhile undertaking the planned research with the available resources and planned sample size. The usual cut-off for deciding whether it is worth undertaking a piece of research is 80% Power. Even if Power for your proposed research is less than 80%, you may decide it is worth continuing. For example, the research may provide opportunities for you to learn methodological approaches and analytical techniques (including statistical analysis) that will be of value in the future. Similarly, if it is a genuinely new area of research in which the measurements that you make have not been collected before, you can regard your research as a pilot that contributes to the understanding of (say) the mean and spread of measurements that might be useful in planning future research, and accept that it will have Power less than 80%.

Study design. Students often jump straight to randomized double-blind placebo-controlled intervention trials for testing hypotheses, but not every study needs to be an intervention trial. In your literature search, look for articles which assess hypotheses in different ways. When you choose your own hypothesis, think about how it can be tested using a variety of study designs. Remember that an intervention trial is often the hardest to set up and complete, especially when the time for research is limited. An intelligently designed cross-sectional study may provide more useful information and greater insight into a research problem than an intervention study that doesn't allow enough time for the impact of the intervention to produce the desired effects.

14.4.4 Write Your Hypothesis

Now write the hypothesis you want to test. Discuss it with your fellow student and your tutor.

Action 2. Develop a realistic hypothesis which you think will be testable within the time and resources available using your chosen study design.

14.4.5 Developing the Study Design, Aims and Objectives

Once you have done your initial reading, written a rationale, and crafted a good hypothesis, you need to decide on your study design and set out your Aims and Objectives. Make sure your study design is not too ambitious and will fit within the time frame. Then write your Aims and Objectives.

Table 14.1 provides an example of Aims and Objectives. These should be clear and concise. You'll get a chance to expand on exactly what you propose to do when you write the Methods section in the next stage of development.

Action 3. Draft the first version of your proposal: title,[6] background, rationale, hypothesis, study design, and aims and objectives. This should be on NOT MORE THAN ONE SIDE OF A4 (250 words). Submit this for review by close of play on Wednesday.[7] You will be given feedback at the next session.

---

[6]The title is important: it should convey in just a few words what the research is about, including the central topic and study design.

[7]The classes were on a Monday morning, so students had two days to do this work.

TABLE 14.1   Examples of Aims and Objectives

Aims and Objectives	Examples
The aims are the main goals that you have set for yourself which include a description of the study design	• To demonstrate associations between alpha-tocopherol intake, blood pressure indices and walking distance in peripheral arterial disease patients using a cross-sectional study design
The objectives are brief but specific descriptions of the main points you hope to be able to demonstrate	• To show an inverse association between dietary alpha-tocopherol intake, wrist–ankle blood pressure ratios and walking distance in a sequential series of 80 nondiabetic PAD patients attending the outpatient clinic at Denmark Hill Hospital.
	• To show an association between serum alpha-tocopherol : cholesterol ratios, blood pressure indices and walking distance in these same patients.
	• To evaluate the strength of the dietary and biochemical associations using correlation and regression analysis, taking age and gender into account.
	• To speculate on the value of intervention with dietary alpha-tocopherol supplements as a means for improving pressure ratios and walking distance in similar patients.

14.5 RESPONSES TO STAGE 1 PROTOCOL DEVELOPMENT

This section summarizes responses to previous first submissions. Read them carefully, reflect mindfully, and rewrite what you have proposed!

- Almost all the studies proposed are too ambitious.
- You have thought of an idea but not really thought about how you are going to find subjects and make the necessary measurements.
- Some of the hypotheses are woolly or unfocused – make them as specific as you can.
- Be clear in your mind which measurements you plan to make, and think about who is going to make them, how long they take to make, how much they might cost – remember that you were instructed to consider only those assays that can be done within the Department. Consult with the Departmental technicians or the member of staff likely to supervise your project to ensure that you can measure what you propose to measure.

- Several students have gone for a randomized double-blind placebo-controlled intervention trial. This may be the Rolls Royce of study designs, but they are difficult to carry out well and very time consuming (probably more than 10 weeks). There are many other designs to consider, so consider looking cross-sectionally at groups that already have the characteristics that you are interested in.
- A common problem with intervention studies is that you have only 10–12 weeks available to recruit, measure, intervene, and re-measure your subjects. You will not be able to see all your subjects in one day or even 1 week, so you must allow for the time it will take to see all your subjects on both occasions. The longer it takes to see all your subjects, the shorter time for your intervention, as you need to allow equal lengths of time at the beginning and end of the field work to see all your subjects at baseline and follow-up. You will need to find a balance between the number of subjects you will be able to see and the length of the intervention, not to mention recruitment time.

- Recruitment can be very time consuming. Unless you have a hospital clinic with a known throughput of patients matching your selection criteria (and a cooperative consultant and medical staff), or a cooperative GP or institution (e.g. school or university), recruitment will be slow. For an intervention study, think in terms of 10 or 20 subjects, especially if taking blood is involved, not 50 or 100. For a cross-sectional study you might be able to see 40 or 50 subjects, maybe more if your main measuring instrument is a short questionnaire.
- Some ideas have been rejected outright as they are too complicated, or the research will take too long. Do not expect to be able to collect faeces, urine, or blood multiple times over extended periods. In fact, forget about collecting faeces, and don't expect to get more than a couple of blood samples or 24-hour urine samples.

Whatever you do, KEEP IT SIMPLE!
Look again at your idea, and ask yourself the following questions:

- Who will do the sampling? How long will it take to recruit subjects? From where are you going to recruit them? Will you get permission to recruit from the sources you think of (e.g. schools, hospital wards or clinics)? How long will it take to get permission? What about parental consent for people under 18?
- Can enough patients with specific characteristics, conditions, or illnesses be identified in the time frame?
- If a clinical study, is the condition or illness adequately specified? Limit variation in subject characteristics (reduce number of potential confounding factors) to improve chances of demonstrating the effect of exposure or treatment on outcome. This may include the severity and cause of the problem being addressed.
- For clinical studies, will permission be given by clinicians or consultants to patients with the specified condition or illness?

- If you need matched subjects (either for treatment vs. placebo, or cases vs. controls) are the matching criteria clearly defined? Will there be enough subjects available in the time to recruit matched groups?
- Are the necessary facilities available (e.g. exercise and breath monitoring equipment for a study on energy expenditure)? Can the patients or subjects get to these facilities or have access as often as required if not under your supervision?
- For home or out of clinic interventions (e.g. diet, physical activity), are subjects likely to comply with the planned interventions? How will compliance be assessed?
- Who will undertake the measurements? Are you competent in the methods to be used, or is this a learning exercise, or will someone help you to make the measurements?
- How long will it take to obtain measurements on each subject? (Remember that for an intervention study you will need to take baseline as well as follow-up measurements).
- Is it feasible to collect the information needed?
- Is your study ethical? If a controlled intervention trial, is it ethical to withhold treatment from the placebo (control) group? Will the control group be wait-listed? Do you need approval from a research ethics committee?
- Will subjects agree to co-operate (giving blood, for example)?
- What are the implications concerning the generalizability of findings if you get poor co-operation rates (few people are willing to take part in the study) or poor compliance rates (subjects do not do what you ask them to do)?
- You will not have time to prepare food for lots of subjects – any alterations in diet will have to be on the subjects' own cognizance, or based on some form of supplementation and then how will you monitor compliance?
- For any study involving dietary analysis, think of how you will collect data and (if a paper record) how long it may take to enter dietary data if the system is not automated – do not

propose to collect 7 day weighed inventories from 100 people – 10 or 20 will take you long enough to enter.

- Ask yourself if the length of any intervention (in most studies not more than a few weeks, probably 6 at most) is long enough to bring about the change that you are hoping to observe. If the aim is to influence iron status, for example, at least 10 weeks of iron supplementation (or similar) would be needed to change Hb level.
- Allow time for analysis and writing up.

Action 4. Re-write what you proposed initially for Stage 1. Now:
   *** Submit your Stage 1 protocol ***

14.5.1 Feedback to Stage 1

When you have submitted your Stage 1 protocol, prepare to consider the comments that come back from your tutor. These will be many and varied and (hopefully) constructive.

The 'killer' comment. If you see a general comment such as 'Think again' or 'You may need to think again', either you need to choose a new topic, or your tutor is doubtful of the rationale behind the hypothesis, or the hypothesis is flawed, or the design is faulty. Whatever the case, a discussion with the course tutor is needed. This underpins why Stage 1 is so short: you want to work with a viable idea and approach.

Be thick-skinned. If what you think is a great idea is rejected, maybe it wasn't such a great idea after all. Argue your case but be humble. Listen. Prepare to change ground. You're here to learn.

Remember that research is collaborative. Long-gone are the days of the lone genius sitting in the laboratory and shouting 'Eureka!' Talk to your tutor, other students, friendly experts, lab technicians, clinicians, patients, subjects, your dog, yourself in the mirror, whatever. Make sure that what you are proposing to do is useful and humane.

Rewrite your initial proposal in light of feedback before you go on to Stage 2.

14.6 STAGE 2: DEVELOPMENT

Having reached the point with Stage 1 that makes you think what you are proposing is a Good Idea, the next stage is to develop the methods and set out the protocol in more detail. In this next stage of writing, there are three golden rules:

- Be concise
- Keep language simple and uncomplicated
- Avoid vague terms (e.g. quite, rather, a lot)

14.6.1 Choosing and Describing the Methods

For a hypothesis to be testable, it must be possible to obtain the necessary information. You must ensure that the variables which you measure will allow you to test your hypothesis (i.e. that they are the *appropriate and relevant* measurements to make), and that it is possible to make those measurements with the resources available.

There are *four principal elements* that you need to consider:

1. **The sample and its size**. Whether conducting an animal or human experiment, you need to think carefully about the species or group in which the measurements are to be made, and how many subjects and observations will be required. Imaginative sampling may spell the success or failure of a research project. For example, in a study to assess the effects of maternal under-nutrition on growth and development, one researcher selected, as a control group, siblings born to the same mothers when they were not undernourished. The aim was to control for the effects of social class and genetic and environmental factors. The time between the two sets of observations was limited to three years (so maternal age was not a major factor). In another example, the researcher excluded subjects whose presence might confound the

outcome (they excluded post-obese subjects in a study comparing metabolic characteristics of lean and obese people).

Think of which subjects you plan to use, from where you will obtain them, how you will obtain them, and how long the sampling procedure is likely to take.

The size of the sample *in part* dictates the **Power** that the study will have.[8] To achieve the desired Power, you may need a sample size greater than one you can acquire in the limited recruitment time available in an undergraduate or MSc research project. So, two steps to be followed are:

a. Make a realistic estimate of the number of observations that you think you will be able to collect with the resources which you have available.

b. Calculate the Power that the study is likely to have.

This may help you decide whether it is worth undertaking the study. If Power is less than 80%, you may not be giving yourself a fair chance (statistically speaking) to test your hypothesis. If you are keen to have a chance of demonstrating a statistically significant finding from your research, and the Power is low, it may be better to abandon your proposed research rather than commit your limited time and resources to something that is unlikely to help you effectively test your hypothesis.

On the other hand, because the protocol is for an undergraduate or MSc research project, the experience of undertaking the research and learning new skills and techniques may themselves make it worthwhile to undertake the project; low Power may be acceptable. And who knows: you might get lucky and generate a statistically significant finding even though the Power *is* low. Power simply indicates the chance of demonstrating a

statistically significant finding (if one exists); higher Power bends the chances of observing such a finding in your favour.

2. **Variables to be measured.** Before you can begin a study, you must know exactly which variables you are going to measure. They must be the ones that will give you the measurements you need to test your hypothesis. If you are measuring nutrients in blood or urine, which form of the metabolite do you need to measure? In which fraction of blood (whole blood, serum [without platelets], plasma [with platelets], specific cells [erythrocytes, monocytes, lymphocytes], membranes or whole cells, etc.)? If you are measuring diet, which is the best method – record (duplicate diet, weighed record, household measures record) or recall (diet history, 24-hour recall, questionnaire); how many days; current or past diet; individual or household; etc.? If you are sampling tissue, which tissue will best reflect the measures you need? If you are measuring grip strength or blood flow, which equipment will you use?

Before you start, you must know the technique or method of analysis that you are going to use to obtain each measurement. This is important both in terms of the equipment or facilities that you will need, and in terms of the errors likely to be associated with each measurement. This in turn will be reflected in the number of observations you will be able to collect. Is it better to have more, less accurate observations, or fewer more accurate observations? The answer will depend on the hypothesis and the resources available.

Decide on which variables you will measure, how many observations per variable per subject (or experimental unit), and how big your sample size will be. Be prepared to justify your choices, particularly with reference to the resources available.

[8]Ask yourself, what else has an impact on Power? If you can't remember, look again at Chapter 12.

3. **Research design and statistical analysis**. Every study must have a design which will dictate how many groups are to be measured, how many observations are to be made per subject (experimental unit) for each variable being measured, and how those observations are to be treated statistically so you can test your hypothesis. This in turn will dictate which statistical test or tests are to be applied to the data.

In terms of protocol development, we have not yet considered the statistical tests you might want to apply to your data. Think instead, at this stage, simply how many groups in which you will want to make observations, and how many observations you will make per subject per variable. Think also of whether you will be looking at differences between group means or medians; whether you want to match subjects, animals, or experimental units between groups (and if so, what your matching criteria will be)[9]; whether you will want to make comparisons between two or more variables (e.g. to see how levels of LDL serum cholesterol vary with intake of medium-chain triglycerides; or if people with different levels of education differ in their opinions about the benefits of vitamin supplements); and if you want to look at changes over time.

Describe the basic design of the research (cross-sectional observations, group comparisons, intervention, etc.), with some detail of the procedures that each subject will undergo.

4. **Ethical approval**. All studies on humans require approval by a committee whose main purpose is to ensure that studies are ethically sound. This includes issues such as the information which people need to be given before agreeing to take part in a study (so-called 'informed consent'); the discomfort or pain involved in any measurements which are made, and whether the procedures to be used are safe, appropriate and necessary; whether the risks (e.g. from X-rays or blood sampling) are justified by the benefits to be derived from the research; clarification of the right of any subject to withdraw from a study without having to give a reason; etc. Ethical guidelines will be available from your institution's research ethics office. If you don't have a research ethics office, or the group of subjects is not from your institution, approach another ethics office that has jurisdiction over the patients or subjects you propose to use in your study. For example, if your study involves patients from a local doctor's general practice, the local health authority will have a research ethics office that can scrutinize and provide approval for your study.

Think about the ethical issues that are likely to arise in conducting the research you are proposing and how you will obtain approval. In relation to animal experiments, find out which institution or government office oversees approval for animal research and standards relating to animal care, welfare, accommodation, and health and safety issues relating to humans handling animals in experiments. Check committee deadlines for submission and replies so that you have approval in time to undertake your research.

14.6.2 The Next Draft of Your Proposal

You can begin to develop your proposal. You probably have a clear enough idea to be able to revise your title so it reflects the hypothesis you wish to test and the design of the study which you are proposing.

---

[9]Choose only one or two matching criteria. If there are more than two, it often becomes difficult to find matches. Other factors that you might want to take into account – possible confounders (factors related to both exposure *and* outcome) – can be taken into account in statistical analysis. This means you need to measure them but not necessarily use them as matching criteria.

Write the next draft of your research proposal. It should include:

- TITLE
- BACKGROUND. Simply list the references which you have used in your initial library search. You will expand this section later.
- HYPOTHESIS
- AIMS, OBJECTIVES AND RATIONALE
- METHODS
  - A clear statement of the study design, and the procedures
  - Sample selection
  - Sample size
  - Key variables to be measured
  - A brief description of what you see as the main ethical issues

Action: Submit your Stage 2 protocol for your tutor's comments. Be willing to engage in discussion and be prepared to change what you plan to do.

14.7 STAGE 3: FULL PROTOCOL

Once you have comments from your tutor for Stage 2, you can develop the full protocol.

Agree with your tutor which sections to include (see the general outline at the start of this chapter). As this is a learning exercise, length might be 2000–2500 words (roughly 8–10 double-spaced A4 pages) but agree this with your tutor. This should encompass everything from Background through References. Other items such as study timeline, data collection sheets, draft questionnaire, consent forms, etc., should be included in the Appendices.

14.7.1 Consider the Following Outline for this Exercise:

- **Title**. In a few words, the title should provide a clear and concise statement of what the research is about and how you plan to carry it out
- **Summary** of proposed project (not more than 150 words)

- **Background**. Draft this in more detail, starting with the references which you have found. The background should provide information about significant work that has been done to date, and how your own project will take the research forward. You should add to the references you found initially, based on your additional reading. Most protocols at this stage should have 10–20 references (don't go overboard). Full citations should appear at the end of the protocol, just ahead of any appendices.
- **Hypothesis**. As agreed with your tutor
- **Rationale**. Why the study needs to be done
- **Study design**. This should be appropriate for a student project
- **Aims and objectives**. A concise list or table that makes the overall stages of the research clear
- **Methods**. This will have several subsections, including:
  - **Sample**. From where, how big, inclusion and exclusion criteria, matching variables, etc.
  - **Measurements**. Explain exactly which measurements you are going to collect and the techniques you will use.
  - **Procedures**. Set out how you are going to collect your measurements, e.g. where you will see subjects, what they will have to do, what you will do to them, and when you will see them. Describe randomization procedures (e.g. assignment to intervention or control, the order of administration of two or more alternative treatments). Ask yourself if the length of any proposed diet record is long enough to enable you to classify subjects correctly into the top or bottom thirds, fourths or fifths of the distribution of intakes (depending on your statistical model). Similarly, ask yourself if the length of any proposed intervention is long enough to produce the desired effects. Evidence from the literature will be important to support your design, so you will need to cite the relevant literature that describes what you

are going to do. The length and nature of an intervention and any assessment (dietary, physical activity, etc.) need to be explicit (and justified in the rationale). The amount of any supplement or treatment should be specified, together with the nature or composition of the placebo (if any).

○ **Statistical analysis**. State and justify which statistical tests you plan to use, the variables you are going to analyze, matching variables, etc. In analysis of variance and multiple regression, state which are the main factors and which are covariates. Define groups for chi-squared analyses, etc.

○ **Power**. Provide an estimate of the Power of the proposed study, making clear the parameters and measurements on which the calculation is based. Specify where the values used in the calculation were obtained from the literature (if they exist, with citations) or how you estimated them.

• **Ethical Issues**. State the risks involved and any ethical issues related to subject safety, confidentiality, and data protection. State where ethical permission would be obtained (you do not need to obtain ethical permission for the purposes of this exercise, but you will if the proposal becomes the basis for your research project).

• **Projected outcomes**. Speculate on the possible outcomes that your project might produce and how they would contribute to the field of research. This is NOT a restatement in a different tense of what you have said in the aims and objectives, but a forecast of the benefits that you see accruing from the work, and any further research that is likely to be needed as a direct consequence of the work undertaken.

• **References**. This should give full citations. Refer to a relevant journal (e.g. The British Journal of Nutrition) for details about how to cite journal articles, books, online resources, etc., and agree the citation style (Vancouver or Harvard) with your tutor.

At this stage, and within the time available, you should consider preparing material for inclusion in the Appendices:

• Study information sheet to be given to subjects before undertaking a study. This should state how the subjects were recruited, the procedures to be undergone, a statement regarding confidentiality, clarification on how to refuse participation or withdraw from the study, and an email address and phone number where the principal researcher can be contacted.
• Consent form. A proforma for this will be available from the ethics committee to which you apply for approval.
• Questionnaire. Draft of proposed form of questions. You do not need to produce a 'finished product', but you should specify the key questions that you propose to ask, or cite relevant literature if the questionnaire has been used in previous research, with any modifications that you propose to make.
• Data sheet or design of the spreadsheet in which you plan to record all your measurements for each subject.

14.8 COMMENTS ON PREVIOUS SUBMISSIONS AT STAGE 3. PLEASE READ THESE CAREFULLY BEFORE COMPLETING STAGE 3.

1. **Originality**. A good protocol explores an original problem. If you are re-testing an existing hypothesis, or repeating a study, you should describe the weaknesses in the work that has been done previously and justify its repetition.

2. **Inclusion and exclusion criteria**. Make sure that you have a 'clean' sample, e.g. if

carrying out a study on hypercholesterolaemic patients, exclude subjects with familial (genetic) hypercholesterolaemia and select only those whose raised cholesterol is likely to be due to environmental factors (diet, body size, etc.).

3. **Confounders**. Make sure that you *measure* any potential confounders. The most common confounders are gender, age, social or educational background, etc. You might have already addressed some of these in the sampling procedure (that is, limiting your sample to a particular subgroup in the population, or using one or two as matching criteria). Confounders may also be medical (e.g. concomitant disease states, disease stage), dietary (e.g. energy or nutrient intakes), physical (weight, height, activity level), etc. The important thing is that you measure them so you can take them into account in your analysis.

4. **Tense**. When writing a protocol, the tense should always be in the future e.g. 'subjects will be selected...', and not in the past e.g. 'subjects were selected...'.

5. **Time available for fieldwork**. Remember that for undergraduates, you probably have only two days per week for 10 weeks to identify the sample and collect measurements, and for MSc students, roughly two months full time.[10] Try and be realistic about what can be done in the time available. Recruitment should take a short time and be feasible. Think about how long you will need to see each subject, remembering that subjects may not always be available exactly when you would like to see them, how long the measurement procedures will take, etc. Be realistic about the time it will take to undertake each step.

6. **Subject motivation and compliance**. Be reasonable in what you ask subjects to do. Carrying out multiple 24-hour urine collections (taking PABA to verify completeness), recording diet for 28 days, undertaking exercise which is over and above what they normally do, altering meal patterns, etc. may not be acceptable to many subjects, who will either drop out from your study or fail to comply with your intervention. You should have a measure of compliance that does not rely solely on what your subject tells you they have done.

7. **Procedures**. All procedures must be in routine use in your department or available in your College at reasonable cost. Make sure you reference your assays with clarity (be specific about equipment models, reagents, etc.) and cite relevant literature. Estimate the number of procedures and assays that you plan to carry out, think about your own experience or how long you imagine each interview or procedure will take, and adjust the numbers accordingly (usually downwards!). Imagine if you yourself would be willing to undergo the procedures which you are asking other people to undergo.

8. **Access to subjects**. Make sure that you could gain access to the subjects you wish to study, e.g. specified weight or BMI group, patients with NIDDM, post surgery, cancer, post chemotherapy, etc.

9. **Covering letter**. Any mailings or approaches to patients will have to go under a letter with a doctor's or tutor's signature to preserve rights of privacy. For example, do not expect GPs or consultants to let you have a list of names, email addresses, and phone numbers. Asking for volunteers via email or postings on Facebook, for example, will also require approval by your institution.

---

[10]These were the time allocations at King's College London. Your institute may have a different programme and therefore time available for undergraduate or MSc research.

10. **Confidentiality**. Subjects' privacy must be preserved.[11] When selecting a sample from a GP list or similar, the name and address of the subject is kept secret by getting the GP to send a letter or email prepared by the researcher. Those subjects who wish to participate then respond direct to the researcher, revealing name and address on a voluntary basis. You may not have access to subjects who have not given prior agreement to be approached.

11. **Subject information sheet**. This should describe how the subjects were selected, how many people will be in the study, what procedures are going to be used, how the data will be used (including a statement about confidentiality), and who will be informed of the outcome. At the same time, it may help to be a bit vague about the hypothesis so as not to alert the subject to a possible intervention which could be self-administered (e.g. extra vitamin supplements). The subject information sheet should not be an invitation to take part in the study (this should be a separate letter), nor a set of instructions for the patient (these should comprise an explicit list of instructions rather than the summary of procedures which appears on the information sheet). At the end of the information sheet

you should include a contact name, address (your institution) and telephone number. **The key things are: keep the language simple; keep the message brief; conceal the true hypothesis (if possible) if it is likely to influence subjects' behaviour or reporting**.

12. **Ethical issues**. This discussion should address the specific procedures which subjects are being asked to carry out or undergo, and not talk generally about the issues. Some form of justification is required to show that any risks are more than compensated for by the potential benefits either to the individuals taking part in your study or to similar groups in the future. 'Wait-listing' in intervention studies can sometimes be used to overcome ethical objections to withholding a potentially beneficial treatment, provided the delay to treatment is not in itself likely to be harmful. The higher the risk for any individual, the more it needs to be shown that the individual can potentially benefit directly from the procedures.

14.9 PRESENTATION OF PROTOCOLS

Each tutor will have specific instructions about the format of the presentation. Students are expected to adhere to these closely. When you submit a 'real' protocol, or a research ethics application, the rules about format are very strict, and deviation from the rules will mean your protocol or application may not be considered by the committee to which you are applying.

14.9.1 Grading Scheme

Overall marks for protocols were awarded using the following scheme for undergraduates and MSc students:

[11]See the latest General Data Protection Regulations (GDPR) for the UK: https://www.gov.uk/government/publications/guide-to-the-general-data-protection-regulation. Accessed October 2019.

In Europe, General Data Protection Regulations must be followed with no exceptions:
https://ec.europa.eu/commission/priorities/justice-and-fundamental-rights/data-protection/2018-reform-eu-data-protection-rules/eu-data-protection-rules_en

Use the relevant information and procedures for the country where the research is taking place. Your own institution will have a summary of relevant procedures to ensure GDPR rules are followed. If your country is outside of Europe, there may be similar data protection legislation in place which must be observed.

Grade	Marks	Criteria
Excellent	70–100	This category is used with great reserve! Only a very exceptional protocol is awarded a mark over 70, and a mark over 80 is almost unheard of. All components are presented to a very high standard.
Good	60–69	Marks in this range are for well presented, competent protocols, with almost all the components at a high standard.
Average	50–59	The protocol contains most of the components asked for at a reasonable standard, but some elements are limited or incomplete.
Below average	40–49	The protocol lacks organization and thought. Many components are incomplete or limited.
Fail	<40	The protocol is messy and incomplete, with little thought or care in its completion.

For MSc students, marks below 50 were regarded as a Fail.

14.9.2 Breakdown of Mark Allocation

Marks were awarded specifically as follows:

Component	Percent of Mark	>70	60–70	50–60	40–50	<40
Summary	5	Excellent	Very clear	Clear	Not clear	Missing
Background	10	Clearly identified relevant problem, concise, well supported by references	Identifies problem, indicates relevance, relevant references	Problem identified, some relevant references	Problem not clearly described, weak references	No problem defined, references not relevant
Hypothesis and Rationale	5	Clear, testable hypothesis justified by clear and concise rationale	Testable hypothesis with good justification	Relevant hypothesis with moderate justification	Poorly stated hypothesis with some justification	Hypothesis not clearly stated or untestable, inadequate justification
Study design, aims and objectives (milestones)	5	Lucid aim and highly relevant objectives	Clear overall aim, relevant objectives	Aim given, objectives not always clear or justified	Aim poorly described, few or no clear objectives	Aim and objectives not clear
Methods (including sampling, procedures, statistical tests, and Power	40	Methods fully described and feasible within the scope of the project, easily understood and replicated; Power calculations	Methods well described; Power calculations given and sample size justified; relevant statistical test chosen, with good justification.	Methods adequately described; Power calculations given but not clear or not well interpreted;	Methods poorly described, replication difficult; Power calculations incorrect, sample size not justified;	Methods not clear or incomplete, impossible to replicate study; Power calculation missing,

(Continued)

(Continued)

Component	Percent of Mark	>70	60–70	50–60	40–50	<40
		clearly set out and justified, relevance to choice of sample size made clear; appropriate statistical test identified with clear justification for choice.		appropriate statistical test chosen with some justification.	statistical test correct but poorly justified.	sample size not justified; statistical test chosen incorrect.
Ethical issues	10	Ethical issues very clearly identified and addressed	Ethical issues well described and addressed	Ethical issues moderately described and addressed	Ethical issues described but not all relevant and not well addressed	Ethical issues omitted or not relevant, not addressed
Projected outcomes	5	Clear and perceptive forecast of benefits likely to accrue from the work done, with strong justification	Likely benefits well described and justified	Likely benefits described but not well justified	Likely benefits poorly described and not justified	Likely benefits not described or justified
Additional material	15	Study information sheet, consent form, data sheet, questionnaire all very clear, well laid out and thought through	Good effort at developing supporting material, well presented	Good outlines of supporting material, presentation less complete	Some supporting material, elements missing, not clearly presented	Little or no supporting material
References	5	Highly relevant references which clarify background and support argument for carrying out the study, consistent method of citation	Mainly relevant references supporting the argument, accurately cited	Adequate references with some support for argument, accurate citations	References weakly support argument; inconsistent citations	Few or irrelevant references which do not support the argument, inaccurate citations

CHAPTER 15

Presenting Results to Different Audiences

Learning Objectives

After studying this chapter, you should be able to:

- Set out results to make your findings clear to different audiences
- Highlight elements of your results that are of particular interest
- Use a variety of approaches to maintain audience attention
- Learn to be economical in your style of presenting

15.1 INTRODUCTION

In Chapter 1, Section 1.7, we looked at basic rules for ensuring that your results are presented in useful and consistent formats. We also clarified that *results* are what you present, based on the analysis of your data, and that you *never* present raw data unless your study warrants a detailed look.

As I pointed out in Chapter 1, if you are talking to a scientific audience, or preparing a scientific paper describing your results, you need to support your findings with relevant statistics. If it is a lay audience, make the story clear and compelling without too many numbers, and rely more on graphs and charts.

This chapter suggests a few modes of presentation that will help your audiences understand your results. It highlights times when points of particular interest can be emphasized, and how to do that. There are no hard and fast rules about how to present results. The aim is to give your story life and character. You wouldn't read a boring novel. Why should you expect your audience to sit through a boring presentation, or your tutor to read a boring report? If you are making a presentation, rehearse it to make sure the timing is right, then present it to a friendly (but critical) group of fellow students or peers before taking it to a wider audience.

Statistics in Nutrition and Dietetics, First Edition. Michael Nelson.
© 2020 John Wiley & Sons Ltd. Published 2020 by John Wiley & Sons Ltd.
Companion website: www.wiley.com/go/nelson/statistics

In preparing presentations, be aware of 'Death by PowerPoint': the type of presentation with an un-varying format (bar chart after bar chart after bar chart, one virtually indistinguishable from the next) which is guaranteed to confuse your audience and send them to sleep. This applies to all presentations, whether 10 minutes or 60 minutes. Don't rush. It is your job to keep your audience engaged and alert. If you are good at telling jokes, tell a (relevant) joke. Do something unexpected with imagery – insert a cartoon, or a picture of your dog[1] – something that will change the pace of your presentation. Sometimes, I simply stop my presentation and ask members of the audience to talk to their neighbour for a minute or stand up and wave their arms about. If your story can be told clearly without PowerPoint (without asking your audience to hold too many ideas or numbers in their heads at one time), don't use PowerPoint.

If you are not experienced with PowerPoint, it is a good idea to find a good tutorial in a book or online. There are lots of useful things that you can do without needing a BA in Graphic Design. But don't make your presentation so glitzy that it overwhelms the import of your results. You have worked hard on your research, so you want your story to be clear and interesting. Clever graphics are no substitute for good science and clear story-telling. There are endless resources that you can access, from *PowerPoint for Dummies* [1] to courses (in classes and online) that will provide lots of useful tips on how to present findings to different types of audience. These can be fun, and it is worth spending a little time learning about presentation skills.

The rest of this chapter is devoted to presenting results in different formats, with different emphases.

15.2 MY ELDER SON'S GROWTH – A SIMPLE TIME TREND ANALYSIS

Between birth and age 18 years, I collected information on my elder son's length and height. Height (length when he was less than two years old) was measured in a standard way [2, 3]. The values for age (years) and height (cm) are shown in Table 15.1.

While it is possible to deduce a relationship bet-ween age and height by looking at the numbers, it is far easier to see how they relate by drawing a scatter-gram (plotting the [x,y] points height [cm] versus age [years]) and then joining the points with short, straight lines (Figure 15.1).

The plot tells us immediately about the general relationship between height and age: as my son got older, he got taller. We could probably have deduced

TABLE 15.1   My Elder Son's Height from 0 to 18 Years

Age (yr)	Height (cm)
0.0	54.0
1.0	72.0
2.0	86.0
3.0	95.0
4.0	103.0
5.0	112.0
6.0	120.0
7.0	129.0
8.0	137.0
8.6	142.0
8.9	142.5
9.4	146.1
9.8	148.6
10.2	151.4
10.7	154.1
11.0	156.0
11.5	159.7
12.0	163.5
12.5	170.0
13.0	176.0
13.4	179.9
13.8	183.0
18.0	190.0

[1]You can tell I am a dog person – I never mention cats, do I?

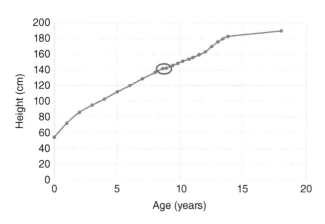

FIGURE 15.1 My son's height (cm) from birth to 18 years.

that from the numbers in the table. What would not have been so easy to see was that he grew very rapidly in the first year of life, and that shortly after his eighth birthday he seemed virtually to stop growing (see the circle on the line at age 8). What happened? Did we stop feeding him? No, of course not. What did happen? We moved house, from the town where he grew up to a new house in London, leaving his friends and school behind. It was probably the stress of moving that caused his growth almost to stop. The impact of stress on growth rate is a well-documented phenomenon [4], but if I hadn't plotted the growth data carefully (as Elsie Widdowson had done in her study years before), it is likely I would not have seen this particular association. The other fact that emerges is that from age 14 to 18 his rate of growth was considerably slower than from age 12 to 14. His maximum adolescent growth spurt arrived more or less when expected (age 12 years) [5] (although it was a bit of shock to discover he was on the 97th centile for height[2]). The plot provided more insight into the data than the table.

When we draw a plot of this type, it is important to follow some standard conventions. First, identify the *independent* variable (the *x* variable, or 'explanatory' variable) and plot it on the horizontal axis. The *dependent* variable (the *y* variable, or 'response' variable) is always plotted on the vertical axis. In this example, we can say that height is dependent upon

age – that is, the older a child is, the taller they are likely to be. It would not make sense to say that age was dependent upon height – that as you got taller, so you got older. We describe this by saying that we have 'plotted *y* against *x*'. The title of the graph is 'My elder son's height (cm) by age (years)', that is, the name of the dependent variable 'by' (or 'according to' or 'versus' or 'vs') the name of the independent variable. The units of measure are given both in the title and in the labels to the axes. You should always follow these conventions when plotting and describing data.

15.3 DISTRIBUTION OF CHILDREN'S AGES ACCORDING TO HOUSEHOLD INCOME – CONTINGENCY TABLES, PIE CHARTS, BAR CHARTS, AND HISTOGRAMS

I carried out a nutrition survey in Cambridge, England. Table 15.2 shows the distribution of the age of children in the survey according to household income.

This 2×2 *contingency table* presents lots of information. First, it shows both number and percentage of children by age group in each income group. Second, it suggests that the distribution of age is contingent upon income. This is confirmed statistically, based on the chi-squared statistic,

TABLE 15.2 Number and Percentage of Children in Cambridge Study According to Age and Income Group

Age (yr)	Income Group			
	High		Low	
	n	%	n	%
0–4	34	23%	47	39%
5–17	115	77%	74	61%
All ages	149	100%	121	100%

Chi-squared = 8.165, *df* = 1, P = 0.004.

[2]Where he stayed – as a fully grown adult he is 190 cm.

degrees of freedom, and P value given below the table. As $P = 0.004$, I would be telling my audience that this was a very statistically significant association between children's age group and income group. This type of presentation would be appropriate in a scientific paper.

If I were presenting my findings to a group of local councillors in the town, I would use a different approach. The relationships shown here are easier to grasp if we present them using pie charts (Figure 15.2).

The shaded areas are proportional to the percentage of children in each age group by income group. It is easy to see straight away that there is a higher proportion of younger children in the lower income group. I have included the percentages (not the numbers) in the chart. I have left out the details of the chi-squared analysis. I might say in a presentation that the association between age and household income group is 'significant' but leave out the words 'very statistically' or maybe not mention stats at all. If the story that you want to tell the councillors is about the differences in the proportions of younger and older children living in households on high and low income and the issues that might present relating to child nutrition, then the pie charts with the percentages highlighted, in a visually attractive format, would be more immediately informative and engaging than the table.

Suppose that you want to illustrate the age distribution in more detail. Table 15.3 provides the information. Rather than a pie-chart, I have chosen to create bar charts to show the numbers of children in four age categories. A bar chart provides a useful visual representation of the numbers by income group. I could use the same approach as in Figure 15.2 and show a bar chart for each income group separately (Figure 15.3a). More helpful, I think, is to put the data into one bar chart so that that comparisons between income groups are more immediately apparent (Figure 15.3b).

Note that the x axis is not a proportional axis – not all of the bars are of equal width in terms of the number of years of age which the bar represents. This graph is a bar-chart, not a histogram. In a histogram, the width of the bars would be proportional to the size of the category. Histograms are most useful for categories of equal size and hence equal width (as shown in Figure 4.4, for example).

15.4 MORE EXAMPLES

The next section looks at examples of tables and graphs from recent publications. The purpose is to

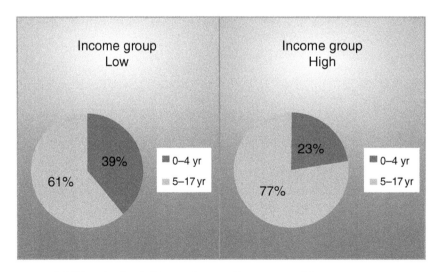

FIGURE 15.2   Percentage of children in Cambridge study according to age and income group.

TABLE 15.3 Number and Percentage of Children in Cambridge Study by Age and Income Group

Age (yr)	Income Group			
	High		Low	
	n	%	*n*	%
0	6	4%	6	5%
1–4	28	19%	41	34%
5–10	62	42%	47	39%
11–17	53	36%	27	22%
All ages	149	100%	121	100%

Chi-squared = 10.17, *df* = 3, P = 0.017.

highlight the features of each table or graph, making sure that the key elements of each are understood. As I said earlier, you might present the same data without the statistical detail to a lay audience and reserve the statistics for a scientific audience.

15.4.1 The Eatwell Guide – Changes Over Time and Stacked Column Bar Charts

The Eatwell Guide [6] (Figure 15.4) is an important public health tool that sets out the balance of a healthy diet using food group guidance.

The Guide has evolved over time, and an examination of the changes [7] showed (among other

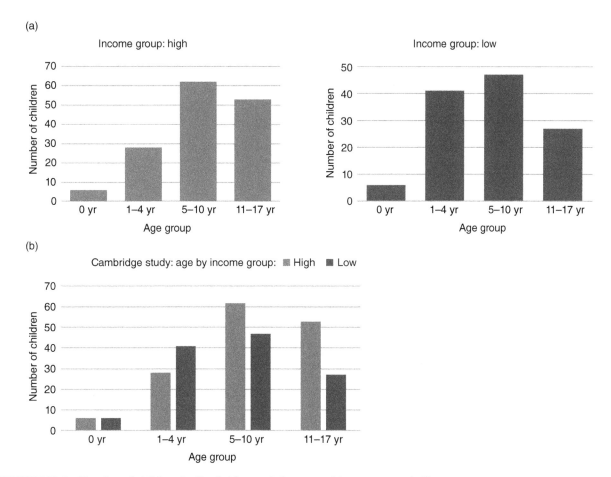

FIGURE 15.3 Number of children in Cambridge study by age and income group (a,b).

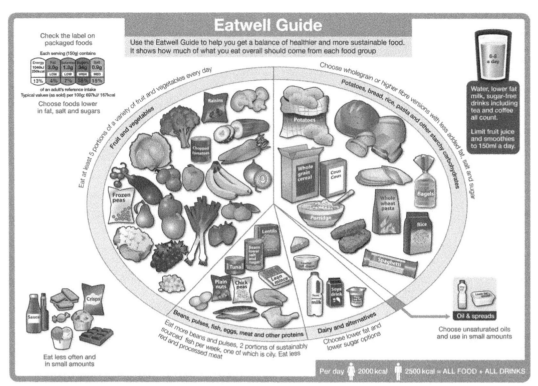

Source: Public Health England 2016

FIGURE 15.4   The Eatwell Guide.

things) how the relative proportions of the food groups changed (Figure 15.5).

Two pieces of information are neatly illustrated in the stacked bar chart: the changes over time; and the way in which the guidance relates to current UK diets. There are no statistical analyses, but the comparisons are immediately evident. Of course, if this were part of a presentation, it would be important to bring to an audience's attention how the underlying advice had changed, particularly in relation to foods high in fat and sugar and the consumption of fruit juice.

15.4.2 Room Service in a Public Hospital – Comparing Means in a Table

This study [8] compared energy and nutrient intake of patients in a public hospital in Australia before and after the transition from a traditional food service to a room service model.[3] While the experimental model is not perfect – there are significant differences between the two groups in patients' mean age and weight and the types of ward in hospital – the table of the main findings provides a good example of simplicity and clarity (Table 15.4).

The results show clear differences in mean energy and protein intake between the two groups.

---

[3]Completing a paper menu (cook fresh, 14-day cycle menu) up to 24 hours prior to meals, which were then collected at a set time by Nutrition Assistant staff. Meals were delivered at set meal times during the day: breakfast between 06.30 hours and 07.30 hours; lunch between 11.45 hours and 12.45 hours; and dinner between 17.00 hours and 18.00 hours. In RS, patients order meals from a single integrated a la carte style menu anytime between 06.30 hours and 19.00 hours by phoning RS representatives in a central call centre. Meals were prepared on demand; the aim was to deliver the meal within 45 minutes of receiving the order.

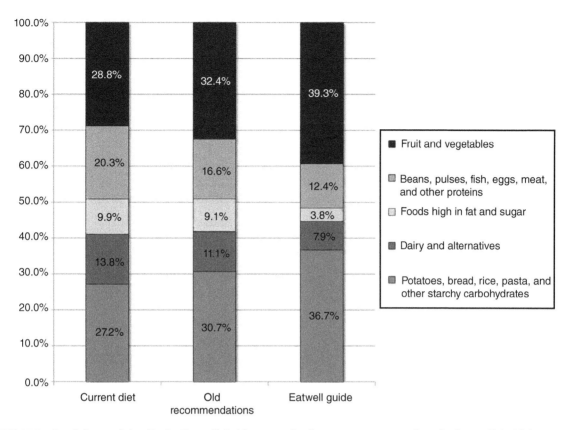

FIGURE 15.5 Breakdown of the diet by Eatwell Guide categories for current consumption, the 'Eatwell Guide' scenario and the 'old recommendations' scenario. *Source:* Reproduced with permission of BMJ Publications.

TABLE 15.4 A Comparison of Energy and Protein Intake (Absolute and Percentage of Requirements) Between two Groups of Adult Inpatients Allocated to either a Traditional Foodservice Model or a Room Service Model

Variable	Traditional Foodservice Model	Room Service	P
n	84	103	
	mean (SD)	mean (SD)	
Average energy intake (kJ/day)	5513 (2112)	6379 (2797)	0.020[a]
Average protein intake (g/day)	52.9 (23.5)	73.9 (32.9)	<0.001[a]
Proportion of EER met (%)	63.5% (26.1%)	78.0% (36.7%)	0.002[a]
Proportion of EPR met (%)	69.7% (35.7%)	99.0% (51.0%)	<0.001[a]

Source: Royal College of Paediatrics and Child Health [5].
EER, estimated energy requirement; EPR, estimated protein requirement.
[a]Independent samples t-test (two-tailed).

The two sample (independent) *t*-test makes clear the statistical significance of the difference. The authors could have carried out an analysis of variance which took into account the potential confounders (age, weight, ward) to provide better evidence of the differences, but the results as they stand (supported by other benefits reported in the published paper such as lower costs and higher levels of patient satisfaction) tell a clear story about the benefits of moving from the traditional to the room service model.

For a lay audience (say, food service managers for whom the statistical details might be of less interest), Figure 15.6 might provide a more engaging format. This is not to suggest that this audience is less intelligent – the simpler graphs might help you to tell your story better and faster, omitting detail that may not be of special interest to your audience.

It is worth noting that most of the field work in this study was completed by students. This is just the type of project which, when well-thought out by students and tutors over time, can produce good data worthy of further analysis and publication.

15.4.3 Impact of Feeding Support on Dysphagic Patients - Comparing Means in a Table with 95% Confidence Intervals

The next study [9] compares the effectiveness of an intervention (targeted feeding assistance to improve the nutritional intake of elderly dysphagic patients in hospital) with a control group. The main findings (Table 15.5) provide more information than the table from the previous study. The authors have included the mean difference and the 95% confidence interval in their reporting. This helpfully shows the size of the impact of the intervention compared with the control group; and lets you know not only the P value but also the likely range of the impact in the parent population from which the samples were drawn (95% CI). Note that where the value for $P > 0.05$, the 95% confidence interval includes zero. This makes for a clearer story, nutritionally and statistically, and gives you a sense of the probable true extent of the impact, taking sampling variation into account.

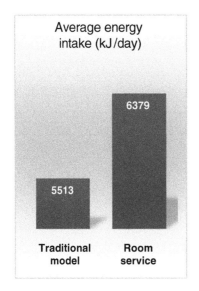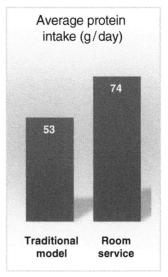

FIGURE 15.6   A comparison of energy and protein intake between two groups of adult inpatients allocated to either a Traditional Foodservice Model or a Room Service Model. *Source:* Reproduced with permission of Elsevier. (Note: origin of bars for Average energy intake is 5000 kJ/day.)

TABLE 15.5   Estimated Energy and Protein Requirements and Total Measured Intake of the Control and Feeding Assistance Groups

		Feeding Assistance Group	Control Group	Difference	P	95% Confidence Interval
n		16	30			
		Mean (SD)	Mean (SD)			
Energy requirements (kJ)		6358 (1323)	6430 (1029)	72	0.84	−781 to 638
Protein requirements (g)		54 (14)	62 (13)	6	0.08	−16 to 0.8
Energy consumed (meals only) (kJ)		3578 (1512)	2242 (1197)	1336	0.002	517 to 2155
Protein consumed (meals only) (g)		36 (21)	21 (13)	15	0.02	2.1 to 26.4

Source: Public Health England in association with the Welsh Government, Food Standards Scotland and the Food Standards Agency in Northern Ireland [6].

15.4.4 Probiotics and Immune Response; Gene-nutrient Interaction and Metabolic Disease – Statistical Findings Shown in a Bar Chart

An interesting paper by Przemska-Kosicka and co-authors [10] reported the effect of a synbiotic on the response to seasonal influenza vaccination in a placebo-controlled intervention trial. They discovered at the end of the study that when subjects were allocated to placebo and intervention groups it resulted in differences in baseline immunological phenotype in both age cohorts and was statistically significant in the older subjects (Figure 15.7). This explained (in part) the differences in response to vaccination in the older cohort. The difference in phenotype was usefully illustrated with a bar chart, with vertical lines showing the limits of the 95% confidence intervals for each group, and an asterisk to indicate where the difference between groups was statistically significant. Where the bars showing the limits of the 95% confidence intervals overlapped (in the 'Young' group), there was no statistically significant difference between the groups; where they did not overlap (in the 'Old' group), there was a statistically significant difference.

Shatwan et al. [11] used the same approach to present findings in their study to investigate the influence of two commonly studied LPL polymorphisms (rs320, HindIII; rs328, S447X) on postprandial lipaemia in 261 participants using a standard sequential meal challenge (Figure 15.8). They provided more information in their figure than did Przemska-Kosicka. They quoted P values rather than just showing the level of significance using an asterisk; and they reported a highly statistically significant interaction from a two-way analysis of variance ($P=0.0004$) showing that there were marked differences in response between men and women (with clarification in the text of the method of statistical analysis).

15.4.5 Fat Versus Carbohydrate Restriction in Type 2 Diabetes Mellitus – Correlation, Individual Change Plots, and Box-and-Whisker Plots

Barbosa-Yanez and co-authors [12] measured endothelial function assessed by flow mediated dilation (FMD) in patients with Type 2 Diabetes Mellitus following a three-week intervention on very low carbohydrate (VLC) or low fat (LF) diets ($n = 15$ and $n = 18$, respectively), together with anthropometry and biochemical markers.

Both regimens resulted in statistically significant reductions in BMI, total body fat, visceral adipose tissue, and intrahepatic lipids. There were no

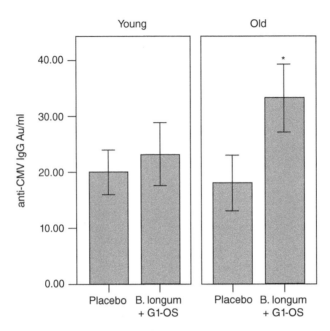

* Difference between treatment groups within age cohort,
Student's independent *t*-tests (*P* < 0.05)

FIGURE 15.7   Baseline levels of anti-CMV IgG differ in younger and older subjects randomized to B. longum + Gl-OS and placebo. *Denotes significant difference between treatment groups within age cohort Student's independent *t*-tests (*P* < 0.05).

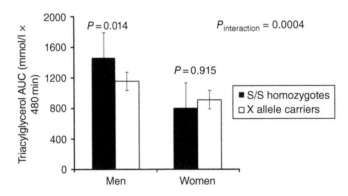

FIGURE 15.8   Mean (SEM) for the area under the curve (AUC) TAG response according to S447X polymorphism after consumption of a test breakfast (49 g fat) at 0 minute and a test lunch (29 g fat) at 330 minutes.

differences in the measurements between the two regimens at baseline or follow-up except for visceral adipose tissue which was statistically significantly greater in the LF group at baseline.

After three weeks, FMD showed positive correlations with protein intake and fat intake in the LF group, and a negative correlation with protein intake

in the VLC group (Figure 15.9). There was no statistically significant correlation with carbohydrate intake in either group. The authors concluded that improvements in FMD may be related to the interplay of fat and protein intake.

This is a clear way of showing associations in a study with a straight-forward model of intervention

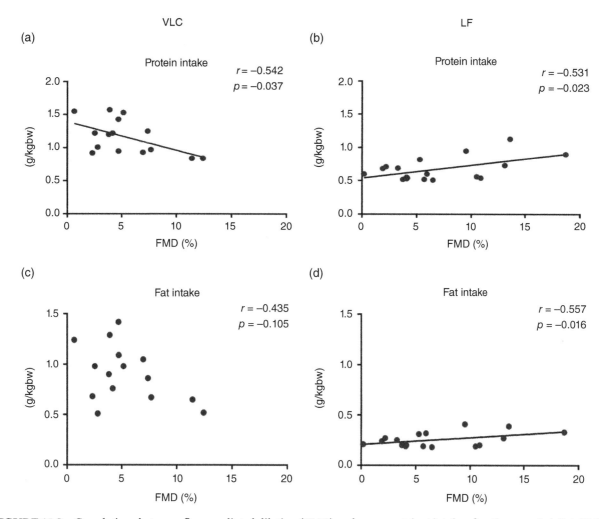

FIGURE 15.9 Correlations between flow mediated dilation (FMD) and macronutrient intake after three weeks' diet. FMD (%) versus protein intake on (a) the very low carbohydrate diet (VLC) and (b) the low fat (LF) diet; FMD (%) versus fat intake on (c) VLC diet and (d) LF diet; after macronutrient intake correction for body weight.

and outcome. The authors use scatterplots to show the linear associations. The correlation statistics are shown in the plots. Ask yourself if these are *important* as well as statistically significant associations (think r^2).[4] Helpfully, the authors restrained themselves from plotting a nonstatistically significant regression line for fat intake versus FMD in the VLC group. They did not include in the text or show in the graph the regression equation for the plotted

lines which would have told you *by how much* FMD changed for each change in g of protein or fat per kg of body weight.

Another useful way the authors showed the changes in FMD was to plot lines for each individual, showing changes from baseline to follow-up by intervention group (Figure 15.10). This makes clear the extent to which changes are similar or different between individuals. The changes in FMD in the LF group appear to be more consistent (generally upward) than in the VLC group. The statistical significance of these changes within the LF group is

[4]Look in Chapter 10 at the Conclusion to Section 10.2.1 to remind yourself about r^2.

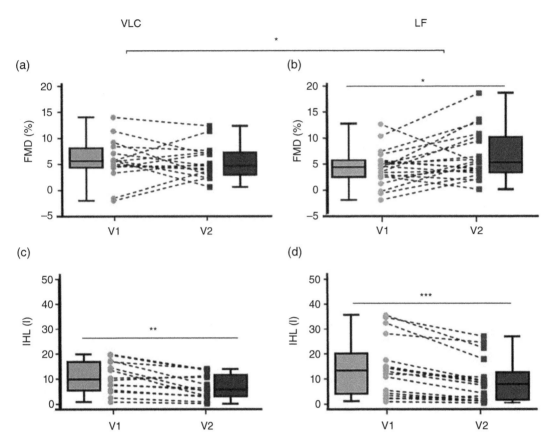

FIGURE 15.10   Boxplots and individual changes in flow mediated dilation (FMD) and intrahepatic lipids (IHL) at baseline (V1) and follow-up (V2). Changes in endothelial function (a) and intra hepatic lipids (c) post-intervention on the very low carbohydrate (VLC) diet ($n = 16$); changes in endothelial function (b) and intra hepatic lipids (d) after 3 weeks on the low fat (LF) diet ($n = 20$). *$P < 0.05$; **$P < 0.01$; ***$P < 0.001$.

indicated by the single asterisk above the horizontal bar, indicating that the change (paired t-test) is statistically significant at the 5% level. The absence of a bar and asterisk above the VLC group indicates no significant change for the group between baseline and follow-up. The bracket connecting both groups and the asterisk above further indicates that the changes were statistically significantly *different* between the groups (again at the 5% level [one asterisk], based on a two-way analysis of variance), greater in the LF compared with the VLC group. In the plots for IHL, the differences between baseline and follow-up are statistically significant at the 1% (two asterisks) and 0.1% level (three asterisks) for the VLC and LF groups, respectively. The absence of a bracket connecting the two groups (and corresponding asterisks) shows that the difference

between the changes in the groups over time was not statistically significant.

Also shown for each set of results are box-and-whisker plots (or box-plots) for each parameter and time point, by diet group. A box-plot shows five characteristic values: minimum, first quartile, median, third quartile, and maximum. The 'whiskers' are plotted at 1.5 times the size of the interquartile range beyond Q1 and Q3 or at the minimum or maximum, whichever is closer to the median. When plotted using Excel or SPSS, extreme values are shown by the use of asterisks appearing above or below the whiskers. Box-plots are simple ways of illustrating the midpoint, interquartile range and extreme values. The authors note in the text that extreme values for FMD were excluded from their analyses, hence there are no asterisks beyond the whiskers.

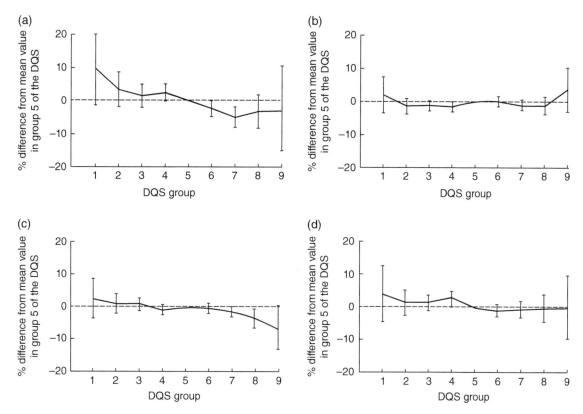

FIGURE 15.11 Percent difference from the mean value in group 5 of the DQS for suPAR (a), BMI (b), total cholesterol (c), and HDL (d). *Source:* Reproduced with permission of Cambridge University Press.

15.4.6 Chronic Inflammation, Diet Quality Score, and Morbidity and Mortality – Analysis of Variance and Risk

For the final example, I want to look at a report by Törnkvist and co-authors [13] on associations between levels of chronic inflammation, diet quality, and risk of cardiovascular disease and mortality in the Danish population. It uses data from 5347 participants in a well-designed cohort study to explore cross-sectional associations between groups with different diet quality scores (DQS), levels of chronic inflammation (suPAR),[5] and BMI, blood lipids, and risks of ischaemic heart disease and

[5] Based on measurements of soluble urokinase plasminogen activator receptor.

stroke incidence and total mortality over time. The paper is rich in statistical analyses that should now be fully within your comprehension. It is interesting in its own right for the analysis of links between diet, a chronic health marker and risks of disease and death, and for the breadth of its statistical analysis.

The authors present mean suPAR, total cholesterol, HDL and BMI values by DQS in a table that shows statistically significant associations (one-way ANOVA) for suPAR and HDL ($P < 0.0001$) but not for total cholesterol ($P = 0.01$) or BMI ($P = 0.27$). They then plot four graphs for these variables (Figure 15.11, suPAR (a), BMI (b), total cholesterol (c), and HDL (d)) showing the percentage difference from the mean value in Group 5 of the DQS (the

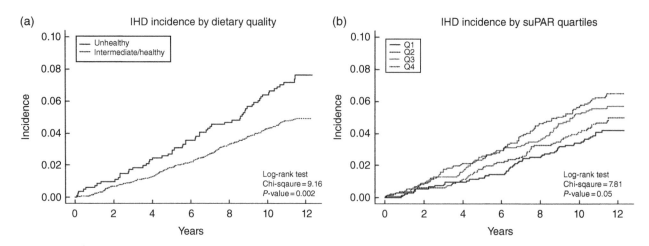

FIGURE 15.12   Survival probability curves for IHD incidence between an unhealthy diet and an intermediate or healthy diet (a) and between sex- and age-specific (≤45 years or >45 years) suPAR quartiles (b) through the follow-up period of approximately 12 years. *Source:* Reproduced with permission of Cambridge University Press.

largest of the groups [$n = 1570$]) for each of the DQS subgroups, together with the 95% confidence intervals. This is an unusual presentation, but it shows neatly how the measurements by DQS groups vary around a central value.

Finally, the authors present the cumulative incidence curves over 12 years for IHD, stroke, and mortality by dichotomized[6] DQS (unhealthy versus intermediate/healthy) and suPAR groups (by quartiles). For purposes of illustration I have used the graphs for IHD (Figure 15.12). The log-rank test looks at the differences in the survival curves between groups, showing statistically significant impact of diet ($P = 0.002$) and suPAR ($P = 0.05$) on the outcomes. The authors have controlled for age, sex, lifestyle factors, and suPAR-adjusted dietary effects when assessing the impact of the dichotomized DQS (a) and suPAR effects adjusted for age, sex, DQS, lifestyle factors, total and HDL cholesterol, blood pressure, prevalent diabetes mellitus, and prevalent CVD as explanatory variables. This reflects the care the authors have taken to present analysis of the impact of diet and suPAR that are unlikely to be explained by potential confounding factors.

I hope that in this final section you feel confident reading about a complex analysis which

addresses the many factors that have been taken into account to obtain a clear understanding of the truth of the hypothesis, and understand the statistical implications. Clearly, a statistician was centrally involved in the design of the analyses. The message here is not to back away from something that looks difficult, but to embrace the complexity with the support of someone who can offer robust guidance.

15.5 CONCLUSION

This chapter has set out numerous examples of ways to present results for different types of audience and with different levels of detail. There are, of course, many other examples in the literature that illustrate ways to present data. When thinking about your own reporting, spend time browsing the literature to find engaging ways of presenting your findings that appeal to you, that fit the model of your data, and that are likely to appeal to your prospective audience. Work with someone who has experience in the field of your research to guide the content and design of your report or presentation: your tutor, a statistician, a researcher familiar with your area of research, and potential members of your audience who can provide feedback on the clarity and intelligibility of what you want to say.

---

[6]Divided into two groups.

In preparing your own research for presentation, be it to fellow students in a seminar, or a written report for grading or publication, or a lay audience, make sure of three things:

1. The story is interesting
2. The story is told clearly
3. The story is truthful

First, as I said at the start of this chapter, no one wants to sit through a boring presentation or read a dull report. More important, if the story is not engaging, you risk losing the attention of your audience or reader. They may never find out the important thing you have to say.

Second, make the story intelligible for your audience. As scientists, we often start a presentation with lots of detail about why we carried out the study (the background and rationale), then put forward the hypothesis and explain the methods, and only then present results and conclusions. This is fine for a scientific meeting, or a written paper for your course or for publication in a scientific journal. A lay audience may not find this format engaging. They may just want to know the headline, why your findings are important, and then some details – more like a newspaper story. Effectively, you state the conclusion at the *start* of your talk or article, then say what you did and why you did it, give a few more details about what you found out, and finally reiterate why the findings are important and their implications. Tailor your presentation to the audience so you hold their attention.

Finally, and most important, tell the truth. Even if there isn't a single test statistic in your presentation, make sure that what you say is truthful, underpinned by the evidence. Statistical analysis helps us understand what is going on in the population. It provides the foundation to help you explain how strong your evidence is. Use the criteria set out by Bradford Hill (Box 1.4) to help structure your evidence.

In this era of 'post-truth' [14], it is more important than ever to be truthful in what we say.

Long live evidence!

The End

(or just the beginning...)

REFERENCES

1. Lowe D. PowerPoint® 2019 for Dummies®. John Wiley and Sons. London. 2018.
2. Public Health England. National Child Measurement Programme: Operational Guidance. Public Health England. London. 2018. https://digital.nhs.uk/services/national-child-measurement-programme/
3. World Health Organization. Training Course on Child Growth Assessment. WHO. Geneva 2008. https://www.who.int/childgrowth/training/module_b_measuring_growth.pdf.
4. Widdowson EM. Mental contentment and physical growth. *Lancet.* 1951;1:1316–1318.
5. Royal College of Paediatrics and Child Health. UK Growth chart 2-18 years BOYS. RCPCH. 2012. https://www.rcpch.ac.uk/resources/uk-who-growth-charts-2-18-years.
6. Public Health England in association with the Welsh Government, Food Standards Scotland and the Food Standards Agency in Northern Ireland. 2016. https://assets.publishing.service.gov.uk/government/uploads/system/uploads/attachment_data/file/528194/Eatwell_guide_greyscale.pdf.
7. Scarborough P, Kaur A, Cobiac L, et al Eatwell Guide: modelling the dietary and cost implications of incorporating new sugar and fibre guidelines *BMJ Open.* 2016;6:e013182. https://bmjopen.bmj.com/content/6/12/e013182
8. McCray S, Maunder K, Barsha L, Mackenzie-Shalders K. Room service in a public hospital improves nutritional intake and increases patient satisfaction while decreasing food waste and cost. *J Human Nutrition Dietetics.* 2018;31,734–741.
9. Wright L, Cotter D, Hickson M. The effectiveness of targeted feeding assistance to improve the nutritional intake of elderly dysphagic patients in hospital. *J Human Nutrition and Dietetics.* 2008;21: 555–562

10. Przemska-Kosicka A, Childs CE, Enani S, Maidens C, Dong H, Bin Dayel I, Tuohy K, Todd S, Gosney MA, Yaqoob P. *Immunity Ageing.* 2016;13(6). https://immunityageing.biomedcentral.com/articles/10.1186/s12979-016-0061-4

11. Shatwan IM, Minihane AM, Williams CM, Lovegrove JA, Jackson KG, Vimaleswaran KS. Impact of lipoprotein lipase gene polymorphism, S447X, on postprandial triacylglycerol and glucose response to sequential meal ingestion. *Int J Mol Sci.* 2016;17(3):397–405. doi: 10.3390/ijms17030397

12. Barbosa-Yañez RL, Dambeck U, Li L, Machann J, Kabisch S, Pfeiffer AFH. Endothelial benefits of fat restriction over carbohydrate restriction in type 2 diabetes mellitus: beyond carbs and fats. *Nutrients* 2018; 10(12): 1859. https://doi.org/10.3390/nu10121859

13. Törnkvist P, Haupt T, Rasmussen L, Ladelund S, Toft U, Pisinger C, Eugen-Olsen J. Soluble urokinase plasminogen activator receptor, a marker of mortality, is linearly associated with dietary quality. *Br J Nutrition.* 1–31.doi:https://doi.org/10.1017/S0007114518003720 https://www.cambridge.org/core/services/aop-cambridge-core/content/view/7B899F6C484A52AC4DC08F3E8D7C5F58/S0007114518003720a.pdf/soluble_urokinase_plasminogen_activator_receptor_a_marker_of_mortality_is_linearly_associated_with_dietary_quality.pdf

14. The Oxford English Dictionary 'word of the year' 2016. https://languages.oup.com/word-of-the-year/word-of-the-year-2016

PART 4

SOLUTIONS TO EXERCISES

Learning Objectives

After doing the exercises at the end of each chapter, you should be confident that:

- You used the right approach to analysis, including formulae and statistical tables
- Your solution is correct, including graphs and tables
- You understand why the solution for each exercise makes sense

Introduction

While teaching the course in statistics for nutrition and dietetics students, I came to two conclusions:

1. Most students have a deep desire to learn
2. Inflicting exams on students can be unfair and distracting

The exercises at the end of each chapter were designed to address these conclusions.

First, for students to learn, the teaching needs to be engaging. Before I designed the course, I read *Freedom to Learn* by Carl Rogers [1]. He depicts many settings in which student-centred activity leads to stronger and better learning outcomes. His least favourite teaching model involves students sitting in a lecture theatre for 50 minutes, listening to an 'expert' drone on, taking copious notes (or none), and then going away to 'learn' what the lecture was about. What a waste of time! The best model, in his view, involves no more than 20 minutes of explication, opportunities for students to get up, move around, and work together, and to use class time to explore the material. At the end of a teaching session, everyone would have had a chance to try out the ideas and techniques and ask questions. It was more like a practical than a lecture.

When we started the course at King's, we set a statistics exam at the end of the year. This was a disaster for two reasons. First, students devoted a disproportionate amount of time studying for the statistics exam instead of revising core topics in nutrition and dietetics. Second, only a handful of students did well in the exams, dragging average

Statistics in Nutrition and Dietetics, First Edition. Michael Nelson.
© 2020 John Wiley & Sons Ltd. Published 2020 by John Wiley & Sons Ltd.
Companion website: www.wiley.com/go/nelson/statistics

grades down. Many students ended up discouraged and downhearted.

Far more effective was to assess performance on the course through completion of the exercises (workings had to be handed in each week) and the protocol development. Each week, work on the exercises was begun in class time, students working in pairs or small groups. They were asked to complete the week's exercises before the next session, and to hand in their work. We would review the answers to the previous week's exercises before starting on a new topic. This provided opportunities to ask questions, clarify concepts, correct misunderstandings, and reinforce learning. Students learned from other students. Everyone was happier, learning improved, and marks were higher. Away with statistics exams, I say!

Chapter 1 The Scientific Method

1.9.1 Rounding and significant digits (Table 1)

For two examples, 13.6652 and 99.4545, the value rounded to two decimal places is different from the one which is achieved in the final column under Sequence. This is because common sense tells us that 13.6652 is more than halfway between 13.66 and 13.67, so should be rounded up, but if a strict sequence of rounding is applied you obtain the lower value. Similarly, 99.4545 is closer to 99.5 than it is to 99.4, so again following the strict sequence of rounding gives us the lower (less correct) value. Follow the rules where you can but use common sense as well. Welcome to the world of statistics!

1.9.2 Interpreting data: does screening save lives? (Table 2)

a. Does screening save lives? Which numbers tell you so?
   Yes, screening saves lives. Rate (deaths per 1000) in Screened group = 1.3/1000. Rate in Control group = 2.0/1000

b. Among the women in the screening group, the death rate from all other causes in the 'Refused' group (38/1000) was almost twice that in the 'Examined' group (21/1000). Did screening cut the death rate in half? Explain briefly.
   No, screening did not cut the death rate in half. Self-selection to refuse screening may be associated with other behaviours likely to increase mortality from other causes (e.g. smoking).

c. Was the study blind?
   No. You know if you are being screened, the researchers know who is being screened, and there is no placebo.

1.9.3 Hypothesis and null hypothesis

In a study designed to assess whether under nutrition is a cause of short stature in poor inner-city children:

a. State the hypothesis (H_1)
   - Undernutrition is a cause of short stature in poor inner-city children
b. State the null hypothesis (H_0)
   - The stature of poor inner-city children is not dependent upon their nutritional status

TABLE 1 Results for Rounding Exercise

Original Value	Rounded to 2 Decimal Places	Rounded to 3 Significant Digits	Sequence
12.2345	12.23	12.2	12.2345→12.234→12.23→12.2
144.5673	144.57	145	144.5673→144.567→144.57→144.6→145
73.665	73.66	73.7	73.665→73.66→73.7
13.6652	13.67	13.7	13.6652→13.665→13.66→13.7
99.4545	99.45	99.5	99.4545→99.454→99.45→99.4

TABLE 2   Impact of Screening for Breast Cancer on 5-year Mortality in 62 000 Women

| | | Cause of Death | | | |
| | | Breast Cancer | | All Other Causes | |
	n	n	Rate/1000	n	Rate/1000
Screening Group					
Examined	20 200	23	1.1	428	21
Refused	10 800	16	1.5	409	38
Total	31 000	39	1.3	837	27
Control group	31 000	63	2.0	879	28

c. Consider:
   i. Confounding factors
     • Parental height; Sibling number; Over-crowding; Infection
     • Household amenities: bath, toilet, fridge, etc.
     • Income; Social class; Education; Parental smoking
     • Age and sex of children in study and comparison groups, etc.
   ii. Sources of systematic bias
     • Measuring devices: height, nutritional intake
     • Sampling frame (see Chapter 2)
     • Observer bias

d. Consider ways to minimize the effects of confounding and systematic bias
Make sure that you measure the confounders and calibrate and validate your measuring instruments (including questionnaires, i.e. make sure that they are telling you what you think they are telling you [validate your method against a reference method with known performance], make comparisons between interviewers to make sure everyone is doing the same thing [account for inter-observer error], etc.)

Chapter 2 Populations and Samples

2.8.1   Weighted means

A town with a population of 100 000 has a social class distribution as shown in Table 3. A sample of 50 households is drawn from each social class, and

TABLE 3   Income by Social Class in a Town with Population = 100 000

Social Class	Number in Town	Number in Sample	Income (£/yr)
I	8 000	50	50 000
II	20 000	50	25 000
III	50 000	50	15 000
IV	15 000	50	10 000
V	7 000	50	8 000

income assessed. Calculate the unweighted and weighted means of income for the town. Explain why the two values differ.

1. **Unweighted mean**: take average of the values for income in the final column:

$$\frac{50\,000 + 25\,000 + 15\,000 + 10\,000 + 8\,000}{5} = 21600$$

2. **Weighted mean**: multiply 'Number in town' times 'Income', take the sum of the products, and divide by the total number of households, e.g.

$$\frac{8000 \times 50000 + 20000 \times 25000 + 50000 \times 15000 + 15000 \times 10000 + 7000 \times 8000}{8000 + 20000 + 50000 + 15000 + 7000}$$
$$= 18560$$

The weighted mean gives a value for average income of £18 560, £3 040 less than the unweighted mean of £21 600. This is because the proportion of people in the town with low incomes is higher than the proportion with high incomes. The weighted mean emphasizes their contribution to the average. The influence of the high incomes in the unweighted mean is reduced.

2.8.2   Mean and standard deviation

Time (in seconds) taken to walk 10 m by 12 patients attending a stroke rehabilitation centre was: 14 18 29 34 22 25 15 22 33 20 11 21

The number of observations: $n = 12$

The average time to walk 10 m is the arithmetic mean of the 12 observations:

$$\bar{x} = \frac{\sum x}{n}$$
$$= \frac{14 + 18 + 29 + 34 + 22 + 25 + 15 + 22 + 33 + 20 + 11 + 21}{12}$$
$$= \frac{264}{12} = 22$$

a. Find the standard deviation (s) the 'long' way:

$$\sqrt{\frac{\sum(x - \bar{x})^2}{n - 1}}$$
$$= \sqrt{\frac{(14 - 22)^2 + (18 - 22)^2 + (29 - 22)^2 + \ldots + (21 - 22)^2}{12 - 1}}$$
$$= \sqrt{\frac{64 + 16 + 49 + \ldots + 1}{12 - 1}} = \sqrt{\frac{578}{11}} = \sqrt{52.545454} = 7.25$$

b. Find the standard deviation (s) the 'short' way:

$$s = \sqrt{\frac{\sum x^2 - (\sum x)^2 / n}{n - 1}}$$
$$= \sqrt{\frac{14^2 + 18^2 + 29^2 + \ldots + 21^2 - (14 + 18 + 29 + \ldots + 21)^2 / 12}{12 - 1}}$$
$$= \sqrt{\frac{6\,386 - (264)^2 / 12}{12 - 1}}$$
$$= \sqrt{\frac{6386 - (69\,696 / 12)}{12 - 1}} = \sqrt{\frac{6\,386 - 5\,808}{12 - 1}} = \sqrt{\frac{578}{11}}$$
$$= \sqrt{52.545\,454} = 7.25$$

As pointed out in the text, the last two steps of the 'long' way and the 'short' way are the same. The beauty of the 'short' way is that there are no intermediate calculations of the difference between the mean and each observation. For example, if I have 100 observations in my sample and delete one (for example, if I decide one of my observations is flawed), I have to calculate the new mean and then redo over a 100 calculations. If I add or delete an observation from my data set and use the 'short' way, I have to redo precisely seven calculations. What's not to like.

2.8.3   Tally

1. Here is what your tally should look like (Table 4):
2. Here is what your histogram should look like (Figure 1):
3. Find the values for mean, standard deviation and median for $n = 100$.

$$\bar{x} = 882 \text{ mg/d}$$
$$s = 300.31 \text{ mg/d}$$
$$\text{median} = 866$$

Because in this example the number of observations is even, the median (by convention) is half way between the two mid-most observations, in this case the 50th and the 51st, equal to 861 and 871, respectively. You know from the tally that the median is somewhere in the 800-899 range, so you need to order only these 13 values.

4. Find the values for mean, standard deviation, and median for the random and systematic samples.

    When I used the Excel function '= randbetween(1,100)' to generate 10 random numbers, the first ten numbers generated were:[1]

03	97	16	12	55	16	84	63	33	57

---

[1] '=rand()' and '=randbetween(value1,value2)' are volatile functions in Excel. This means that every time you change *anything* on the spreadsheet you are working in, the random number values will change. If you want to preserve a set of random values for future reference, you need to highlight it, press control-C, and then paste it as text (right click in the cell in the spreadsheet where you want to save the values and select the paste symbol with the '123' subscript).

TABLE 4   Tally of Calcium Intakes (mg/d) in 100 Cambridge Women age 18–53 Years

Calcium Intake (mg) per day	Tally	Frequency	Cumulative Frequency
300	///	3	3
400	/////	5	8
500	///// ////	9	17
600	///// ///// //	12	29
700	///// ///// ///// //	17	46
800	///// ///// ///	13	59
900	///// /////	10	69
1000	///// //	7	76
1100	///// ///	8	84
1200	/////	5	89
1300	///// //	7	96
1400		0	96
1500	/	1	97
1600	///	3	100

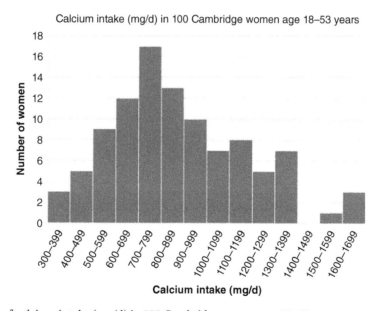

FIGURE 1   Histogram of calcium intake (mg/d) in 100 Cambridge women age 18–53 years.

These identify the subjects to be included in my random sample. As the number 16 appears twice,[2] and we want to sample 'without replacement' (that is, we don't want to use the same subject's result twice), only nine subjects have been identified uniquely. We need to generate another random number (the number 18 came up) to obtain the 10th subject.

The 10 values for calcium intake for these subjects are therefore:

| 1241 | 505 | 730 | 743 | 904 | 1335 | 1688 | 697 | 596 | 545 |

[2]There is a way to select random samples in Excel so that the numbers are generated using the 'without replacement' paradigm. Have a look at this helpful website for how to do this and other useful things in Excel: https://www.ablebits.com.

The statistics are given in the second column in Table 5, below.

TABLE 5   Summary Statistics for Selected Samples of 10 Observations Drawn from Calcium Intakes (mg/d) in 100 Cambridge Women Aged 18–53 years

Term	Random Sample	Systematic Sample	
		Starting Point: Subject 6	Starting Point: Subject 5
n	10	10	10
Σx	8 984	8 691	7 913
Σx^2	9 466 890	8 390 383	6 966 171
$\bar{x}$	898.4	869.1	791.3
s	393.8	305.0	279.8

For the 1 in 10 systematic sample, the random number generated for the starting point was subject 6. The 10 subjects are therefore subjects number 6, 16, 26, 36, and so on to the end of the data set. The statistics are given in the third column in Table 5, above.

I repeated the exercise using another randomly generated number, 5. Thus, subject 5 was the first subject in the systematic sample, the next subjects being numbers 15, 25, and so on up to subject 95. The statistics are given in the fourth column in Table 5, above. Note the marked differences in the computed statistics.

Try the exercise for yourself using your own randomly generated number (but not 5 or 6 – they've been used already).

Chapter 3 Principles of Measurement

3.9.1   Measurement scales

For each of the following variables, name the type of measurement scale – Nominal (N), Ordinal (O), Interval (I), or Ratio (R) and state whether the variables are Qualitative (Q), Quantitative and Discrete (D), or Quantitative and Continuous (C) (Table 6):

There is more than one answer for rank and colour because they can be defined in different ways. Not all numbers (zip codes, car registration numbers) behave mathematically like real or rational numbers. They are (effectively) labels.

TABLE 6   Exercise on Measurement Scales

Variable	Nominal (N) Ordinal (O) Interval (I) Ratio (R)	Qualitative (Q) Quantitative and Discrete (D) Quantitative and Continuous (C)
Age at last birthday	R	D
Exact age	R	C
Sex (gender)	N	Q
Car registration number	N	Q
Height to nearest inch	R	D
Exact height (cm)	R	C
Weight at last birthday	R	C
Race	N	Q
Place of birth	N	Q
Rank:		
1. Numeric	O	D
2. Military	O	Q
Iron intake (mg/d)	R	C
Colour		
3. Hue	N	Q
4. Wavelength	R	C
Postal codes	N	Q
IQ scores	O	D

Some numbers (like an IQ score) may have a mathematical definition ('average' IQ is defined as 100) but no mathematical properties other than rank. You cannot say, for example, that someone with an IQ of 120 is 'twice as smart' as someone with an IQ of 60, or that the difference in intelligence (or whatever IQ measures) between two people with IQs of 80 and 90 is the same as the difference in intelligence between two people with IQs of 100 and 110.

3.9.2   Exercise on reliability, validity, and error

When you consider your measurement per group, it helps to prepare a table so that you can summarize your collective thoughts. Prepare a table with six columns, like the one below.

Variable	Methods to Assess:		Sources of:		How to Measure and Minimize Error and Bias
	Reliability	Validity	Error	Bias	

Of course, once you have filled in the rows for a couple of variables and considered how to minimize error and bias, you discover that the process is never ending: when you identify sources of error and bias, you realize that you are going to have to establish the reliability and validity of measures of error and bias. Have fun!

Chapter 4 Probability and Types of Distribution

4.6.1

a. Give two formulae for the standard normal deviate

$$u = \frac{x - \mu}{\sigma}$$

$$u = \frac{\bar{x} - \mu}{\sigma/\sqrt{n}} = \frac{\bar{x} - \mu}{SE}$$

b. For a variable x which follows the normal distribution, what is the probability that x lies beyond the following values of u in one direction ($\frac{1}{2}P$) and in both directions (P)?

u	1.645	1.96	2.326	2.576	2.88	3.291
In one direction: $\frac{1}{2}P$:	0.05	0.025	0.01	0.005	0.002	0.0005
In both directions P:	0.10	0.05	0.02	0.01	0.004	0.001

Note that where u is given to three decimal places, you are going to need to interpolate the values in the table. For example, 1.645 is five-tenths of the way between 1.64 and 1.65. When $u = 1.64$, $\frac{1}{2}P = 0.0505$. When $u = 1.65$, $\frac{1}{2}P = 0.0495$. Five-tenths of the way

between these two values gives us a value for $\frac{1}{2}P$ based on the following equation:

$$\frac{1}{2}P = 0.0505 - (0.0505 - 0.0495) \times \frac{5}{10}$$

$$= 0.0505 - 0.001 \times \frac{5}{10} = 0.0505 - 0.0005 = 0.05$$

Use the same technique to find the values for $\frac{1}{2}P$ for the other values for u with three decimal places.

4.6.2

Assume $\mu = 882$ and $\sigma = 300.3$. Using the standard normal deviate, find:

a. The percentage below 700 mg/d, the UK Reference Nutrient Intake (RNI)
b. The percentage below 1000 mg/d, the US Dietary Reference Intakes (DRI):
c. The percentage above 525 mg/d, the UK Estimated Average Requirement (EAR)

From the first formula in 4.6.1(a), the value for u for subjects with calcium intakes less than 700 mg/d would be:

$$u = \frac{700 - 882}{300.3} = -0.606$$

that is, 700 is 0.606 standard normal deviates below the mean, 882. As there are no negative values in the table in Appendix A2, we take the absolute value of our computed value for u and apply common sense to find the answer we are looking for.

I'm going to be lazy for a minute, and round 0.606 to 0.61. (If I want the interpolated value for

0.606, I can do it later.) The area under the curve which is *more than* 0.61 standard normal deviates from the mean (shown by the shaded region) is 0.2709 as a proportion of the total area, or 27.1%. Because my computed value for u was negative, I can assume that the percentage of women with intakes *below* 700 mg/d is 27.1%, that is, in the tail to the *left* of the mean. The actual *number* of women who reported calcium intakes below 700 mg/d was 29 (see Table 4), or 29%, compared with my mathematical model which suggests that 27.1% would have intakes below 700 mg/d. So, the model provides a reasonably good reflection of what was actually observed.

For women with intakes below 1000 mg/d,

$$u = \frac{1000 - 882}{300.3} = 0.393$$

From Appendix A2, I see that for $u = 0.39$ (I'm being lazy again), $\frac{1}{2}P = 0.3483$. So, the model predicts that roughly 35% of women have intakes *above* 1000 mg/d. My question was, what percentage of women have intakes below 1000 mg/d. As the total area under the curve is 100%, the percentage of women with intakes *below* 1000 mg/d is 100% − 35% = 65%. When I counted in the tally (Table 4), the number of women in my sample with intakes below 1000 mg/d was $n = 69$. So again, the model provides a good reflection of the actual distribution.

Finally, to find the number of women with intakes above the EAR (525 mg/d), I find the value for $\frac{1}{2}P$ when

$$u = \frac{525 - 882}{300.3} = -1.188$$

(call it −1.19) which is 0.1170, or 11.7%. As in the previous example, the area under the curve that I am interested in is not the value given in the table (which tells us the percentage of women with intakes *below* 525 mg/d) but the percentage of women with intakes above 525 mg/d, which this time will be 100% − 11.7% = 88.3%. If I look at the counts in Table 4 and Figure 2 (the histogram with a normal curve superimposed), I see that the number reporting intakes below 500 mg/d ($n = 11$) is agrees well with the model.

4.6.3

If the standard deviation (σ) of weekly sweet consumption is about 3 ounces, he can find the standard error for the different sample sizes using Equation 4.1, $SE = \sqrt{\sigma^2/n}$, or its simplified version $SE = \sigma/\sqrt{n}$

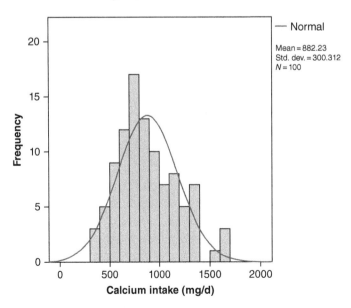

FIGURE 2 Histogram of calcium intake (mg/d) in 100 Cambridge women age 18–53 years with normal curve superimposed.

For each value of n, the SE is as follows:

n	25	100	625
SE	0.6	0.3	0.12

As n increases, the size of the error around the estimate of the mean decreases. So large samples are likely to provide a better estimate of the true population mean than small samples. Note, however, that because SE is related to the inverse of the square root of n, reducing the size of the SE to gain better precision when estimating the true population mean is expensive (in terms of sample size). Our dental epidemiologist would have to have a four-fold increase in sample size to reduce the size of the SE by half; a 25-fold increase in sample size is needed to reduce SE to one-fifth of its former value. We will come back to this discussion in Chapter 12.

Chapter 5   Confidence Intervals and Significance Testing

5.5.1

You have the following information
$\bar{x} = 4.5391$, $\mu = 4.5$, $\sigma = 1.28$, $n = 2000$.

a. The limits of the 95% confidence interval around μ for a sample of this size is given by the equation
$$\mu \pm u\left(\sigma/\sqrt{n}\right) = 4.5 \pm u\left(1.28/\sqrt{2000} = 4.5 \pm 0.056\right)$$

b. The limits of the 95% confidence interval are therefore 4.444 and 4.556. This includes the value for the sample mean $\bar{x} = 4.5391$. The sample mean is therefore included in the 95% of the values for samples of $n = 2000$ that we expect to see around $\mu = 4.5$

c. We can compute our test statistic u to find out if our sample mean is an unlikely observation:
$$u = \frac{\bar{x} - \mu}{\sigma/\sqrt{n}} = \frac{4.5391 - 4.5}{1.28/\sqrt{2000}} = \frac{0.0391}{0.0286} = 1.366$$

d. $u < 1.96$, so we accept the null hypothesis. There is no strong evidence to suggest that random digits generated by the computer do *not* have a mean of 4.5.

e. The exact value for P can be found from the normal table (Appendix A2). When $u = 1.366$, $\frac{1}{2}P = 0.086$, so $P = 2 \times 0.086 = 0.172$. We can say that $P > 0.05$. We accept the null hypothesis.

5.5.2

Again, we look at what we know. The mean level of prothrombin in the normal population is 20.0 mg/100 ml of plasma and the standard deviation is 4 mg/100 ml. A sample of 40 patients showing vitamin K deficiency has a mean prothrombin level of 18.50 mg/100 ml.
$$\mu = 20 \text{ mg}/100 \text{ ml}, \quad \sigma = 4 \text{ mg}/100 \text{ ml}, \quad n = 40,$$
$$\bar{x} = 18.5 \text{ mg}/100 \text{ ml}$$

a. Find u using
$$u = \frac{\bar{x} - \mu}{\sigma/\sqrt{n}} = \frac{18.5 - 20}{4/\sqrt{40}} = -2.372$$

From the Normal table, we see that when $u = -2.37$, $\frac{1}{2}P = 0.008\,89$, so $P = 0.017\,78$. We can say that P is between 0.01 and 0.05, or between 1% and 5%, or that $0.01 < P < 0.05$. It is therefore *unlikely* that the sample comes from the general population. Our conclusion expressed in English could be, 'The probability of drawing a sample of 40 subjects with a mean prothrombin of 18.5 mg/100 ml from a population with mean prothrombin of 20 mg/100 ml and standard deviation 4 mg/100 ml is between 1% and 5%. I therefore reject the null hypothesis. I conclude that this group of patients has a prothrombin level lower than the normal population, statistically significant at the 5% level'.

b. What are the limits within which we would expect to see the mean prothrombin level for all patients with vitamin K deficiency? We have enough information to calculate the 95% confidence limits for μ around the sample mean $\bar{x}$ (i.e. where we would expect to find the true mean for the population from which this sample was drawn). If the 95% CI for μ around $\bar{x}$ does not contain the mean value for the population of patients with normal vitamin K levels, we can conclude (statistically speaking) that the population from which the vitamin K deficient patients were drawn is not the same as the population of patients with normal vitamin K levels.

The formula for finding the 95% CI for μ around $\bar{x}$ is:

$$\bar{x} \pm u\frac{\sigma}{\sqrt{n}} = 18.5 \pm 1.96\frac{4}{\sqrt{40}} = 18.5 \pm 1.96 \times 0.63$$
$$= 18.5 \pm 1.24$$

We will be right 95% of the time in saying that the limits of the prothrombin levels for the population mean of patients with vitamin K deficiency are 17.26 and 19.74 mg/100 ml. As these limits do not include 20 mg/100 ml, the population mean for patients with normal vitamin K levels, we can conclude with a 95% level of confidence that this sample was drawn from a different population.

5.5.3

As in the previous exercise, we must ask ourselves 'What do we know?'
$\bar{x} = 11.5$ seconds, $s = 0.7$ seconds, $n = 30$

a. The equation for finding the 95% confidence interval for μ around $\bar{x}$ is:
$\bar{x} \pm t(s/\sqrt{n})$. This is different from the equation used in the previous exercise, as we know s, not σ. We are therefore obliged to use t rather than u for our multiplier to find the 95% CI. If we look up the value for t in Appendix A3 for $\nu = n - 1 = 30 - 1 = 29$ and $P = 0.05$, we find $t_{\nu = 29, P = 0.05} = 2.045$. So, our equation is:

$$\bar{x} \pm t_{\nu=29,P=0.05} \frac{s}{\sqrt{n}} = 11.5 \pm 2.045 \frac{0.7}{\sqrt{30}}$$
$$= 11.5 \pm 2.045 \times 0.128 = 11.5 \pm 0.262$$

which yields 11.24 and 11.76 as the limits of the 95% C.I. We would be right 95% of the time in thinking that the true population mean for this group of runners lies somewhere within this interval.

b. What is the probability that this group of 30 athletes has been drawn from the group of world class runners in which the average sprint time for 100 m is 11.1 seconds? We can answer this question in two ways.
   i. First, we see that the 95% CI for this group of runners, 11.24 seconds and 11.76 seconds, does not include the mean for the world class runners, 11.1 seconds. We could reasonably conclude that the observed sample came from a population different from the population of world-class runners.

   ii. We can calculate the test statistic t using the information that we have about our two groups of athletes and the following equation:

$$t = \frac{\bar{x} - \mu}{s / \sqrt{n}} = \frac{11.5 - 11.1}{0.7 / \sqrt{30}} = \frac{0.4}{0.128} = 3.13$$

Now look up this value up in the Appendix A3, the t table. You will find that when $\nu = 29$, 3.13 falls between the columns headed 0.01 and 0.001. The probability of this group of runners coming from the world class group is between 1 in 100 and 1 in 1000. It seems highly unlikely ($0.001 < P < 0.01$) that our group of runners came from the world class group. They will have to work a little harder.

Chapter 6 Two Sample Comparisons for Normal Distributions: The t-test

6.4.1

Patient anxiety scores

This fits the model for a paired t-test. We have repeat measures in the same subjects on two different treatments. Assume that the underlying distribution of anxiety scores is normal. Higher scores indicate a greater level of anxiety.

The null hypothesis assumes that the drug is no better than the placebo, that the average scores in both sets of observations should be the same, that there is no difference between treatments, and that the average of the differences in the scores in the parent population from which the patients are drawn is zero: $\mu = 0$.

Follow the test procedure set out in Box 6.4. The steps to finding the solution are set out below:

1. Take the difference between each pair of observations (Table 7).
   • **Note!! Take the difference in the same direction for EVERY pair!**
   • **Note!! The sign of the difference is important!**

TABLE 7   Anxiety Scores in Patients with Anorexia

Patient	Anxiety Score			
	Drug	Placebo	Drug–Placebo (d)	d^2
1	19	22	−3	9
2	11	18	−7	49
3	14	17	−3	9
4	17	19	−2	4
5	23	22	1	1
6	11	12	−1	1
7	15	14	1	1
8	19	11	8	64
9	11	19	−8	64
10	8	7	1	1
Sum (Σ)	148	161	−13	203
Mean	14.8	16.1	−1.3	

2. Calculate the mean and standard deviation of the differences.

Find d^2 for each pair of differences. Find the sum of d and d^2 (Table 7).

Find the standard deviation of the difference in scores using the "short" method:

$$s = \sqrt{\frac{\Sigma d^2 - \left(\Sigma d\right)^2 / n}{n-1}} = \sqrt{\frac{203 - \left(-13\right)^2 / 10}{10-1}}$$

$$= \sqrt{\frac{203 - 16.9}{9}} = \sqrt{\frac{186.1}{9}} = \sqrt{20.7} = 4.55$$

3. Calculate the value for t, where $t = (\bar{d} - \mu)/SE = (\bar{d} - 0)/(s/\sqrt{n})$

This assumes that the null hypothesis is true ($\mu = 0$), and that there is no difference in the effect of the drug compared with the placebo.

$$t = \frac{\bar{d} - \mu}{SE} = \frac{-1.3 - 0}{4.55 / \sqrt{10}} = \frac{-1.3}{1.44} = -0.904$$

4. Compare the calculated value for t with the value in Appendix A3 for $v = 9$ and $P = 0.05$. The value in the table is 2.262. As the calculated value is negative, I ignore the sign for the purposes of looking it up in the t table. As the absolute value of calculated value (0.904) is *less than* the value in the table, we accept H_0.

The level of anxiety when taking the drug is no different (statistically speaking) compared with the placebo, although the initial impression is that the drug appears to be more effective at relieving anxiety.

6.4.2

Smoking knowledge

This also fits the model of a paired t-test. This time, we have measures of learning in subjects matched for age and sex who have had two different exposures relating to learning about smoking, video learning and discussion for Group A, and traditional lecturing for Group B. Again, assume that the underlying distribution of scores is normal.

The null hypothesis assumes that the two teaching methods will yield the same result. There will be no difference in learning between methods, and that the average of the differences in the knowledge scores in the parent population from which the pupils are drawn is zero: $\mu = 0$.

The approach will be the same as in the previous example (Box 6.4). The steps to finding the solution are set out below:

1. Take the difference between each pair of observations (Table 8).
2. Calculate the mean and standard deviation of the differences.

Find d^2 for each pair of differences. Find the sum of d and d^2.

TABLE 8   Knowledge Scores Comparing Different Teaching Methods

Pair	Group A (Video)	Group B (Formal)	Difference (d) (A – B)	d²
1	51	37	14	196
2	48	53	–5	25
3	35	39	–4	16
4	60	46	14	196
5	57	51	6	36
6	64	60	4	16
7	71	50	21	441
8	63	41	22	484
9	55	33	22	484
10	50	45	5	25
Sum (Σ)	554	455	99	1919
Mean	55.4	45.5	9.9	

Find the standard deviation of the difference in scores using the 'short' method:

$$s = \sqrt{\frac{\sum d^2 - \left(\sum d\right)^2 / n}{n-1}} = \sqrt{\frac{1919 - \left(99\right)^2 / 10}{10-1}}$$

$$= \sqrt{\frac{1919 - 980.1}{9}} = \sqrt{\frac{938.9}{9}} = \sqrt{104.3} = 10.214$$

3. Calculate the value for t, where $t = (\bar{d} - \mu)/SE = (\bar{d} - 0)/(s/\sqrt{n})$

   This assumes that the null hypothesis is true, and that there is no difference in the impact of the teaching methods.

$$t = \frac{\bar{d} - \mu}{SE} = \frac{9.9 - 0}{10.214 / \sqrt{10}} = \frac{9.9}{3.23} = 3.07$$

4. Compare the calculated value for t with the value in Appendix A3 for $\nu = 9$ and $P = 0.05$.

   The value in the table is 2.262. As the calculated value is *greater than* the value in the table, we reject H_0.

As the value for $p < 0.05$, we can reject the null hypothesis at the 5% level and conclude that the difference between methods results in a significantly greater score for the group who received the Video teaching (Group A).

We can go a step further. As $\nu = 9$, and the calculated value for $t = 3.07$, we see that the calculated value falls between the tabulated values for $P = 0.02$ (2.821) and $P = 0.01$ (3.250). Thus, we can say that $0.02 > P > 0.01$ and reject the null hypothesis at the 2% level.

6.4.3

Weight gain in babies

These data fit the model for an unpaired t-test. There are two similar groups (although we don't appear to have been given information about the age or sex of the babies, so there may be an issue with the differences between the group characteristics).

We will follow the test procedure set out in Box 6.7.

1. Calculate the mean and standard deviation for each set of observations (Table 9).

2. Calculate the difference between the means:

   $1290\,g - 842\,g = 448\,g$

   It appears that the breast-fed babies are growing faster on average than the bottle-fed babies.

3. Calculate the value for the pooled standard deviation s_0.

$$s_0 = \sqrt{\frac{\sum_1 x^2 - \left(\sum_1 x\right)^2 / n_1 + \sum_2 x^2 - \left(\sum_2 x\right)^2 / n_2}{n_1 + n_2 - 2}}$$

$$= \sqrt{\frac{17\,850\,000 - (12\,900^2/10) + 4\,492\,500 - (5050^2/6)}{10 + 6 - 2}}$$

$$= 322$$

TABLE 9   Growth in Babies from Guatemala between 4 and 12 Weeks Either Breast or Bottle Fed

	Breast	Bottle	(Breast)²	(Bottle)²
	1 600	600	2 560 000	360 000
	1 500	800	2 250 000	640 000
	600	750	360 000	562 500
	1 000	700	1 000 000	490 000
	1 100	1 000	1 210 000	1 000 000
	1 700	1 200	2 890 000	1 440 000
	900		810 000	
	1 500		2 250 000	
	1 400		1 960 000	
	1 600		2 560 000	
n	10	6		
Sum ($\sum$)	12 900	5 050	17 850 000	4 492 500
Mean	1 290	842	1 785 000	748 750
SD	366.5	220.0		

4. Calculate the value for t, where

$$t = \frac{\bar{x}_1 - \bar{x}_2}{SE} = \frac{\bar{x}_1 - \bar{x}_2}{s_0\sqrt{(1/n_1)+(1/n_2)}}$$

$$= \frac{1290 - 842}{322\sqrt{(1/10)+(1/6)}} = \frac{448}{166} = 2.69$$

Remember that $t = (\bar{x}_1 - \bar{x}_2)/SE$, the difference between the means divided by the standard error of the difference between the means, where $SE = s_0\sqrt{(1/n_1)+(1/n_2)}$.

5. Compare the calculated value for t with the value in Appendix A3. When $\nu = 10 + 6 - 2 = 14$ and $P = 0.05$ the tabulated value for $t = 2.145$. The calculated value was 2.69. As the calculated value is greater than the value in the table, we can reject H_0. We conclude that in babies from a Guatemalan village, breast fed babies grow faster between 4 weeks and 12 weeks than bottle-fed babies.

6. If the null hypothesis is rejected, decide the level at which to reject H_0. The value for t is between the values in the table for $P = 0.02$ and $P = 0.01$. We can conclude that $0.02 > P > 0.01$ and say that the finding is significant at the 2% level.

Chapter 7 Nonparametric Two-sample Tests

7.6.1

As we are in the chapter concerning nonparametric two-sample tests, we will assume that the unpaired data comparing two treatments for pressure areas (bed sores) are not from a normally distributed population (otherwise we would be using the paired t-test).

The null hypothesis says that there is no difference in the median healing score between the two groups.

The model (Box 7.3) for the Mann–Whitney test says:

1. There is one variable, not normally distributed (pressure area score)
2. Two groups of observations, independently drawn from patients receiving one of two treatments.
3. Observations are *not* paired between samples.
4. The score is ordinal (higher scores denote worse outcome than lower scores, but the interval is not necessarily the same between scores)
5. Test to see if the difference between the sample medians in the two groups is different from zero.

Our data fit the model.
The test procedure (Box 7.4) says:

1. Combine results for both groups and rank, keeping note of which result (and rank) belongs to which group (Table 10)
2. Calculate the sum of the ranks for each group separately (R_1 and R_2)
3. Check your sums
   $R_1 + R_2 = \frac{1}{2}(n_1 + n_2)(n_1 + n_2 + 1)$
   $126 + 45 = \frac{1}{2}(12 + 6)(12 + 6 + 1) = \frac{1}{2}(18)(19)$
   $171 = 171$

TABLE 10   Scores for Pressure Scores in two Groups of Hospital Patients given Two Different Treatments

Treatment A		Treatment B	
Score	Rank	Score	Rank
	1		1
2	2		
	3		3
	4		4
6	5.5		
6	5.5		
7	9		
7	9		
7	9		
7	9		
	7		9
	8		14
	8		14
8	14		
8	14		
8	14		
9	17.5		
9	17.5		
Median = 7	$R_1 = 126$	Median = 5.5	$R_2 = 45$

4. Calculate the Wilcoxon U statistic
$$U_1 = n_1 n_2 + n_2(n_2 + 1)/2 - R_2 = 48$$
$$U_2 = n_1 n_2 + n_1(n_1 + 1)/2 - R_1 = 24$$

5. Check your sums
$$U_1 + U_2 = n_1 \times n_2$$
$$48 + 24 = 12 \times 6 = 72$$

6. Compare the calculated value for U with the tabulated value in Appendix A4 for n_1 and n_2.
The test statistic is $U = \min(U_1, U_2) = 24$
If the calculated value for U is less than or equal to the value in the table, reject the null hypothesis.

The value in the table for sample sizes of $n_1 = 12$ and $n_2 = 6$ (or the other way around) is $U_{12,6,P=0.05} = 14$. The calculated value is greater than the tabulated

value, so we accept H_0. We conclude that there is no statistically significant difference between the median scores for the two treatments: 7 and 5.5.

7.6.2

a. H_0: There is no difference between heights measured using procedure A and procedure B.
b. A *quick test* would be the Wilcoxon sign test. For each pair of observations (Table 11), see if the value for A is greater than the value for B. Of the 20 data pairs, there are 14 times when A > B, 4 times when A < B, and 2 ties. So we can say $R+ = 14$, $R- = 4$, $n = 18$ and $R = \min(R+, R-) = 4$. From the table for R (Appendix A6), when $n = 18$, we can reject H_0 at $P < 0.05$ when the calculated value for R is *less than or equal to* 4, or at $P < 0.01$ when the calculated value for R is *less than or equal to* 3.
As the calculated value for R is equal to the tabulated value for $n = 18$ at $P = 0.05$, we can reject the null hypothesis and say that Procedure A gives statistically significantly greater measurements ($P < 0.05$).
c. As the data are paired, we can test the data using the Wilcoxon signed-rank test.

The test procedure says:

1. Find the differences between the height measurements (see Table 11)
2. Rank the differences, *ignoring* the sign, and *ignoring* the zeros
3. Find the sum of the ranks of the positive differences ($R+$) and the sum of the ranks of the negative differences ($R-$)
$R+ = 151$, $R- = 20$, and n (the number of non-zero differences) $= 18$.
Check that $R+ + R- = n(n+1)/2$.
$151 + 20 = 171 = 18 \times 19/2$.
4. Find $T = \min(R+, R-) = 20$.
5. Compare calculated test statistic T with tabulated value in Appendix A5 for $n =$ number of nonzero differences. As the calculated value is *less than* that given in the table at $P = 0.01$ ($T_{n=18,P=0.01} = 28$), we can reject the null hypothesis at the 1% level.

While there is a statistically significant difference between the two methods, the median difference is

TABLE 11   Estimates of Child Height using Two Different Assessment Methods

Child	A	B	Difference	Modulus	Rank	Ranks Positive Differences	Ranks Negative Differences
1	108.4	108.2	0.2	0.2	6	6	
2	109.0	109.0	0.0				
3	111.0	110.0	1.0	1	15.5	15.5	
4	110.3	110.5	−0.2	0.2	6		6
5	109.8	108.6	1.2	1.2	17.5	17.5	
6	113.1	111.9	1.2	1.2	17.5	17.5	
7	115.2	114.8	0.4	0.4	10	10	
8	112.5	112.6	−0.1	0.1	2		2
9	106.3	106.3	0.0				
10	109.9	109.7	0.2	0.2	6	6	
11	108.8	108.6	0.2	0.2	6	6	
12	110.7	110.0	0.7	0.7	12.5	12.5	
13	112.0	112.4	−0.4	0.4	10		10
14	111.6	111.7	−0.1	0.1	2		2
15	109.9	108.9	1.0	1	15.5	15.5	
16	106.7	106.0	0.7	0.7	12.5	12.5	
17	113.5	113.3	0.2	0.2	6	6	
18	110.0	109.9	0.1	0.1	2	2	
19	111.2	110.3	0.9	0.9	14	14	
20	109.7	109.3	0.4	0.4	10	10	
Median	110.2	110.0				R+=151	R−=20

only 0.2 cm (2 mm). You will need to have a discussion with your field director about whether detecting this difference is worth the extra time it will take to use method A to collect the height data.

Chapter 8 Contingency Tables, Chi-squared, and Fisher's Exact Test

8.7.1

The data (Table 12) fit the model for a 2×2 contingency table. To calculate the χ^2 test statistic, follow the test procedure in the steps below.

1. Find the values for E for every cell (row total times column total divided by N: $E_{ij} = r_i c_j / N$)
2. Take the difference between O and E for every cell
3. Square the values for $O - E$ in every cell
4. Divide the square of $O - E$ by E: $(O - E)^2 / E$
5. Add together the values for the standardized deviations for all cells in the table:

$$\chi^2 = \sum \left[\frac{(O-E)^2}{E} \right]$$

6. Find the value for χ^2 in Appendix A7 for $\nu = 1$ and $P = 0.05$

The results of the calculations are shown in Table 12

$$\chi^2 = \sum \left[\frac{(O-E)^2}{E} \right] = 0.933 + 1.716 + 2.36 + 4.34 = 9.349$$

$$\nu = (p-1)(q-1) = (2-1)(2-1) = 1$$

In Appendix A7, find the intersection of the row headed $\nu = 1$ and the column headed $P = 0.05$. The value for $\chi^2_{\nu=1, P=0.05} = 3.841$. Our calculated value for $\chi^2 = 9.349$. As the calculated value is *greater than* the tabulated value, we can reject the null hypothesis at the 5% level. We can say that there is a statistically significant difference between men and women in the way they perceive the need for change in dietary habits as they grow older.

TABLE 12   Numbers of Women and Men Who Thought Changes in Dietary Habits would be Necessary as they Grew Older

		Women	Men	
Yes	O	125	52	$r_1 = 177$
	E	114.66	62.34	
	$\frac{(O-E)^2}{E}$	0.933	1.716	
	$\frac{O-E}{\sqrt{E}}$	0.97	−1.31	
No	O	35	35	$r_2 = 70$
	E	45.34	24.66	
	$\frac{(O-E)^2}{E}$	2.36	4.34	
	$\frac{O-E}{\sqrt{E}}$	−1.54	2.08	
		$c_1 = 160$	$c_2 = 87$	$N = 247$

Can we reject the null hypothesis with greater confidence? From Appendix A7, we see that $\chi^2_{\nu=1, P=0.01} = 6.63$, $\chi^2_{\nu=1, P=0.005} = 7.879$, and $\chi^2_{\nu=1, P=0.001} = 10.83$. Our calculated value for $\chi^2 = 9.349$. We can reject H_0 at $P < 0.005$, the 0.5% level.

The largest value for the standardized residual, $(O-E)/\sqrt{E} = 2.08$, was for the men who thought that no change would be necessary. This is where the strength of the association lies. 50% more men than expected ($O = 35$, $E = 24.66$) thought that no change would be necessary. Silly men.

8.7.2

This is a $p \times q$ table. We follow the same test procedure as in the previous example. The results are shown in Table 13.

$$\chi^2 = \sum \left[\frac{(O-E)^2}{E} \right] = 14.062$$

$$\nu = (p-1)(q-1) = (2-1)(4-1) = 1 \times 3 = 3$$

In Appendix A7, find the intersection of the row headed $\nu = 3$ and the column headed $P = 0.05$. The value for $\chi^2_{\nu=3, P=0.05} = 7.815$. Our calculated value for $\chi^2 = 14.062$. As the calculated value is *greater than* the tabulated value, we can reject the null hypothesis at the 5% level. We can say that there is a statistically significant difference in nutritional status three months postsurgery according to whether or not dietetic support was provided at home.

As before, we can look further across the columns in Appendix A7 to see if we can reject the null hypothesis with greater confidence. For our calculated value for $\chi^2 = 14.062$, we find that $0.001 < P < 0.005$. We can reject H_0 at the 0.5% level. Lastly, if we look at the values for the standardized residual, $(O-E)/\sqrt{E}$, we see that the cells with the largest values are for those with either good nutritional status or malnourished. We might say that the chances of being malnourished are highest for those who declined nutritional support. There may be a host of reasons for this, such as nutritional status on

TABLE 13   Number of Patients Who Had Nutritional Status Assessed Three Months Post-discharge: Nutritional Status Versus Accepting Or Declining Nutritional Support At Home Post-surgery

		Nutritional Status				
		Good	Moderate	Poor	Malnourished	
Dietetic support						
Accepted	O	19	10	8	5	$r_1 = 42$
	E	13.13	7.88	10.50	10.50	
	$\dfrac{(O-E)^2}{E}$	2.630	0.573	0.595	2.881	
	$\dfrac{O-E}{\sqrt{E}}$	1.62	0.76	−0.77	−1.70	
Declined	O	6	5	12	15	$r_2 = 38$
	E	11.88	7.13	9.50	9.50	
	$\dfrac{(O-E)^2}{E}$	2.907	0.634	0.658	3.184	
	$\dfrac{O-E}{\sqrt{E}}$	−1.70	−0.80	0.81	1.78	
		$c_1 = 25$	$c_2 = 15$	$c_3 = 20$	$c_4 = 20$	$N = 80$

discharge, type or extent of surgery, or attitude to diet and health, but we would need a different type of analysis to take these factors into account.

8.7.3

Table 14 shows the numbers of girls with anaemia according to their menarchial status and the expected values for a chi-squared analysis. Two of the values for E in the table are less than 5. This violates the assumptions set out in Box 8.1 that no value for E should be less than 5. An uncorrected chi-squared analysis is likely to lead to misleading conclusion regarding the probability of menarchial status being associated with anaemia. If we were to go ahead with an uncorrected calculation of the test statistic, we would find that $\chi^2 = 3.993$ and we would

end up rejecting the null hypothesis at the 5% level because the tabulated value for $\chi^2_{\nu=1,\, P = 0.05} = 3.841$ and our calculated value is greater than the tabulated value. Given the limitations of the test, we are at risk of making a Type I Error.

There are two alternative approaches to this statistical analysis. The first is to use Yates' correction. Using the shortcut method based on the observed values and the row and column totals (Equation 8.5), we find that:

$$\chi^2_{Yates,2\times2} = \frac{N\left(|ad - bc| - N/2\right)^2}{r_1 r_2 c_1 c_2}$$

$$= \frac{45\left(|5 \times 26 - 2 \times 12| - 45/2\right)^2}{17 \times 28 \times 7 \times 38} = 2.478$$

TABLE 14   Presence of Anaemia in Adolescent Girls According to Menarchial Status

Menarchial status		Anaemic			
		Yes		No	
		n	%	n	%
Started periods	O	5	29.4%	12	70.6%
	E	2.64		14.36	
Not yet started	O	2	7.1%	26	92.9%
	E	4.36		23.64	

TABLE 15   Probabilities of Anaemia in Adolescent Girls According to Menarchial Status (Girls Who Were Anaemic and Had Started their Periods) Based on Fisher's Exact Test for Three Values of **a** Equal to 5, 6, or 7 in Table 8.17

a	P
5	0.0515
6	0.0076
7	0.0004
Area under the tail	0.0596

Difference in the fourth decimal place of the sum of the areas under the tail is due to rounding

This value is well below the tabulated value for $\chi^2_{v=1,\,P=0.05} = 3.841$, and we would accept the null hypothesis, saying that the probability of observing what we observed had a probability greater than 5%, that is, $P > 0.05$.

We know, however, that Yates' correction is very conservative, statistically speaking. As a slightly less conservative alternative, we can apply Fisher's Exact Test to the 2×2 table. Using the formula given in Equation 8.6, we generate the results shown in Table 15. The total probability of getting a value of $a = 5$ *or greater* is 0.0596. We say '*or greater*' to make the test include the tail of the distribution of probabilities. Don't forget, however, this is the area under one tail of the distribution, so in fact we are

saying $\tfrac{1}{2}P = 0.0596$. To make it equivalent to a two-tailed test, we need to double the value, that is, $P = 2 \times 0.0596 = 0.1192$. Again, as for the Yates' correction, you would accept H_0, as $P > 0.05$.

Chapter 9 McNemar's Test

9.4.1 Walking ability

Model

McNemar's test is appropriate for analysis of the results presented in Table 9.4 (p. 203), as we are

---

Box 1 Model for McNemar's Test: Status in Individuals Before and After an Intervention

1. Sample is random and independent
2. There is one non-normal variable ('walking ability') which can take one of two values: 'Moderate to no restriction' or 'Unable to walk or severe restriction'
3. Results show status in individuals before and after an intervention (surgery)
4. Core values are arranged in a table with two rows and two columns
5. The values in tables are counts

---

looking at a change in classification in a before-and-after situation, i.e. before and after surgery (Box 1).

Test procedure and conclusion

As $b + c \leq 20$ we calculate the test statistic $T_2 = b = 1$ and look up the value for P in the binomial table for $n = b + c = 4$, $p = 0.5$. The value for $P = 0.3125$, which times 2 (for a two-tailed test) gives $P = 0.625$. So, as P is not less than 0.05, we accept H_0 and say that surgery has no effect on walking ability in this group of patients.

9.4.2 Gastro-oesophageal Reflux Disease

The model and table would look as follows (Box 2; Table 16):

Model

> ### Box 2 Model for McNemar's Test: Status in Individuals in a Cross-over Trial
>
> 1. Sample is random and independent
> 2. There is one nonnormal variable which can take one of two values: satisfied or not satisfied
> 3. Results show status in individuals on each of two treatments
> 4. Core values are arranged in a table with two rows and two columns
> 5. The values in tables are COUNTS!

TABLE 16   Patients Prescribed Drug A and Drug B for Gastro-oesophageal Reflux Disease (GORD) in a Randomized Cross-over study

		Drug A	
		Satisfied	Not Satisfied
Drug B	Satisfied	150	20
	Not Satisfied	30	50

Test procedure and conclusion

As $b + c > 20$, find test statistic T_1:

$$T_1 = \frac{(b-c)^2}{b+c} = \frac{(20-30)^2}{20+30} = \frac{-10^2}{50} = \frac{100}{50} = 2.0$$

If we look up this value in the χ^2 table with one degree of freedom, we find that $0.100 < P < 0.250$. As $P > 0.05$, we accept H_0 and say that there was no difference in the number of subjects satisfied on the two drugs.

9.4.3   Debate on Salt and Hypertension

If one quarter of each group changed their minds, it means four people moved from thinking salt is 'causative' to being 'in doubt' and 21 people moved from being 'in doubt' to thinking salt is 'causative'. The data fit the model for McNemar's test to assess change of status before and after an intervention (Box 3).

The results are summarized in the 2×2 contingency table shown in Table 17.

Model

> ### Box 3 Model for McNemar's Test: Status in Individuals Before and After an Intervention
>
> 1. Sample is random and independent
> 2. There is one non-normal variable which can take one of two values: 'For' or 'Against'
> 3. Results show status ('Opinion') in individuals before and after an intervention (public debate on salt and hypertension)
> 4. Core values are arranged in a table with two rows and two columns
> 5. The values in tables are counts

TABLE 17   Opinion of 100 Members of the Public on the Role of Salt in Hypertension Before and After A Public Debate

			After Debate	
		Total Before	Causative	In doubt
Before debate	Causative	16	[a] 12	[b] 4
	In doubt	84	[c] 21	[d] 63

Test procedure and conclusion

Because $b + c > 20$, find T_1:

$$T_1 = \frac{(b-c)^2}{b+c} = \frac{(4-21)^2}{4+21} = \frac{-17^2}{25} = \frac{289}{25} = 11.56$$

Look up this value in the χ^2 table with 1 degree of freedom $\chi^2_{v=1, P=0.001} = 10.83$; the result is highly statistically significant at the 0.1% level. The debate has had a substantial impact on public opinion regard the role of salt in the causation of hypertension.

Chapter 10 Association: Correlation and Regression

10.5.1

The relationship between age and dietitian salaries in the NHS is appears to be linear (Table 18. I made these numbers up). The degree of association between the variables can be seen by graphing the points in a scattergram and calculating the Pearson product-moment correlation coefficient and finding the best-fit line through the points using simple linear regression.

Assume that the variables are normally distributed. The test procedure is straightforward and relies simply on doing the sums correctly, as shown in the calculations in Table 18 and the steps in the test procedure that follows.

Test procedure

1. *Find the sum of x, the sum of x^2, the sum of y, and sum of y^2, that is: Σx, Σx^2, Σy, Σy^2*
2. *Multiply the values of each x,y pair together and find the sum of the products: Σxy*
3. *Calculate the sum of squares in x, the sum of squares in y, and the sum of squares in xy, as follows:*

$$S_{xx} = \Sigma x^2 - \frac{(\Sigma x)^2}{n} = 16528 - \frac{211600}{14} = 1413.7$$

$$S_{yy} = \Sigma y^2 - \frac{(\Sigma y)^2}{n} = 9834 - \frac{131044}{14} = 473.7$$

$$S_{xy} = \Sigma xy - \frac{\Sigma x \Sigma y}{n} = 12687 - \frac{460 \times 362}{14} = 792.7$$

TABLE 18 Typical Dietitian Salaries in the NHS in England, By Age (From Dietetic Support Workers to Senior and Specialist Dietitians), and Statistical Workings

Age (yr)	Salary (£1000/yr)			
x	y	x^2	y^2	xy
19	15	361	225	285
21	18	441	324	378
23	20	529	400	460
24	22	576	484	528
26	24	676	576	624
29	24	841	576	696
30	25	900	625	750
32	27	1024	729	864
33	27	1089	729	891
35	28	1225	784	980
44	30	1936	900	1320
45	31	2025	961	1395
48	35	2304	1225	1680
51	36	2601	1296	1836
Σx=460	Σy=362	Σx^2=16528	Σy^2=9834	Σxy=12687

4. *Find the value for the Pearson correlation coefficient r:*

$$r = \frac{S_{xy}}{\sqrt{S_{xx}S_{yy}}} = \frac{792.7}{\sqrt{1413.7 \times 473.7}} = 0.969$$

Correlation of Age and Salary:

$r = 0.969$

$r^2 = 0.938$, that is, 94% of the variation in salary is explained by age

These findings suggest that there is a strong correlation between age and salary. The null hypothesis would say that there is no relationship between x and y, hence the correlation would be equal to zero. To find the statistical significance of the Pearson correlation coefficient r (that is, whether it *is* statistically significantly different from zero), calculate t and look up the value in Appendix A3 with $\nu = n - 2 = 14 - 2 = 12$ degrees of freedom.

$$t = r\sqrt{\frac{n-2}{1-r^2}} = 0.969\sqrt{\frac{14-2}{1-0.969^2}} = 13.51$$

The tabulated value for $t_{\nu=12,P=0.05} = 2.179$. As our calculated value for t is greater than the tabulated value, we can reject H_0 and say that there is a statistically significant correlation between age and salary. Furthermore, $t_{\nu=12,P=0.001} = 4.318$, so we can reject H_0 at the 0.1% level.

For the regression equation:

$$b = \frac{S_{xy}}{S_{xx}} = \frac{792.7}{1413.7} = 0.561$$

$$a = \bar{y} - b\bar{x} = \frac{362}{14} - 0.561 \times \frac{460}{14} = 7.43$$

The regression equation is:

$$\text{Income} = 7.43 + 0.561\,\text{Age}$$

So, for every year of age, a dietitian working in the NHS can expect to earn an additional £561 per year. We know from the discussion in Chapter 10 that the statistical significance of b is the same as r, so we don't need to do that calculation again.

The findings are presented as a scatterplot in Figure 3a, together with the regression line, its equation and r^2 (all of which is provided courtesy of Excel graphics if you click on the data points and click on Trendline). The alternate output from SPSS is shown in Figure 3b. It includes the 95% C.I. for the regression line.

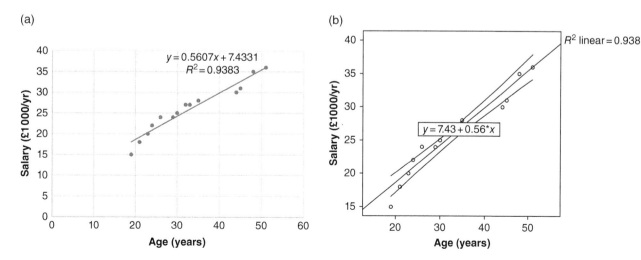

FIGURE 3   (a) Salary (£1000/year) versus age (years) in dieticians working in the NHS (Excel output). (b) Salary (£1000/year) versus age (years) in dieticians working in the NHS (SPSS output).

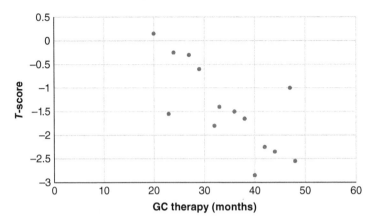

FIGURE 4　Bone-density (*T*-score) versus glucocorticoid therapy (months) in 14 women treated for inflammatory bowel disease (IBD).

10.5.2

Table 19 shows the results for the test procedure set out below for the data on glucocorticoid therapy (months) and bone-density (*T*-score) in 14 women treated for inflammatory bowel disease (IBD).

Test procedure

1. Rank the values for each variable separately
2. Find the difference (*d*) between the ranks for each *x,y* pair
3. Square the difference (*d²*) to get rid of the sign
4. Find the sum of the squares of the differences $\Sigma d^2 = 772$
5. Find ρ using the formula:

$$\rho = 1 - \frac{6\Sigma d^2}{n^3 - n} = 1 - \frac{6 \times 772}{14^3 - 14} = -0.697$$

There appears to be a good negative rank correlation between the duration of glucocorticoid treatment in months with *T*-score for bone density in women treated for IBD (Figure 4). 'Good' in this sense means more than 'moderate' but less than 'strong'.

Is the correlation statistically significant (i.e., can we reject H_0 which says that $\rho = 0$)? We refer to Appendix A8. The tabulated value for $\rho_{n=14, P=0.05} = 0.538$ for the two-tailed test (which is the one we want, because H_0 made no assumptions about the direction of the association between

TABLE 19　Glucocorticoid Therapy (Months) and Bone-density (*T*-score) in 14 Women Treated for Inflammatory Bowel Disease (IBD)

GC therapy (months)	T-score	Rank GC	Rank T-score	d	d²
20	0.15	1	14	-13	169
23	-1.55	2	7	-5	25
24	-0.25	3	13	-10	100
27	-0.3	4	12	-8	64
29	-0.6	5	11	-6	36
32	-1.8	6	5	1	1
33	-1.4	7	9	-2	4
36	-1.5	8	8	0	0
38	-1.65	9	6	3	9
40	-2.85	10	1	9	81
42	-2.25	11	4	7	49
44	-2.35	12	3	9	81
47	-1	13	10	3	9
48	-2.55	14	2	12	144

treatment and bone density). As the table consists only of positive values, we compare the absolute value of the calculated value for $\rho = -0.697$ with the value in the table. We can ignore the sign because in a two-tailed test we just want to know *how far away* we are from what the null hypothesis says we should see, $\rho = 0$, not the direction. As the absolute value of the calculated value for ρ is greater than the tabulated value (0.538), we can reject the null hypothesis at the 5% level. Next question, can we reject the null hypothesis with greater confidence? The values in the table are $\rho_{n\ =14,P\ =0.01} = 0.679$ and $\rho_{n\ =14,P\ =0.005} = 0.723$, so because our value for $\rho = -0.697$, we can reject H_0 at the 1% level.

Chapter 11 Analysis of Variance

The data in Table 20 show results for estimated carbohydrate intake (g/d) in four groups of amateur cyclists who are convinced that their performance is related to their 'carbs'. There do not seem to be great differences, but to keep harmony in the club it seemed worth the effort to measure their carbohydrate intake and do a simple statistical analysis of the results. The data appear to satisfy the model for one-way analysis of variance. We will use SPSS to undertake the analysis.

Model:

1. k groups, where $k > 2$
2. n_i observations in groups, $n_i > 1$

TABLE 20   Carbohydrate Intake (g/d) in Four Groups of Cyclists

	Carbohydrate Intake (g/d)			
Group	1	2	3	4
	279	378	172	381
	338	275	335	346
	334	412	335	340
	198	265	282	471
	303	286	250	318

3. Random selection from normal population
4. Observations in different groups are independent, i.e. no pairing or matching
5. Variances of groups are equal
6. H_0: No differences between group means

The data in SPSS need to be set out in two columns: the first column shows the group number; the second column shows the carbohydrate intakes for each person in the group (so two columns and 20 rows). The data are set out in the file: 'ch11e01.sav'.

The menu sequence is Analyze>Compare Means>Oneway ANOVA. You need to indicate the

Oneway

Carbohydrate (g/d)

Descriptives

	N	Mean	Std. deviation	Std. error	95% confidence interval for mean		Minimum	Maximum
					Lower bound	Upper bound		
1	5	290.40	56.994	25.488	219.63	361.17	198	338
2	5	323.20	67.050	29.986	239.95	406.45	265	412
3	5	274.80	67.976	30.400	190.40	359.20	172	335
4	5	371.20	60.197	26.921	296.46	445.94	318	471
Total	20	314.90	69.277	15.491	282.48	347.32	172	471

ANOVA

Carbohydrate (g/d)

	Sum of squares	df	Mean square	F	Sig.
Between groups	27 234.200	3	9078.067	2.271	0.119
Within groups	63 953.600	16	3997.100		
Total	91 187.800	19			

FIGURE 5   One-way analysis of variance of carbohydrate intake (g/d) in four groups of amateur cyclists.
Source: Reproduced with permission of International Business Machines Corporation.

Factor (Group) and the independent variable (CHO – carbohydrate intake). Click on Options, then tick Descriptives to produce a summary table. The syntax is in 'ch11e01.sps'.

The results look like this (Figure 5):

Group 4 (the one with the highest level of performance) does have a higher mean carbohydrate intake (Descriptives). But from the ANOVA table, we see that $P = 0.119$. As $P > 0.05$, we accept the null hypothesis that there are no differences between the group means.

Take a moment to look up the computed F statistic in Appendix A9 just to satisfy yourself that for the degrees of freedom in the numerator ($v_1 = 3$) and the denominator ($v_2 = 16$), the calculated value (2.271) is less than the tabulated value for F at $P_{3,16,0.05} = 3.24$. Also, have a look at the upper and lower bounds for the 95% confidence intervals for all four groups in the Descriptives. There are no groups for which the 95% confidence intervals do not overlap. This is further evidence that the groups could all have been drawn from the same population whose mean carbohydrate intake is 314.9 g/d with a standard deviation of 69.3 g/d. No *post hoc* tests are required.

REFERENCE

1. Rogers, Carl. *Freedom to Learn for the 80's*. Princeton. Merrill. 2nd Revised edition. 31 December 1983

Probabilities (*P*) of the Binomial Distribution for *n*, *r*, and *p* (Based on Sample Proportions) or π (Proportion in the Population)

Statistics in Nutrition and Dietetics, First Edition. Michael Nelson.
© 2020 John Wiley & Sons Ltd. Published 2020 by John Wiley & Sons Ltd.
Companion website: www.wiley.com/go/nelson/statistics

n	r	p= 0.05	0.10	0.15	0.20	0.25	0.30	0.35	0.40	0.45	0.50
		P									
1	0	0.9500	0.9000	0.8500	0.8000	0.7500	0.7000	0.6500	0.6000	0.5500	0.5000
	1	1.0000	1.0000	1.0000	1.0000	1.0000	1.0000	1.0000	1.0000	1.0000	1.0000
2	0	0.9025	0.8100	0.7225	0.6400	0.5625	0.4900	0.4225	0.3600	0.3025	0.2500
	1	0.9975	0.9900	0.9775	0.9600	0.9375	0.9100	0.8775	0.8400	0.7975	0.7500
	2	1.0000	1.0000	1.0000	1.0000	1.0000	1.0000	1.0000	1.0000	1.0000	1.0000
3	0	0.8574	0.7290	0.6141	0.5120	0.4219	0.3430	0.2746	0.2160	0.1664	0.1250
	1	0.9928	0.9720	0.9393	0.8960	0.8438	0.7840	0.7183	0.6480	0.5748	0.5000
	2	0.9999	0.9990	0.9966	0.9920	0.9844	0.9730	0.9571	0.9360	0.9089	0.8750
	3	1.0000	1.0000	1.0000	1.0000	1.0000	1.0000	1.0000	1.0000	1.0000	1.0000
4	0	0.8145	0.6561	0.5220	0.4096	0.3164	0.2401	0.1785	0.1296	0.0915	0.0625
	1	0.9860	0.9477	0.8905	0.8192	0.7383	0.6517	0.5630	0.4752	0.3910	0.3125
	2	0.9995	0.9963	0.9880	0.9728	0.9492	0.9163	0.8735	0.8208	0.7585	0.6875
	3	1.0000	0.9999	0.9995	0.9984	0.9961	0.9919	0.9850	0.9744	0.9590	0.9375
	4	1.0000	1.0000	1.0000	1.0000	1.0000	1.0000	1.0000	1.0000	1.0000	1.0000
5	0	0.7738	0.5905	0.4437	0.3277	0.2373	0.1681	0.1160	0.0778	0.0503	0.0313
	1	0.9774	0.9185	0.8352	0.7373	0.6328	0.5282	0.4284	0.3370	0.2562	0.1875
	2	0.9988	0.9914	0.9734	0.9421	0.8965	0.8369	0.7648	0.6826	0.5931	0.5000
	3	1.0000	0.9995	0.9978	0.9933	0.9844	0.9692	0.9460	0.9130	0.8688	0.8125
	4	1.0000	1.0000	0.9999	0.9997	0.9990	0.9976	0.9947	0.9898	0.9815	0.9688
	5	1.0000	1.0000	1.0000	1.0000	1.0000	1.0000	1.0000	1.0000	1.0000	1.0000
6	0	0.7351	0.5314	0.3771	0.2621	0.1780	0.1176	0.0754	0.0467	0.0277	0.0156
	1	0.9672	0.8857	0.7765	0.6554	0.5339	0.4202	0.3191	0.2333	0.1636	0.1094
	2	0.9978	0.9842	0.9527	0.9011	0.8306	0.7443	0.6471	0.5443	0.4415	0.3438
	3	0.9999	0.9987	0.9941	0.9830	0.9624	0.9295	0.8826	0.8208	0.7447	0.6563
	4	1.0000	0.9999	0.9996	0.9984	0.9954	0.9891	0.9777	0.9590	0.9308	0.8906
	5	1.0000	1.0000	1.0000	0.9999	0.9998	0.9993	0.9982	0.9959	0.9917	0.9844
	6	1.0000	1.0000	1.0000	1.0000	1.0000	1.0000	1.0000	1.0000	1.0000	1.0000

n	*r*	*p*= 0.55	0.60	0.65	0.70	0.75	0.80	0.85	0.90	0.95
		P								
1	0	0.4500	0.4000	0.3500	0.3000	0.2500	0.2000	0.1500	0.1000	0.0500
	1	1.0000	1.0000	1.0000	1.0000	1.0000	1.0000	1.0000	1.0000	1.0000
2	0	0.2025	0.1600	0.1225	0.0900	0.0625	0.0400	0.0225	0.0100	0.0025
	1	0.6975	0.6400	0.5775	0.5100	0.4375	0.3600	0.2775	0.1900	0.0975
	2	1.0000	1.0000	1.0000	1.0000	1.0000	1.0000	1.0000	1.0000	1.0000
3	0	0.0911	0.0640	0.0429	0.0270	0.0156	0.0080	0.0034	0.0010	0.0001
	1	0.4253	0.3520	0.2818	0.2160	0.1563	0.1040	0.0608	0.0280	0.0073
	2	0.8336	0.7840	0.7254	0.6570	0.5781	0.4880	0.3859	0.2710	0.1426
	3	1.0000	1.0000	1.0000	1.0000	1.0000	1.0000	1.0000	1.0000	1.0000
4	0	0.0410	0.0256	0.0150	0.0081	0.0039	0.0016	0.0005	0.0001	0.0000
	1	0.2415	0.1792	0.1265	0.0837	0.0508	0.0272	0.0120	0.0037	0.0005
	2	0.6090	0.5248	0.4370	0.3483	0.2617	0.1808	0.1095	0.0523	0.0140
	3	0.9085	0.8704	0.8215	0.7599	0.6836	0.5904	0.4780	0.3439	0.1855
	4	1.0000	1.0000	1.0000	1.0000	1.0000	1.0000	1.0000	1.0000	1.0000
5	0	0.0185	0.0102	0.0053	0.0024	0.0010	0.0003	0.0001	0.0000	0.0000
	1	0.1312	0.0870	0.0540	0.0308	0.0156	0.0067	0.0022	0.0005	0.0000
	2	0.4069	0.3174	0.2352	0.1631	0.1035	0.0579	0.0266	0.0086	0.0012
	3	0.7438	0.6630	0.5716	0.4718	0.3672	0.2627	0.1648	0.0815	0.0226
	4	0.9497	0.9222	0.8840	0.8319	0.7627	0.6723	0.5563	0.4095	0.2262
	5	1.0000	1.0000	1.0000	1.0000	1.0000	1.0000	1.0000	1.0000	1.0000
6	0	0.0083	0.0041	0.0018	0.0007	0.0002	0.0001	0.0000	0.0000	0.0000
	1	0.0692	0.0410	0.0223	0.0109	0.0046	0.0016	0.0004	0.0001	0.0000
	2	0.2553	0.1792	0.1174	0.0705	0.0376	0.0170	0.0059	0.0013	0.0001
	3	0.5585	0.4557	0.3529	0.2557	0.1694	0.0989	0.0473	0.0159	0.0022
	4	0.8364	0.7667	0.6809	0.5798	0.4661	0.3446	0.2235	0.1143	0.0328
	5	0.9723	0.9533	0.9246	0.8824	0.8220	0.7379	0.6229	0.4686	0.2649
	6	1.0000	1.0000	1.0000	1.0000	1.0000	1.0000	1.0000	1.0000	1.0000

(Continued)

(Continued)

n	r	p=	0.05	0.10	0.15	0.20	0.25	0.30	0.35	0.40	0.45	0.50
		P										
7	0		0.6983	0.4783	0.3206	0.2097	0.1335	0.0824	0.0490	0.0280	0.0152	0.0078
	1		0.9556	0.8503	0.7166	0.5767	0.4449	0.3294	0.2338	0.1586	0.1024	0.0625
	2		0.9962	0.9743	0.9262	0.8520	0.7564	0.6471	0.5323	0.4199	0.3164	0.2266
	3		0.9998	0.9973	0.9879	0.9667	0.9294	0.8740	0.8002	0.7102	0.6083	0.5000
	4		1.0000	0.9998	0.9988	0.9953	0.9871	0.9712	0.9444	0.9037	0.8471	0.7734
	5		1.0000	1.0000	0.9999	0.9996	0.9987	0.9962	0.9910	0.9812	0.9643	0.9375
	6		1.0000	1.0000	1.0000	1.0000	0.9999	0.9998	0.9994	0.9984	0.9963	0.9922
	7		1.0000	1.0000	1.0000	1.0000	1.0000	1.0000	1.0000	1.0000	1.0000	1.0000
8	0		0.6634	0.4305	0.2725	0.1678	0.1001	0.0576	0.0319	0.0168	0.0084	0.0039
	1		0.9428	0.8131	0.6572	0.5033	0.3671	0.2553	0.1691	0.1064	0.0632	0.0352
	2		0.9942	0.9619	0.8948	0.7969	0.6785	0.5518	0.4278	0.3154	0.2201	0.1445
	3		0.9996	0.9950	0.9786	0.9437	0.8862	0.8059	0.7064	0.5941	0.4770	0.3633
	4		1.0000	0.9996	0.9971	0.9896	0.9727	0.9420	0.8939	0.8263	0.7396	0.6367
	5		1.0000	1.0000	0.9998	0.9988	0.9958	0.9887	0.9747	0.9502	0.9115	0.8555
	6		1.0000	1.0000	1.0000	0.9999	0.9996	0.9987	0.9964	0.9915	0.9819	0.9648
	7		1.0000	1.0000	1.0000	1.0000	1.0000	0.9999	0.9998	0.9993	0.9983	0.9961
	8		1.0000	1.0000	1.0000	1.0000	1.0000	1.0000	1.0000	1.0000	1.0000	1.0000
9	0		0.6302	0.3874	0.2316	0.1342	0.0751	0.0404	0.0207	0.0101	0.0046	0.0020
	1		0.9288	0.7748	0.5995	0.4362	0.3003	0.1960	0.1211	0.0705	0.0385	0.0195
	2		0.9916	0.9470	0.8591	0.7382	0.6007	0.4628	0.3373	0.2318	0.1495	0.0898
	3		0.9994	0.9917	0.9661	0.9144	0.8343	0.7297	0.6089	0.4826	0.3614	0.2539
	4		1.0000	0.9991	0.9944	0.9804	0.9511	0.9012	0.8283	0.7334	0.6214	0.5000
	5		1.0000	0.9999	0.9994	0.9969	0.9900	0.9747	0.9464	0.9006	0.8342	0.7461
	6		1.0000	1.0000	1.0000	0.9997	0.9987	0.9957	0.9888	0.9750	0.9502	0.9102
	7		1.0000	1.0000	1.0000	1.0000	0.9999	0.9996	0.9986	0.9962	0.9909	0.9805
	8		1.0000	1.0000	1.0000	1.0000	1.0000	1.0000	0.9999	0.9997	0.9992	0.9980
	9		1.0000	1.0000	1.0000	1.0000	1.0000	1.0000	1.0000	1.0000	1.0000	1.0000

n	r	p=	0.55	0.60	0.65	0.70	0.75	0.80	0.85	0.90	0.95
		P									
7	0		0.0037	0.0016	0.0006	0.0002	0.0001	0.0000	0.0000	0.0000	0.0000
	1		0.0357	0.0188	0.0090	0.0038	0.0013	0.0004	0.0001	0.0000	0.0000
	2		0.1529	0.0963	0.0556	0.0288	0.0129	0.0047	0.0012	0.0002	0.0000
	3		0.3917	0.2898	0.1998	0.1260	0.0706	0.0333	0.0121	0.0027	0.0002
	4		0.6836	0.5801	0.4677	0.3529	0.2436	0.1480	0.0738	0.0257	0.0038
	5		0.8976	0.8414	0.7662	0.6706	0.5551	0.4233	0.2834	0.1497	0.0444
	6		0.9848	0.9720	0.9510	0.9176	0.8665	0.7903	0.6794	0.5217	0.3017
	7		1.0000	1.0000	1.0000	1.0000	1.0000	1.0000	1.0000	1.0000	1.0000
8	0		0.0017	0.0007	0.0002	0.0001	0.0000	0.0000	0.0000	0.0000	0.0000
	1		0.0181	0.0085	0.0036	0.0013	0.0004	0.0001	0.0000	0.0000	0.0000
	2		0.0885	0.0498	0.0253	0.0113	0.0042	0.0012	0.0002	0.0000	0.0000
	3		0.2604	0.1737	0.1061	0.0580	0.0273	0.0104	0.0029	0.0004	0.0000
	4		0.5230	0.4059	0.2936	0.1941	0.1138	0.0563	0.0214	0.0050	0.0004
	5		0.7799	0.6846	0.5722	0.4482	0.3215	0.2031	0.1052	0.0381	0.0058
	6		0.9368	0.8936	0.8309	0.7447	0.6329	0.4967	0.3428	0.1869	0.0572
	7		0.9916	0.9832	0.9681	0.9424	0.8999	0.8322	0.7275	0.5695	0.3366
	8		1.0000	1.0000	1.0000	1.0000	1.0000	1.0000	1.0000	1.0000	1.0000
9	0		0.0008	0.0003	0.0001	0.0000	0.0000	0.0000	0.0000	0.0000	0.0000
	1		0.0091	0.0038	0.0014	0.0004	0.0001	0.0000	0.0000	0.0000	0.0000
	2		0.0498	0.0250	0.0112	0.0043	0.0013	0.0003	0.0000	0.0000	0.0000
	3		0.1658	0.0994	0.0536	0.0253	0.0100	0.0031	0.0006	0.0001	0.0000
	4		0.3786	0.2666	0.1717	0.0988	0.0489	0.0196	0.0056	0.0009	0.0000
	5		0.6386	0.5174	0.3911	0.2703	0.1657	0.0856	0.0339	0.0083	0.0006
	6		0.8505	0.7682	0.6627	0.5372	0.3993	0.2618	0.1409	0.0530	0.0084
	7		0.9615	0.9295	0.8789	0.8040	0.6997	0.5638	0.4005	0.2252	0.0712
	8		0.9954	0.9899	0.9793	0.9596	0.9249	0.8658	0.7684	0.6126	0.3698
	9		1.0000	1.0000	1.0000	1.0000	1.0000	1.0000	1.0000	1.0000	1.0000

(Continued)

n	r	p=	0.05	0.10	0.15	0.20	0.25	0.30	0.35	0.40	0.45	0.50
		P										
10	0		0.5987	0.3487	0.1969	0.1074	0.0563	0.0282	0.0135	0.0060	0.0025	0.0010
	1		0.9139	0.7361	0.5443	0.3758	0.2440	0.1493	0.0860	0.0464	0.0233	0.0107
	2		0.9885	0.9298	0.8202	0.6778	0.5256	0.3828	0.2616	0.1673	0.0996	0.0547
	3		0.9990	0.9872	0.9500	0.8791	0.7759	0.6496	0.5138	0.3823	0.2660	0.1719
	4		0.9999	0.9984	0.9901	0.9672	0.9219	0.8497	0.7515	0.6331	0.5044	0.3770
	5		1.0000	0.9999	0.9986	0.9936	0.9803	0.9527	0.9051	0.8338	0.7384	0.6230
	6		1.0000	1.0000	0.9999	0.9991	0.9965	0.9894	0.9740	0.9452	0.8980	0.8281
	7		1.0000	1.0000	1.0000	0.9999	0.9996	0.9984	0.9952	0.9877	0.9726	0.9453
	8		1.0000	1.0000	1.0000	1.0000	1.0000	0.9999	0.9995	0.9983	0.9955	0.9893
	9		1.0000	1.0000	1.0000	1.0000	1.0000	1.0000	1.0000	0.9999	0.9997	0.9990
	10		1.0000	1.0000	1.0000	1.0000	1.0000	1.0000	1.0000	1.0000	1.0000	1.0000
11	0		0.5688	0.3138	0.1673	0.0859	0.0422	0.0198	0.0088	0.0036	0.0014	0.0005
	1		0.8981	0.6974	0.4922	0.3221	0.1971	0.1130	0.0606	0.0302	0.0139	0.0059
	2		0.9848	0.9104	0.7788	0.6174	0.4552	0.3127	0.2001	0.1189	0.0652	0.0327
	3		0.9984	0.9815	0.9306	0.8389	0.7133	0.5696	0.4256	0.2963	0.1911	0.1133
	4		0.9999	0.9972	0.9841	0.9496	0.8854	0.7897	0.6683	0.5328	0.3971	0.2744
	5		1.0000	0.9997	0.9973	0.9883	0.9657	0.9218	0.8513	0.7535	0.6331	0.5000
	6		1.0000	1.0000	0.9997	0.9980	0.9924	0.9784	0.9499	0.9006	0.8262	0.7256
	7		1.0000	1.0000	1.0000	0.9998	0.9988	0.9957	0.9878	0.9707	0.9390	0.8867
	8		1.0000	1.0000	1.0000	1.0000	0.9999	0.9994	0.9980	0.9941	0.9852	0.9673
	9		1.0000	1.0000	1.0000	1.0000	1.0000	1.0000	0.9998	0.9993	0.9978	0.9941
	10		1.0000	1.0000	1.0000	1.0000	1.0000	1.0000	1.0000	1.0000	0.9998	0.9995
	11		1.0000	1.0000	1.0000	1.0000	1.0000	1.0000	1.0000	1.0000	1.0000	1.0000
12	0		0.5404	0.2824	0.1422	0.0687	0.0317	0.0138	0.0057	0.0022	0.0008	0.0002
	1		0.8816	0.6590	0.4435	0.2749	0.1584	0.0850	0.0424	0.0196	0.0083	0.0032
	2		0.9804	0.8891	0.7358	0.5583	0.3907	0.2528	0.1513	0.0834	0.0421	0.0193
	3		0.9978	0.9744	0.9078	0.7946	0.6488	0.4925	0.3467	0.2253	0.1345	0.0730
	4		0.9998	0.9957	0.9761	0.9274	0.8424	0.7237	0.5833	0.4382	0.3044	0.1938
	5		1.0000	0.9995	0.9954	0.9806	0.9456	0.8822	0.7873	0.6652	0.5269	0.3872
	6		1.0000	0.9999	0.9993	0.9961	0.9857	0.9614	0.9154	0.8418	0.7393	0.6128
	7		1.0000	1.0000	0.9999	0.9994	0.9972	0.9905	0.9745	0.9427	0.8883	0.8062
	8		1.0000	1.0000	1.0000	0.9999	0.9996	0.9983	0.9944	0.9847	0.9644	0.9270
	9		1.0000	1.0000	1.0000	1.0000	1.0000	0.9998	0.9992	0.9972	0.9921	0.9807
	10		1.0000	1.0000	1.0000	1.0000	1.0000	1.0000	0.9999	0.9997	0.9989	0.9968
	11		1.0000	1.0000	1.0000	1.0000	1.0000	1.0000	1.0000	1.0000	0.9999	0.9998
	12		1.0000	1.0000	1.0000	1.0000	1.0000	1.0000	1.0000	1.0000	1.0000	1.0000

n	r	p=	0.55	0.60	0.65	0.70	0.75	0.80	0.85	0.90	0.95
		P									
10	0		0.0003	0.0001	0.0000	0.0000	0.0000	0.0000	0.0000	0.0000	0.0000
	1		0.0045	0.0017	0.0005	0.0001	0.0000	0.0000	0.0000	0.0000	0.0000
	2		0.0274	0.0123	0.0048	0.0016	0.0004	0.0001	0.0000	0.0000	0.0000
	3		0.1020	0.0548	0.0260	0.0106	0.0035	0.0009	0.0001	0.0000	0.0000
	4		0.2616	0.1662	0.0949	0.0473	0.0197	0.0064	0.0014	0.0001	0.0000
	5		0.4956	0.3669	0.2485	0.1503	0.0781	0.0328	0.0099	0.0016	0.0001
	6		0.7340	0.6177	0.4862	0.3504	0.2241	0.1209	0.0500	0.0128	0.0010
	7		0.9004	0.8327	0.7384	0.6172	0.4744	0.3222	0.1798	0.0702	0.0115
	8		0.9767	0.9536	0.9140	0.8507	0.7560	0.6242	0.4557	0.2639	0.0861
	9		0.9975	0.9940	0.9865	0.9718	0.9437	0.8926	0.8031	0.6513	0.4013
	10		1.0000	1.0000	1.0000	1.0000	1.0000	1.0000	1.0000	1.0000	1.0000
11	0		0.0002	0.0000	0.0000	0.0000	0.0000	0.0000	0.0000	0.0000	0.0000
	1		0.0022	0.0007	0.0002	0.0000	0.0000	0.0000	0.0000	0.0000	0.0000
	2		0.0148	0.0059	0.0020	0.0006	0.0001	0.0000	0.0000	0.0000	0.0000
	3		0.0610	0.0293	0.0122	0.0043	0.0012	0.0002	0.0000	0.0000	0.0000
	4		0.1738	0.0994	0.0501	0.0216	0.0076	0.0020	0.0003	0.0000	0.0000
	5		0.3669	0.2465	0.1487	0.0782	0.0343	0.0117	0.0027	0.0003	0.0000
	6		0.6029	0.4672	0.3317	0.2103	0.1146	0.0504	0.0159	0.0028	0.0001
	7		0.8089	0.7037	0.5744	0.4304	0.2867	0.1611	0.0694	0.0185	0.0016
	8		0.9348	0.8811	0.7999	0.6873	0.5448	0.3826	0.2212	0.0896	0.0152
	9		0.9861	0.9698	0.9394	0.8870	0.8029	0.6779	0.5078	0.3026	0.1019
	10		0.9986	0.9964	0.9912	0.9802	0.9578	0.9141	0.8327	0.6862	0.4312
	11		1.0000	1.0000	1.0000	1.0000	1.0000	1.0000	1.0000	1.0000	1.0000
12	0		0.0001	0.0000	0.0000	0.0000	0.0000	0.0000	0.0000	0.0000	0.0000
	1		0.0011	0.0003	0.0001	0.0000	0.0000	0.0000	0.0000	0.0000	0.0000
	2		0.0079	0.0028	0.0008	0.0002	0.0000	0.0000	0.0000	0.0000	0.0000
	3		0.0356	0.0153	0.0056	0.0017	0.0004	0.0001	0.0000	0.0000	0.0000
	4		0.1117	0.0573	0.0255	0.0095	0.0028	0.0006	0.0001	0.0000	0.0000
	5		0.2607	0.1582	0.0846	0.0386	0.0143	0.0039	0.0007	0.0001	0.0000
	6		0.4731	0.3348	0.2127	0.1178	0.0544	0.0194	0.0046	0.0005	0.0000
	7		0.6956	0.5618	0.4167	0.2763	0.1576	0.0726	0.0239	0.0043	0.0002
	8		0.8655	0.7747	0.6533	0.5075	0.3512	0.2054	0.0922	0.0256	0.0022
	9		0.9579	0.9166	0.8487	0.7472	0.6093	0.4417	0.2642	0.1109	0.0196
	10		0.9917	0.9804	0.9576	0.9150	0.8416	0.7251	0.5565	0.3410	0.1184
	11		0.9992	0.9978	0.9943	0.9862	0.9683	0.9313	0.8578	0.7176	0.4596
	12		1.0000	1.0000	1.0000	1.0000	1.0000	1.0000	1.0000	1.0000	1.0000

(Continued)

(Continued)

n	r	p=	0.05	0.10	0.15	0.20	0.25	0.30	0.35	0.40	0.45	0.50
		P										
13	0		0.5133	0.2542	0.1209	0.0550	0.0238	0.0097	0.0037	0.0013	0.0004	0.0001
	1		0.8646	0.6213	0.3983	0.2336	0.1267	0.0637	0.0296	0.0126	0.0049	0.0017
	2		0.9755	0.8661	0.6920	0.5017	0.3326	0.2025	0.1132	0.0579	0.0269	0.0112
	3		0.9969	0.9658	0.8820	0.7473	0.5843	0.4206	0.2783	0.1686	0.0929	0.0461
	4		0.9997	0.9935	0.9658	0.9009	0.7940	0.6543	0.5005	0.3530	0.2279	0.1334
	5		1.0000	0.9991	0.9925	0.9700	0.9198	0.8346	0.7159	0.5744	0.4268	0.2905
	6		1.0000	0.9999	0.9987	0.9930	0.9757	0.9376	0.8705	0.7712	0.6437	0.5000
	7		1.0000	1.0000	0.9998	0.9988	0.9944	0.9818	0.9538	0.9023	0.8212	0.7095
	8		1.0000	1.0000	1.0000	0.9998	0.9990	0.9960	0.9874	0.9679	0.9302	0.8666
	9		1.0000	1.0000	1.0000	1.0000	0.9999	0.9993	0.9975	0.9922	0.9797	0.9539
	10		1.0000	1.0000	1.0000	1.0000	1.0000	0.9999	0.9997	0.9987	0.9959	0.9888
	11		1.0000	1.0000	1.0000	1.0000	1.0000	1.0000	1.0000	0.9999	0.9995	0.9983
	12		1.0000	1.0000	1.0000	1.0000	1.0000	1.0000	1.0000	1.0000	1.0000	0.9999
	13		1.0000	1.0000	1.0000	1.0000	1.0000	1.0000	1.0000	1.0000	1.0000	1.0000
14	0		0.4877	0.2288	0.1028	0.0440	0.0178	0.0068	0.0024	0.0008	0.0002	0.0001
	1		0.8470	0.5846	0.3567	0.1979	0.1010	0.0475	0.0205	0.0081	0.0029	0.0009
	2		0.9699	0.8416	0.6479	0.4481	0.2811	0.1608	0.0839	0.0398	0.0170	0.0065
	3		0.9958	0.9559	0.8535	0.6982	0.5213	0.3552	0.2205	0.1243	0.0632	0.0287
	4		0.9996	0.9908	0.9533	0.8702	0.7415	0.5842	0.4227	0.2793	0.1672	0.0898
	5		1.0000	0.9985	0.9885	0.9561	0.8883	0.7805	0.6405	0.4859	0.3373	0.2120
	6		1.0000	0.9998	0.9978	0.9884	0.9617	0.9067	0.8164	0.6925	0.5461	0.3953
	7		1.0000	1.0000	0.9997	0.9976	0.9897	0.9685	0.9247	0.8499	0.7414	0.6047
	8		1.0000	1.0000	1.0000	0.9996	0.9978	0.9917	0.9757	0.9417	0.8811	0.7880
	9		1.0000	1.0000	1.0000	1.0000	0.9997	0.9983	0.9940	0.9825	0.9574	0.9102
	10		1.0000	1.0000	1.0000	1.0000	1.0000	0.9998	0.9989	0.9961	0.9886	0.9713
	11		1.0000	1.0000	1.0000	1.0000	1.0000	1.0000	0.9999	0.9994	0.9978	0.9935
	12		1.0000	1.0000	1.0000	1.0000	1.0000	1.0000	1.0000	0.9999	0.9997	0.9991
	13		1.0000	1.0000	1.0000	1.0000	1.0000	1.0000	1.0000	1.0000	1.0000	0.9999
	14		1.0000	1.0000	1.0000	1.0000	1.0000	1.0000	1.0000	1.0000	1.0000	1.0000

n	r	p=	0.55	0.60	0.65	0.70	0.75	0.80	0.85	0.90	0.95
		P									
13	0		0.0000	0.0000	0.0000	0.0000	0.0000	0.0000	0.0000	0.0000	0.0000
	1		0.0005	0.0001	0.0000	0.0000	0.0000	0.0000	0.0000	0.0000	0.0000
	2		0.0041	0.0013	0.0003	0.0001	0.0000	0.0000	0.0000	0.0000	0.0000
	3		0.0203	0.0078	0.0025	0.0007	0.0001	0.0000	0.0000	0.0000	0.0000
	4		0.0698	0.0321	0.0126	0.0040	0.0010	0.0002	0.0000	0.0000	0.0000
	5		0.1788	0.0977	0.0462	0.0182	0.0056	0.0012	0.0002	0.0000	0.0000
	6		0.3563	0.2288	0.1295	0.0624	0.0243	0.0070	0.0013	0.0001	0.0000
	7		0.5732	0.4256	0.2841	0.1654	0.0802	0.0300	0.0075	0.0009	0.0000
	8		0.7721	0.6470	0.4995	0.3457	0.2060	0.0991	0.0342	0.0065	0.0003
	9		0.9071	0.8314	0.7217	0.5794	0.4157	0.2527	0.1180	0.0342	0.0031
	10		0.9731	0.9421	0.8868	0.7975	0.6674	0.4983	0.3080	0.1339	0.0245
	11		0.9951	0.9874	0.9704	0.9363	0.8733	0.7664	0.6017	0.3787	0.1354
	12		0.9996	0.9987	0.9963	0.9903	0.9762	0.9450	0.8791	0.7458	0.4867
	13		1.0000	1.0000	1.0000	1.0000	1.0000	1.0000	1.0000	1.0000	1.0000
14	0		0.0000	0.0000	0.0000	0.0000	0.0000	0.0000	0.0000	0.0000	0.0000
	1		0.0003	0.0001	0.0000	0.0000	0.0000	0.0000	0.0000	0.0000	0.0000
	2		0.0022	0.0006	0.0001	0.0000	0.0000	0.0000	0.0000	0.0000	0.0000
	3		0.0114	0.0039	0.0011	0.0002	0.0000	0.0000	0.0000	0.0000	0.0000
	4		0.0426	0.0175	0.0060	0.0017	0.0003	0.0000	0.0000	0.0000	0.0000
	5		0.1189	0.0583	0.0243	0.0083	0.0022	0.0004	0.0000	0.0000	0.0000
	6		0.2586	0.1501	0.0753	0.0315	0.0103	0.0024	0.0003	0.0000	0.0000
	7		0.4539	0.3075	0.1836	0.0933	0.0383	0.0116	0.0022	0.0002	0.0000
	8		0.6627	0.5141	0.3595	0.2195	0.1117	0.0439	0.0115	0.0015	0.0000
	9		0.8328	0.7207	0.5773	0.4158	0.2585	0.1298	0.0467	0.0092	0.0004
	10		0.9368	0.8757	0.7795	0.6448	0.4787	0.3018	0.1465	0.0441	0.0042
	11		0.9830	0.9602	0.9161	0.8392	0.7189	0.5519	0.3521	0.1584	0.0301
	12		0.9971	0.9919	0.9795	0.9525	0.8990	0.8021	0.6433	0.4154	0.1530
	13		0.9998	0.9992	0.9976	0.9932	0.9822	0.9560	0.8972	0.7712	0.5123
	14		1.0000	1.0000	1.0000	1.0000	1.0000	1.0000	1.0000	1.0000	1.0000

(Continued)

(Continued)

n	r	p=	0.05	0.10	0.15	0.20	0.25	0.30	0.35	0.40	0.45	0.50
		P										
15	0		0.4633	0.2059	0.0874	0.0352	0.0134	0.0047	0.0016	0.0005	0.0001	0.0000
	1		0.8290	0.5490	0.3186	0.1671	0.0802	0.0353	0.0142	0.0052	0.0017	0.0005
	2		0.9638	0.8159	0.6042	0.3980	0.2361	0.1268	0.0617	0.0271	0.0107	0.0037
	3		0.9945	0.9444	0.8227	0.6482	0.4613	0.2969	0.1727	0.0905	0.0424	0.0176
	4		0.9994	0.9873	0.9383	0.8358	0.6865	0.5155	0.3519	0.2173	0.1204	0.0592
	5		0.9999	0.9978	0.9832	0.9389	0.8516	0.7216	0.5643	0.4032	0.2608	0.1509
	6		1.0000	0.9997	0.9964	0.9819	0.9434	0.8689	0.7548	0.6098	0.4522	0.3036
	7		1.0000	1.0000	0.9994	0.9958	0.9827	0.9500	0.8868	0.7869	0.6535	0.5000
	8		1.0000	1.0000	0.9999	0.9992	0.9958	0.9848	0.9578	0.9050	0.8182	0.6964
	9		1.0000	1.0000	1.0000	0.9999	0.9992	0.9963	0.9876	0.9662	0.9231	0.8491
	10		1.0000	1.0000	1.0000	1.0000	0.9999	0.9993	0.9972	0.9907	0.9745	0.9408
	11		1.0000	1.0000	1.0000	1.0000	1.0000	0.9999	0.9995	0.9981	0.9937	0.9824
	12		1.0000	1.0000	1.0000	1.0000	1.0000	1.0000	0.9999	0.9997	0.9989	0.9963
	13		1.0000	1.0000	1.0000	1.0000	1.0000	1.0000	1.0000	1.0000	0.9999	0.9995
	14		1.0000	1.0000	1.0000	1.0000	1.0000	1.0000	1.0000	1.0000	1.0000	1.0000
	15		1.0000	1.0000	1.0000	1.0000	1.0000	1.0000	1.0000	1.0000	1.0000	1.0000
16	0		0.4401	0.1853	0.0743	0.0281	0.0100	0.0033	0.0010	0.0003	0.0001	0.0000
	1		0.8108	0.5147	0.2839	0.1407	0.0635	0.0261	0.0098	0.0033	0.0010	0.0003
	2		0.9571	0.7892	0.5614	0.3518	0.1971	0.0994	0.0451	0.0183	0.0066	0.0021
	3		0.9930	0.9316	0.7899	0.5981	0.4050	0.2459	0.1339	0.0651	0.0281	0.0106
	4		0.9991	0.9830	0.9209	0.7982	0.6302	0.4499	0.2892	0.1666	0.0853	0.0384
	5		0.9999	0.9967	0.9765	0.9183	0.8103	0.6598	0.4900	0.3288	0.1976	0.1051
	6		1.0000	0.9995	0.9944	0.9733	0.9204	0.8247	0.6881	0.5272	0.3660	0.2272
	7		1.0000	0.9999	0.9989	0.9930	0.9729	0.9256	0.8406	0.7161	0.5629	0.4018
	8		1.0000	1.0000	0.9998	0.9985	0.9925	0.9743	0.9329	0.8577	0.7441	0.5982
	9		1.0000	1.0000	1.0000	0.9998	0.9984	0.9929	0.9771	0.9417	0.8759	0.7728
	10		1.0000	1.0000	1.0000	1.0000	0.9997	0.9984	0.9938	0.9809	0.9514	0.8949
	11		1.0000	1.0000	1.0000	1.0000	1.0000	0.9997	0.9987	0.9951	0.9851	0.9616
	12		1.0000	1.0000	1.0000	1.0000	1.0000	1.0000	0.9998	0.9991	0.9965	0.9894
	13		1.0000	1.0000	1.0000	1.0000	1.0000	1.0000	1.0000	0.9999	0.9994	0.9979
	14		1.0000	1.0000	1.0000	1.0000	1.0000	1.0000	1.0000	1.0000	0.9999	0.9997
	15		1.0000	1.0000	1.0000	1.0000	1.0000	1.0000	1.0000	1.0000	1.0000	1.0000
	16		1.0000	1.0000	1.0000	1.0000	1.0000	1.0000	1.0000	1.0000	1.0000	1.0000

n	r	p= 0.55	0.60	0.65	0.70	0.75	0.80	0.85	0.90	0.95
		P								
15	0	0.0000	0.0000	0.0000	0.0000	0.0000	0.0000	0.0000	0.0000	0.0000
	1	0.0001	0.0000	0.0000	0.0000	0.0000	0.0000	0.0000	0.0000	0.0000
	2	0.0011	0.0003	0.0001	0.0000	0.0000	0.0000	0.0000	0.0000	0.0000
	3	0.0063	0.0019	0.0005	0.0001	0.0000	0.0000	0.0000	0.0000	0.0000
	4	0.0255	0.0093	0.0028	0.0007	0.0001	0.0000	0.0000	0.0000	0.0000
	5	0.0769	0.0338	0.0124	0.0037	0.0008	0.0001	0.0000	0.0000	0.0000
	6	0.1818	0.0950	0.0422	0.0152	0.0042	0.0008	0.0001	0.0000	0.0000
	7	0.3465	0.2131	0.1132	0.0500	0.0173	0.0042	0.0006	0.0000	0.0000
	8	0.5478	0.3902	0.2452	0.1311	0.0566	0.0181	0.0036	0.0003	0.0000
	9	0.7392	0.5968	0.4357	0.2784	0.1484	0.0611	0.0168	0.0022	0.0001
	10	0.8796	0.7827	0.6481	0.4845	0.3135	0.1642	0.0617	0.0127	0.0006
	11	0.9576	0.9095	0.8273	0.7031	0.5387	0.3518	0.1773	0.0556	0.0055
	12	0.9893	0.9729	0.9383	0.8732	0.7639	0.6020	0.3958	0.1841	0.0362
	13	0.9983	0.9948	0.9858	0.9647	0.9198	0.8329	0.6814	0.4510	0.1710
	14	0.9999	0.9995	0.9984	0.9953	0.9866	0.9648	0.9126	0.7941	0.5367
	15	1.0000	1.0000	1.0000	1.0000	1.0000	1.0000	1.0000	1.0000	1.0000
16	0	0.0000	0.0000	0.0000	0.0000	0.0000	0.0000	0.0000	0.0000	0.0000
	1	0.0001	0.0000	0.0000	0.0000	0.0000	0.0000	0.0000	0.0000	0.0000
	2	0.0006	0.0001	0.0000	0.0000	0.0000	0.0000	0.0000	0.0000	0.0000
	3	0.0035	0.0009	0.0002	0.0000	0.0000	0.0000	0.0000	0.0000	0.0000
	4	0.0149	0.0049	0.0013	0.0003	0.0000	0.0000	0.0000	0.0000	0.0000
	5	0.0486	0.0191	0.0062	0.0016	0.0003	0.0000	0.0000	0.0000	0.0000
	6	0.1241	0.0583	0.0229	0.0071	0.0016	0.0002	0.0000	0.0000	0.0000
	7	0.2559	0.1423	0.0671	0.0257	0.0075	0.0015	0.0002	0.0000	0.0000
	8	0.4371	0.2839	0.1594	0.0744	0.0271	0.0070	0.0011	0.0001	0.0000
	9	0.6340	0.4728	0.3119	0.1753	0.0796	0.0267	0.0056	0.0005	0.0000
	10	0.8024	0.6712	0.5100	0.3402	0.1897	0.0817	0.0235	0.0033	0.0001
	11	0.9147	0.8334	0.7108	0.5501	0.3698	0.2018	0.0791	0.0170	0.0009
	12	0.9719	0.9349	0.8661	0.7541	0.5950	0.4019	0.2101	0.0684	0.0070
	13	0.9934	0.9817	0.9549	0.9006	0.8029	0.6482	0.4386	0.2108	0.0429
	14	0.9990	0.9967	0.9902	0.9739	0.9365	0.8593	0.7161	0.4853	0.1892
	15	0.9999	0.9997	0.9990	0.9967	0.9900	0.9719	0.9257	0.8147	0.5599
	16	1.0000	1.0000	1.0000	1.0000	1.0000	1.0000	1.0000	1.0000	1.0000

(Continued)

(Continued)

n	r	p=	0.05	0.10	0.15	0.20	0.25	0.30	0.35	0.40	0.45	0.50
		P										
17	0		0.4181	0.1668	0.0631	0.0225	0.0075	0.0023	0.0007	0.0002	0.0000	0.0000
	1		0.7922	0.4818	0.2525	0.1182	0.0501	0.0193	0.0067	0.0021	0.0006	0.0001
	2		0.9497	0.7618	0.5198	0.3096	0.1637	0.0774	0.0327	0.0123	0.0041	0.0012
	3		0.9912	0.9174	0.7556	0.5489	0.3530	0.2019	0.1028	0.0464	0.0184	0.0064
	4		0.9988	0.9779	0.9013	0.7582	0.5739	0.3887	0.2348	0.1260	0.0596	0.0245
	5		0.9999	0.9953	0.9681	0.8943	0.7653	0.5968	0.4197	0.2639	0.1471	0.0717
	6		1.0000	0.9992	0.9917	0.9623	0.8929	0.7752	0.6188	0.4478	0.2902	0.1662
	7		1.0000	0.9999	0.9983	0.9891	0.9598	0.8954	0.7872	0.6405	0.4743	0.3145
	8		1.0000	1.0000	0.9997	0.9974	0.9876	0.9597	0.9006	0.8011	0.6626	0.5000
	9		1.0000	1.0000	1.0000	0.9995	0.9969	0.9873	0.9617	0.9081	0.8166	0.6855
	10		1.0000	1.0000	1.0000	0.9999	0.9994	0.9968	0.9880	0.9652	0.9174	0.8338
	11		1.0000	1.0000	1.0000	1.0000	0.9999	0.9993	0.9970	0.9894	0.9699	0.9283
	12		1.0000	1.0000	1.0000	1.0000	1.0000	0.9999	0.9994	0.9975	0.9914	0.9755
	13		1.0000	1.0000	1.0000	1.0000	1.0000	1.0000	0.9999	0.9995	0.9981	0.9936
	14		1.0000	1.0000	1.0000	1.0000	1.0000	1.0000	1.0000	0.9999	0.9997	0.9988
	15		1.0000	1.0000	1.0000	1.0000	1.0000	1.0000	1.0000	1.0000	1.0000	0.9999
	16		1.0000	1.0000	1.0000	1.0000	1.0000	1.0000	1.0000	1.0000	1.0000	1.0000
	17		1.0000	1.0000	1.0000	1.0000	1.0000	1.0000	1.0000	1.0000	1.0000	1.0000
18	0		0.3972	0.1501	0.0536	0.0180	0.0056	0.0016	0.0004	0.0001	0.0000	0.0000
	1		0.7735	0.4503	0.2241	0.0991	0.0395	0.0142	0.0046	0.0013	0.0003	0.0001
	2		0.9419	0.7338	0.4797	0.2713	0.1353	0.0600	0.0236	0.0082	0.0025	0.0007
	3		0.9891	0.9018	0.7202	0.5010	0.3057	0.1646	0.0783	0.0328	0.0120	0.0038
	4		0.9985	0.9718	0.8794	0.7164	0.5187	0.3327	0.1886	0.0942	0.0411	0.0154
	5		0.9998	0.9936	0.9581	0.8671	0.7175	0.5344	0.3550	0.2088	0.1077	0.0481
	6		1.0000	0.9988	0.9882	0.9487	0.8610	0.7217	0.5491	0.3743	0.2258	0.1189
	7		1.0000	0.9998	0.9973	0.9837	0.9431	0.8593	0.7283	0.5634	0.3915	0.2403
	8		1.0000	1.0000	0.9995	0.9957	0.9807	0.9404	0.8609	0.7368	0.5778	0.4073
	9		1.0000	1.0000	0.9999	0.9991	0.9946	0.9790	0.9403	0.8653	0.7473	0.5927
	10		1.0000	1.0000	1.0000	0.9998	0.9988	0.9939	0.9788	0.9424	0.8720	0.7597
	11		1.0000	1.0000	1.0000	1.0000	0.9998	0.9986	0.9938	0.9797	0.9463	0.8811
	12		1.0000	1.0000	1.0000	1.0000	1.0000	0.9997	0.9986	0.9942	0.9817	0.9519
	13		1.0000	1.0000	1.0000	1.0000	1.0000	1.0000	0.9997	0.9987	0.9951	0.9846
	14		1.0000	1.0000	1.0000	1.0000	1.0000	1.0000	1.0000	0.9998	0.9990	0.9962
	15		1.0000	1.0000	1.0000	1.0000	1.0000	1.0000	1.0000	1.0000	0.9999	0.9993
	16		1.0000	1.0000	1.0000	1.0000	1.0000	1.0000	1.0000	1.0000	1.0000	0.9999
	17		1.0000	1.0000	1.0000	1.0000	1.0000	1.0000	1.0000	1.0000	1.0000	1.0000
	18		1.0000	1.0000	1.0000	1.0000	1.0000	1.0000	1.0000	1.0000	1.0000	1.0000

n	r	p=	0.55	0.60	0.65	0.70	0.75	0.80	0.85	0.90	0.95
		P									
17	0		0.0000	0.0000	0.0000	0.0000	0.0000	0.0000	0.0000	0.0000	0.0000
	1		0.0000	0.0000	0.0000	0.0000	0.0000	0.0000	0.0000	0.0000	0.0000
	2		0.0003	0.0001	0.0000	0.0000	0.0000	0.0000	0.0000	0.0000	0.0000
	3		0.0019	0.0005	0.0001	0.0000	0.0000	0.0000	0.0000	0.0000	0.0000
	4		0.0086	0.0025	0.0006	0.0001	0.0000	0.0000	0.0000	0.0000	0.0000
	5		0.0301	0.0106	0.0030	0.0007	0.0001	0.0000	0.0000	0.0000	0.0000
	6		0.0826	0.0348	0.0120	0.0032	0.0006	0.0001	0.0000	0.0000	0.0000
	7		0.1834	0.0919	0.0383	0.0127	0.0031	0.0005	0.0000	0.0000	0.0000
	8		0.3374	0.1989	0.0994	0.0403	0.0124	0.0026	0.0003	0.0000	0.0000
	9		0.5257	0.3595	0.2128	0.1046	0.0402	0.0109	0.0017	0.0001	0.0000
	10		0.7098	0.5522	0.3812	0.2248	0.1071	0.0377	0.0083	0.0008	0.0000
	11		0.8529	0.7361	0.5803	0.4032	0.2347	0.1057	0.0319	0.0047	0.0001
	12		0.9404	0.8740	0.7652	0.6113	0.4261	0.2418	0.0987	0.0221	0.0012
	13		0.9816	0.9536	0.8972	0.7981	0.6470	0.4511	0.2444	0.0826	0.0088
	14		0.9959	0.9877	0.9673	0.9226	0.8363	0.6904	0.4802	0.2382	0.0503
	15		0.9994	0.9979	0.9933	0.9807	0.9499	0.8818	0.7475	0.5182	0.2078
	16		1.0000	0.9998	0.9993	0.9977	0.9925	0.9775	0.9369	0.8332	0.5819
	17		1.0000	1.0000	1.0000	1.0000	1.0000	1.0000	1.0000	1.0000	1.0000
18	0		0.0000	0.0000	0.0000	0.0000	0.0000	0.0000	0.0000	0.0000	0.0000
	1		0.0000	0.0000	0.0000	0.0000	0.0000	0.0000	0.0000	0.0000	0.0000
	2		0.0001	0.0000	0.0000	0.0000	0.0000	0.0000	0.0000	0.0000	0.0000
	3		0.0010	0.0002	0.0000	0.0000	0.0000	0.0000	0.0000	0.0000	0.0000
	4		0.0049	0.0013	0.0003	0.0000	0.0000	0.0000	0.0000	0.0000	0.0000
	5		0.0183	0.0058	0.0014	0.0003	0.0000	0.0000	0.0000	0.0000	0.0000
	6		0.0537	0.0203	0.0062	0.0014	0.0002	0.0000	0.0000	0.0000	0.0000
	7		0.1280	0.0576	0.0212	0.0061	0.0012	0.0002	0.0000	0.0000	0.0000
	8		0.2527	0.1347	0.0597	0.0210	0.0054	0.0009	0.0001	0.0000	0.0000
	9		0.4222	0.2632	0.1391	0.0596	0.0193	0.0043	0.0005	0.0000	0.0000
	10		0.6085	0.4366	0.2717	0.1407	0.0569	0.0163	0.0027	0.0002	0.0000
	11		0.7742	0.6257	0.4509	0.2783	0.1390	0.0513	0.0118	0.0012	0.0000
	12		0.8923	0.7912	0.6450	0.4656	0.2825	0.1329	0.0419	0.0064	0.0002
	13		0.9589	0.9058	0.8114	0.6673	0.4813	0.2836	0.1206	0.0282	0.0015
	14		0.9880	0.9672	0.9217	0.8354	0.6943	0.4990	0.2798	0.0982	0.0109
	15		0.9975	0.9918	0.9764	0.9400	0.8647	0.7287	0.5203	0.2662	0.0581
	16		0.9997	0.9987	0.9954	0.9858	0.9605	0.9009	0.7759	0.5497	0.2265
	17		1.0000	0.9999	0.9996	0.9984	0.9944	0.9820	0.9464	0.8499	0.6028
	18		1.0000	1.0000	1.0000	1.0000	1.0000	1.0000	1.0000	1.0000	1.0000

(Continued)

(Continued)

n	r	p=	0.05	0.10	0.15	0.20	0.25	0.30	0.35	0.40	0.45	0.50
		P										
19	0		0.3774	0.1351	0.0456	0.0144	0.0042	0.0011	0.0003	0.0001	0.0000	0.0000
	1		0.7547	0.4203	0.1985	0.0829	0.0310	0.0104	0.0031	0.0008	0.0002	0.0000
	2		0.9335	0.7054	0.4413	0.2369	0.1113	0.0462	0.0170	0.0055	0.0015	0.0004
	3		0.9868	0.8850	0.6841	0.4551	0.2631	0.1332	0.0591	0.0230	0.0077	0.0022
	4		0.9980	0.9648	0.8556	0.6733	0.4654	0.2822	0.1500	0.0696	0.0280	0.0096
	5		0.9998	0.9914	0.9463	0.8369	0.6678	0.4739	0.2968	0.1629	0.0777	0.0318
	6		1.0000	0.9983	0.9837	0.9324	0.8251	0.6655	0.4812	0.3081	0.1727	0.0835
	7		1.0000	0.9997	0.9959	0.9767	0.9225	0.8180	0.6656	0.4878	0.3169	0.1796
	8		1.0000	1.0000	0.9992	0.9933	0.9713	0.9161	0.8145	0.6675	0.4940	0.3238
	9		1.0000	1.0000	0.9999	0.9984	0.9911	0.9674	0.9125	0.8139	0.6710	0.5000
	10		1.0000	1.0000	1.0000	0.9997	0.9977	0.9895	0.9653	0.9115	0.8159	0.6762
	11		1.0000	1.0000	1.0000	1.0000	0.9995	0.9972	0.9886	0.9648	0.9129	0.8204
	12		1.0000	1.0000	1.0000	1.0000	0.9999	0.9994	0.9969	0.9884	0.9658	0.9165
	13		1.0000	1.0000	1.0000	1.0000	1.0000	0.9999	0.9993	0.9969	0.9891	0.9682
	14		1.0000	1.0000	1.0000	1.0000	1.0000	1.0000	0.9999	0.9994	0.9972	0.9904
	15		1.0000	1.0000	1.0000	1.0000	1.0000	1.0000	1.0000	0.9999	0.9995	0.9978
	16		1.0000	1.0000	1.0000	1.0000	1.0000	1.0000	1.0000	1.0000	0.9999	0.9996
	17		1.0000	1.0000	1.0000	1.0000	1.0000	1.0000	1.0000	1.0000	1.0000	1.0000
	18		1.0000	1.0000	1.0000	1.0000	1.0000	1.0000	1.0000	1.0000	1.0000	1.0000
	19		1.0000	1.0000	1.0000	1.0000	1.0000	1.0000	1.0000	1.0000	1.0000	1.0000

n	r	p=	0.55	0.60	0.65	0.70	0.75	0.80	0.85	0.90	0.95
		P									
19	0		0.0000	0.0000	0.0000	0.0000	0.0000	0.0000	0.0000	0.0000	0.0000
	1		0.0000	0.0000	0.0000	0.0000	0.0000	0.0000	0.0000	0.0000	0.0000
	2		0.0001	0.0000	0.0000	0.0000	0.0000	0.0000	0.0000	0.0000	0.0000
	3		0.0005	0.0001	0.0000	0.0000	0.0000	0.0000	0.0000	0.0000	0.0000
	4		0.0028	0.0006	0.0001	0.0000	0.0000	0.0000	0.0000	0.0000	0.0000
	5		0.0109	0.0031	0.0007	0.0001	0.0000	0.0000	0.0000	0.0000	0.0000
	6		0.0342	0.0116	0.0031	0.0006	0.0001	0.0000	0.0000	0.0000	0.0000
	7		0.0871	0.0352	0.0114	0.0028	0.0005	0.0000	0.0000	0.0000	0.0000
	8		0.1841	0.0885	0.0347	0.0105	0.0023	0.0003	0.0000	0.0000	0.0000
	9		0.3290	0.1861	0.0875	0.0326	0.0089	0.0016	0.0001	0.0000	0.0000
	10		0.5060	0.3325	0.1855	0.0839	0.0287	0.0067	0.0008	0.0000	0.0000
	11		0.6831	0.5122	0.3344	0.1820	0.0775	0.0233	0.0041	0.0003	0.0000
	12		0.8273	0.6919	0.5188	0.3345	0.1749	0.0676	0.0163	0.0017	0.0000
	13		0.9223	0.8371	0.7032	0.5261	0.3322	0.1631	0.0537	0.0086	0.0002
	14		0.9720	0.9304	0.8500	0.7178	0.5346	0.3267	0.1444	0.0352	0.0020
	15		0.9923	0.9770	0.9409	0.8668	0.7369	0.5449	0.3159	0.1150	0.0132
	16		0.9985	0.9945	0.9830	0.9538	0.8887	0.7631	0.5587	0.2946	0.0665
	17		0.9998	0.9992	0.9969	0.9896	0.9690	0.9171	0.8015	0.5797	0.2453
	18		1.0000	0.9999	0.9997	0.9989	0.9958	0.9856	0.9544	0.8649	0.6226
	19		1.0000	1.0000	1.0000	1.0000	1.0000	1.0000	1.0000	1.0000	1.0000

(Continued)

(Continued)

n	r	p=	0.05	0.10	0.15	0.20	0.25	0.30	0.35	0.40	0.45	0.50
		P										
20	0		0.3585	0.1216	0.0388	0.0115	0.0032	0.0008	0.0002	0.0000	0.0000	0.0000
	1		0.7358	0.3917	0.1756	0.0692	0.0243	0.0076	0.0021	0.0005	0.0001	0.0000
	2		0.9245	0.6769	0.4049	0.2061	0.0913	0.0355	0.0121	0.0036	0.0009	0.0002
	3		0.9841	0.8670	0.6477	0.4114	0.2252	0.1071	0.0444	0.0160	0.0049	0.0013
	4		0.9974	0.9568	0.8298	0.6296	0.4148	0.2375	0.1182	0.0510	0.0189	0.0059
	5		0.9997	0.9887	0.9327	0.8042	0.6172	0.4164	0.2454	0.1256	0.0553	0.0207
	6		1.0000	0.9976	0.9781	0.9133	0.7858	0.6080	0.4166	0.2500	0.1299	0.0577
	7		1.0000	0.9996	0.9941	0.9679	0.8982	0.7723	0.6010	0.4159	0.2520	0.1316
	8		1.0000	0.9999	0.9987	0.9900	0.9591	0.8867	0.7624	0.5956	0.4143	0.2517
	9		1.0000	1.0000	0.9998	0.9974	0.9861	0.9520	0.8782	0.7553	0.5914	0.4119
	10		1.0000	1.0000	1.0000	0.9994	0.9961	0.9829	0.9468	0.8725	0.7507	0.5881
	11		1.0000	1.0000	1.0000	0.9999	0.9991	0.9949	0.9804	0.9435	0.8692	0.7483
	12		1.0000	1.0000	1.0000	1.0000	0.9998	0.9987	0.9940	0.9790	0.9420	0.8684
	13		1.0000	1.0000	1.0000	1.0000	1.0000	0.9997	0.9985	0.9935	0.9786	0.9423
	14		1.0000	1.0000	1.0000	1.0000	1.0000	1.0000	0.9997	0.9984	0.9936	0.9793
	15		1.0000	1.0000	1.0000	1.0000	1.0000	1.0000	1.0000	0.9997	0.9985	0.9941
	16		1.0000	1.0000	1.0000	1.0000	1.0000	1.0000	1.0000	1.0000	0.9997	0.9987
	17		1.0000	1.0000	1.0000	1.0000	1.0000	1.0000	1.0000	1.0000	1.0000	0.9998
	18		1.0000	1.0000	1.0000	1.0000	1.0000	1.0000	1.0000	1.0000	1.0000	1.0000
	19		1.0000	1.0000	1.0000	1.0000	1.0000	1.0000	1.0000	1.0000	1.0000	1.0000
	20		1.0000	1.0000	1.0000	1.0000	1.0000	1.0000	1.0000	1.0000	1.0000	1.0000

For values of n > 20, search the internet for 'Binomial Table n =?', where '?' is the value for n for which you need probabilities. There will be lots to choose from. You will then be able to find the P value for 'n choose r' for the value of p that you want to test. The most common variation in the nomenclature in the tables online is to use the letter 'x' instead of 'r'.

n	r	p=	0.55	0.60	0.65	0.70	0.75	0.80	0.85	0.90	0.95
		P									
20	0		0.0000	0.0000	0.0000	0.0000	0.0000	0.0000	0.0000	0.0000	0.0000
	1		0.0000	0.0000	0.0000	0.0000	0.0000	0.0000	0.0000	0.0000	0.0000
	2		0.0000	0.0000	0.0000	0.0000	0.0000	0.0000	0.0000	0.0000	0.0000
	3		0.0003	0.0000	0.0000	0.0000	0.0000	0.0000	0.0000	0.0000	0.0000
	4		0.0015	0.0003	0.0000	0.0000	0.0000	0.0000	0.0000	0.0000	0.0000
	5		0.0064	0.0016	0.0003	0.0000	0.0000	0.0000	0.0000	0.0000	0.0000
	6		0.0214	0.0065	0.0015	0.0003	0.0000	0.0000	0.0000	0.0000	0.0000
	7		0.0580	0.0210	0.0060	0.0013	0.0002	0.0000	0.0000	0.0000	0.0000
	8		0.1308	0.0565	0.0196	0.0051	0.0009	0.0001	0.0000	0.0000	0.0000
	9		0.2493	0.1275	0.0532	0.0171	0.0039	0.0006	0.0000	0.0000	0.0000
	10		0.4086	0.2447	0.1218	0.0480	0.0139	0.0026	0.0002	0.0000	0.0000
	11		0.5857	0.4044	0.2376	0.1133	0.0409	0.0100	0.0013	0.0001	0.0000
	12		0.7480	0.5841	0.3990	0.2277	0.1018	0.0321	0.0059	0.0004	0.0000
	13		0.8701	0.7500	0.5834	0.3920	0.2142	0.0867	0.0219	0.0024	0.0000
	14		0.9447	0.8744	0.7546	0.5836	0.3828	0.1958	0.0673	0.0113	0.0003
	15		0.9811	0.9490	0.8818	0.7625	0.5852	0.3704	0.1702	0.0432	0.0026
	16		0.9951	0.9840	0.9556	0.8929	0.7748	0.5886	0.3523	0.1330	0.0159
	17		0.9991	0.9964	0.9879	0.9645	0.9087	0.7939	0.5951	0.3231	0.0755
	18		0.9999	0.9995	0.9979	0.9924	0.9757	0.9308	0.8244	0.6083	0.2642
	19		1.0000	1.0000	0.9998	0.9992	0.9968	0.9885	0.9612	0.8784	0.6415
	20		1.0000	1.0000	1.0000	1.0000	1.0000	1.0000	1.0000	1.0000	1.0000

Areas in the Tail of the Normal Distribution

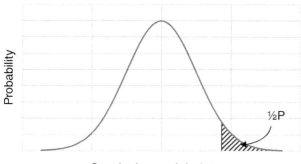

Standard normal deviate, *u*

Areas correspond to the value for u, the standard normal deviate.

To find u, add the value in the first column to the value in the top row.

The probabilities given in the body of the table are for $\frac{1}{2}P$, the 'one-tail' probabilities. For 'two-tail' probabilities, double the values in the table.

Statistics in Nutrition and Dietetics, First Edition. Michael Nelson.
© 2020 John Wiley & Sons Ltd. Published 2020 by John Wiley & Sons Ltd.
Companion website: www.wiley.com/go/nelson/statistics

u	0.00	0.01	0.02	0.03	0.04	0.05	0.06	0.07	0.08	0.09
½P										
0.0	0.500 0	0.496 0	0.492 0	0.488 0	0.484 0	0.480 1	0.476 1	0.472 1	0.468 1	0.464 1
0.1	0.460 2	0.456 2	0.452 2	0.448 3	0.444 3	0.440 4	0.436 4	0.432 5	0.428 6	0.424 7
0.2	0.420 7	0.416 8	0.412 9	0.409 0	0.405 2	0.401 3	0.397 4	0.393 6	0.389 7	0.385 9
0.3	0.382 1	0.378 3	0.374 5	0.370 7	0.366 9	0.363 2	0.359 4	0.355 7	0.352 0	0.348 3
0.4	0.344 6	0.340 9	0.337 2	0.333 6	0.330 0	0.326 4	0.322 8	0.319 2	0.315 6	0.312 1
0.5	0.308 5	0.305 0	0.301 5	0.298 1	0.294 6	0.291 2	0.287 7	0.284 3	0.281 0	0.277 6
0.6	0.274 3	0.270 9	0.267 6	0.264 3	0.261 1	0.257 8	0.254 6	0.251 4	0.248 3	0.245 1
0.7	0.242 0	0.238 9	0.235 8	0.232 7	0.229 6	0.226 6	0.223 6	0.220 6	0.217 7	0.214 8
0.8	0.211 9	0.209 0	0.206 1	0.203 3	0.200 5	0.197 7	0.194 9	0.192 2	0.189 4	0.186 7
0.9	0.184 1	0.181 4	0.178 8	0.176 2	0.173 6	0.171 1	0.168 5	0.166 0	0.163 5	0.161 1
1.0	0.158 7	0.156 2	0.153 9	0.151 5	0.149 2	0.146 9	0.144 6	0.142 3	0.140 1	0.137 9
1.1	0.135 7	0.133 5	0.131 4	0.129 2	0.127 1	0.125 1	0.123 0	0.121 0	0.119 0	0.117 0
1.2	0.115 1	0.113 1	0.111 2	0.109 3	0.107 5	0.105 6	0.103 8	0.102 0	0.100 3	0.098 5
1.3	0.096 8	0.095 1	0.093 4	0.091 8	0.090 1	0.088 5	0.086 9	0.085 3	0.083 8	0.082 3
1.4	0.080 8	0.079 3	0.077 8	0.076 4	0.074 9	0.073 5	0.072 1	0.070 8	0.069 4	0.068 1
1.5	0.066 8	0.065 5	0.064 3	0.063 0	0.061 8	0.060 6	0.059 4	0.058 2	0.057 1	0.055 9
1.6	0.054 8	0.053 7	0.052 6	0.051 6	0.050 5	0.049 5	0.048 5	0.047 5	0.046 5	0.045 5
1.7	0.044 6	0.043 6	0.042 7	0.041 8	0.040 9	0.040 1	0.039 2	0.038 4	0.037 5	0.036 7
1.8	0.035 9	0.035 1	0.034 4	0.033 6	0.032 9	0.032 2	0.031 4	0.030 7	0.030 1	0.029 4
1.9	0.028 7	0.028 1	0.027 4	0.026 8	0.026 2	0.025 6	0.025 0	0.024 4	0.023 9	0.023 3
2.0	0.022 75	0.022 22	0.021 69	0.021 18	0.020 68	0.020 18	0.019 70	0.019 23	0.018 76	0.018 31
2.1	0.017 86	0.017 43	0.017 00	0.016 59	0.016 18	0.015 78	0.015 39	0.015 00	0.014 63	0.014 26
2.2	0.013 90	0.013 55	0.013 21	0.012 87	0.012 55	0.012 22	0.011 91	0.011 60	0.011 30	0.011 01
2.3	0.010 72	0.010 44	0.010 17	0.009 90	0.009 64	0.009 39	0.009 14	0.008 89	0.008 66	0.008 42
2.4	0.008 20	0.007 98	0.007 76	0.007 55	0.007 34	0.007 14	0.006 95	0.006 76	0.006 57	0.006 39
2.5	0.006 21	0.006 04	0.005 87	0.005 70	0.005 54	0.005 39	0.005 23	0.005 08	0.004 94	0.004 80
2.6	0.004 66	0.004 53	0.004 40	0.004 27	0.004 15	0.004 02	0.003 91	0.003 79	0.003 68	0.003 57
2.7	0.003 47	0.003 36	0.003 26	0.003 17	0.003 07	0.002 98	0.002 89	0.002 80	0.002 72	0.002 64
2.8	0.002 56	0.002 48	0.002 40	0.002 33	0.002 26	0.002 19	0.002 12	0.002 05	0.001 99	0.001 93
2.9	0.001 87	0.001 81	0.001 75	0.001 69	0.001 64	0.001 59	0.001 54	0.001 49	0.001 44	0.001 39
3.0	0.001 35	0.001 31	0.001 26	0.001 22	0.001 18	0.001 14	0.001 11	0.001 07	0.001 04	0.001 00
3.1	0.000 97	0.000 94	0.000 90	0.000 87	0.000 84	0.000 82	0.000 79	0.000 76	0.000 74	0.000 71
3.2	0.000 69	0.000 66	0.000 64	0.000 62	0.000 60	0.000 58	0.000 56	0.000 54	0.000 52	0.000 50
3.3	0.000 48	0.000 47	0.000 45	0.000 43	0.000 42	0.000 40	0.000 39	0.000 38	0.000 36	0.000 35
3.4	0.000 34	0.000 32	0.000 31	0.000 30	0.000 29	0.000 28	0.000 27	0.000 26	0.000 25	0.000 24
3.5	0.000 23	0.000 22	0.000 22	0.000 21	0.000 20	0.000 19	0.000 19	0.000 18	0.000 17	0.000 17
3.6	0.000 16	0.000 15	0.000 15	0.000 14	0.000 14	0.000 13	0.000 13	0.000 12	0.000 12	0.000 11
3.7	0.000 11	0.000 10	0.000 10	0.000 10	0.000 09	0.000 09	0.000 08	0.000 08	0.000 08	0.000 08
3.8	0.000 07	0.000 07	0.000 07	0.000 06	0.000 06	0.000 06	0.000 06	0.000 05	0.000 05	0.000 05
3.9	0.000 05	0.000 05	0.000 04	0.000 04	0.000 04	0.000 04	0.000 04	0.000 04	0.000 03	0.000 03
4.0	0.000 03	0.000 03	0.000 03	0.000 03	0.000 03	0.000 03	0.000 02	0.000 02	0.000 02	0.000 02

Areas in the Tail of the *t* Distribution

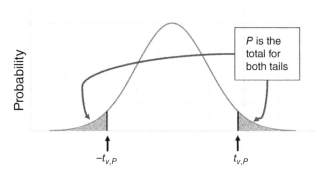

Values for *t* for given levels of:

- *P* (the shaded area in both tails)
- Percentage of the area under the curve in both tails
- The width of the confidence interval
- ν (degrees of freedom).

	0.5	0.4	0.3	0.2	0.1	0.05	0.02	0.01	0.001
Probability (P) of greater value for t in both directions	0.5	0.4	0.3	0.2	0.1	0.05	0.02	0.01	0.001
Percentage of the area under the curve in both tails	50%	40%	30%	20%	10%	5%	2%	1%	0.1%
Width of confidence interval						95%	98%	99%	99.9%
Degrees of freedom, ν									
1	1.000	1.376	1.963	3.078	6.314	12.706	31.821	63.657	636.619
2	0.816	1.080	1.386	1.886	2.920	4.303	6.965	9.925	31.598
3	0.765	0.978	1.250	1.638	2.353	3.182	4.541	5.841	12.924

(Continued)

Statistics in Nutrition and Dietetics, First Edition. Michael Nelson.
© 2020 John Wiley & Sons Ltd. Published 2020 by John Wiley & Sons Ltd.
Companion website: www.wiley.com/go/nelson/statistics

(Continued)

Probability (P) of greater value for t in both directions	0.5	0.4	0.3	0.2	0.1	0.05	0.02	0.01	0.001
Percentage of the area under the curve in both tails	50%	40%	30%	20%	10%	5%	2%	1%	0.1%
Width of confidence interval						95%	98%	99%	99.9%
4	0.741	0.941	1.190	1.533	2.132	2.776	3.747	4.604	8.610
5	0.727	0.920	1.156	1.476	2.015	2.571	3.365	4.032	6.869
6	0.718	0.906	1.134	1.440	1.943	2.447	3.143	3.707	5.959
7	0.711	0.896	1.119	1.415	1.895	2.365	2.998	3.499	5.408
8	0.706	0.889	1.108	1.397	1.860	2.306	2.896	3.355	5.041
9	0.703	0.883	1.100	1.383	1.833	2.262	2.821	3.250	4.781
10	0.700	0.879	1.093	1.372	1.812	2.228	2.764	3.169	4.587
11	0.697	0.876	1.088	1.363	1.796	2.201	2.718	3.106	4.437
12	0.695	0.873	1.083	1.356	1.782	2.179	2.681	3.055	4.318
13	0.694	0.870	1.079	1.350	1.771	2.160	2.650	3.012	4.221
14	0.692	0.868	1.076	1.345	1.761	2.145	2.624	2.977	4.140
15	0.691	0.866	1.074	1.341	1.753	2.131	2.602	2.947	4.073
16	0.690	0.865	1.071	1.337	1.746	2.120	2.583	2.921	4.015
17	0.689	0.863	1.069	1.333	1.740	2.110	2.567	2.898	3.965
18	0.688	0.862	1.067	1.330	1.734	2.101	2.552	2.878	3.922
19	0.688	0.861	1.066	1.328	1.729	2.093	2.539	2.861	3.883
20	0.687	0.860	1.064	1.325	1.725	2.086	2.528	2.845	3.850
21	0.686	0.859	1.063	1.323	1.721	2.080	2.518	2.831	3.819
22	0.686	0.858	1.061	1.321	1.717	2.074	2.508	2.819	3.792
23	0.685	0.858	1.060	1.319	1.714	2.069	2.500	2.807	3.767
24	0.685	0.857	1.059	1.318	1.711	2.064	2.492	2.797	3.745
25	0.684	0.856	1.058	1.316	1.708	2.060	2.485	2.787	3.725
26	0.684	0.856	1.058	1.315	1.706	2.056	2.479	2.779	3.707
27	0.684	0.855	1.057	1.314	1.703	2.052	2.473	2.771	3.690
28	0.683	0.855	1.056	1.313	1.701	2.048	2.467	2.763	3.674
29	0.683	0.854	1.055	1.311	1.699	2.045	2.462	2.756	3.659
30	0.683	0.854	1.055	1.310	1.697	2.042	2.457	2.750	3.646
40	0.681	0.851	1.050	1.303	1.684	2.021	2.423	2.704	3.551
50	0.679	0.849	1.047	1.299	1.676	2.009	2.403	2.678	3.496
60	0.679	0.848	1.045	1.296	1.671	2.000	2.390	2.660	3.460
80	0.678	0.846	1.043	1.292	1.664	1.990	2.374	2.639	3.416
100	0.677	0.845	1.042	1.290	1.660	1.984	2.364	2.626	3.390
120	0.677	0.845	1.041	1.289	1.658	1.980	2.358	2.617	3.373
∞	**0.674**	**0.842**	**1.036**	**1.282**	**1.645**	**1.960**	**2.326**	**2.576**	**3.291**

Values in bold signify the convergence at infinite sample size of the values for the two-tailed t distribution with the values for the two-tailed u distribution.

Wilcoxon U Statistic (Mann–Whitney Test)

Values for U for given levels of:

- P (0.05 and 0.01, two-tailed)
- n_1 and n_2

Computed values of U *less than or equal to* the values in the table are statistically significant at the given value for P.

P = 0.05

$n_1 \backslash n_2$	2	3	4	5	6	7	8	9	10	11	12	13	14	15	16	17	18	19	20
2							0	0	0	0	1	1	1	1	1	2	2	2	2
3				0	1	1	2	2	3	3	4	4	5	5	6	6	7	7	8
4			0	1	2	3	4	4	5	6	7	8	9	10	11	11	12	13	14
5		0	1	2	3	5	6	7	8	9	11	12	13	14	15	17	18	19	20
6		1	2	3	5	6	8	10	11	13	14	16	17	19	21	22	24	25	27
7		1	3	5	6	8	10	12	14	16	18	20	22	24	26	28	30	32	34
8	0	2	4	6	8	10	13	15	17	19	22	24	26	29	31	34	36	38	41
9	0	2	4	7	10	12	15	17	20	23	26	28	31	34	37	39	42	45	48
10	0	3	5	8	11	14	17	20	23	26	29	33	36	39	42	45	48	52	55

(Continued)

Statistics in Nutrition and Dietetics, First Edition. Michael Nelson.
© 2020 John Wiley & Sons Ltd. Published 2020 by John Wiley & Sons Ltd.
Companion website: www.wiley.com/go/nelson/statistics

(Continued)

P = 0.05

n_1\ n_2	2	3	4	5	6	7	8	9	10	11	12	13	14	15	16	17	18	19	20
11	0	3	6	9	13	16	19	23	26	30	33	37	40	44	47	51	55	58	62
12	1	4	7	11	14	18	22	26	29	33	37	41	45	49	53	57	61	65	69
13	1	4	8	12	16	20	24	28	33	37	41	45	50	54	59	63	67	72	76
14	1	5	9	13	17	22	26	31	36	40	45	50	55	59	64	69	74	78	83
15	1	5	10	14	19	24	29	34	39	44	49	54	59	64	70	75	80	85	90
16	1	6	11	15	21	26	31	37	42	47	53	59	64	70	75	81	86	92	98
17	2	6	11	17	22	28	34	39	45	51	57	63	69	75	81	87	93	99	105
18	2	7	12	18	24	30	36	42	48	55	61	67	74	80	86	93	99	106	112
19	2	7	13	19	25	32	38	45	52	58	65	72	78	85	92	99	106	113	119
20	2	8	14	20	27	34	41	48	55	62	69	76	83	90	98	105	112	119	127

P = 0.01

n_1\ n_2	2	3	4	5	6	7	8	9	10	11	12	13	14	15	16	17	18	19	20
2																		0	0
3								0	0	0	1	1	1	2	2	2	2	3	3
4					0	0	1	1	2	2	3	3	4	5	5	6	6	7	8
5				0	1	1	2	3	4	5	6	7	7	8	9	10	11	12	13
6			0	1	2	3	4	5	6	7	9	10	11	12	13	15	16	17	18
7			0	1	3	4	6	7	9	10	12	13	15	16	18	19	21	22	24
8			1	2	4	6	7	9	11	13	15	17	18	20	22	24	26	28	30
9		0	1	3	5	7	9	11	13	16	18	20	22	24	27	29	31	33	36
10		0	2	4	6	9	11	13	16	18	21	24	26	29	31	34	37	39	42
11		0	2	5	7	10	13	16	18	21	24	27	30	33	36	39	42	45	48
12		1	3	6	9	12	15	18	21	24	27	31	34	37	41	44	47	51	54
13		1	3	7	10	13	17	20	24	27	31	34	38	42	45	49	53	57	60
14		1	4	7	11	15	18	22	26	30	34	38	42	46	50	54	58	63	67
15		2	5	8	12	16	20	24	29	33	37	42	46	51	55	60	64	69	73
16		2	5	9	13	18	22	27	31	36	41	45	50	55	60	65	70	74	79
17		2	6	10	15	19	24	29	34	39	44	49	54	60	65	70	75	81	86
18		2	6	11	16	21	26	31	37	42	47	53	58	64	70	75	81	87	92
19	0	3	7	12	17	22	28	33	39	45	51	57	63	69	74	81	87	93	99
20	0	3	8	13	18	24	30	36	42	48	54	60	67	73	79	86	92	99	105

Source: With permission: Real-Statistics.com.

Wilcoxon *T* Statistic

Values for *T* for given levels of:
- *P* (0.05, 0.02 and 0.01, two-tailed)
- *n* – number of non-zero differences

Computed values of *T less than or equal to* the values in the table are statistically significant.

n	P		
	0.05	0.02	0.01
7	2	0	—
8	4	2	0
9	6	3	2
10	8	5	3
11	11	7	5
12	14	10	7
13	17	13	10
14	21	16	13

n	P		
	0.05	0.02	0.01
15	25	20	16
16	30	24	20
17	35	28	23
18	40	33	28
19	46	38	32
20	52	43	38
21	59	49	43
22	66	56	49
23	73	62	55
24	81	69	61
25	89	77	68

Source: https://cehd.gmu.edu/assets/dimitrovbook/
Wilcoxon%20matched-pairs%20T-distribution.pdf.
__ Statistic unreliable.

Statistics in Nutrition and Dietetics, First Edition. Michael Nelson.
© 2020 John Wiley & Sons Ltd. Published 2020 by John Wiley & Sons Ltd.
Companion website: www.wiley.com/go/nelson/statistics

Sign Test Statistic R

Values for *R* for given levels of:

- *P* (0.05 and 0.01, two-tailed)
- *n* – number of non-zero differences

Computed values of *R* *less than or equal to* the values in the table are statistically significant.

	P	
n	0.05	0.01
6	0	—
7	0	—
8	0	0
9	1	0
10	1	0
11	1	0
12	2	1
13	2	1

	P	
n	0.05	0.01
14	2	1
15	3	2
16	3	2
17	4	2
18	4	3
19	4	3
20	5	3
21	5	4
22	5	4
23	6	4
24	6	5
25	7	5

— Statistic unreliable.

Statistics in Nutrition and Dietetics, First Edition. Michael Nelson.
© 2020 John Wiley & Sons Ltd. Published 2020 by John Wiley & Sons Ltd.
Companion website: www.wiley.com/go/nelson/statistics

Percentages in the Tail of the Chi-Squared Distribution

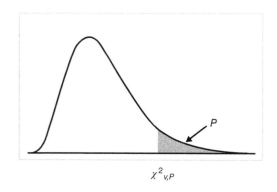

$$\chi^2_{\nu,P}$$

Values for χ^2 for given levels of:

- P (the shaded area in the right-hand tail)
- Percentage of the area under the curve in one tail
- ν (degrees of freedom)

	Probability (P) of greater value for χ^2 in one direction										
	0.95	0.9	0.75	0.5	0.25	0.1	0.05	0.025	0.01	0.005	0.001
Percentage of the area under the curve in one tail	95.0%	90.0%	75.0%	50.0%	25.0%	10.0%	5.0%	2.5%	1.0%	0.5%	0.1%
Degrees of freedom, ν											
1	0.004	0.016	0.102	0.455	1.323	2.706	3.841	5.024	6.635	7.879	10.828
2	0.103	0.211	0.575	1.386	2.773	4.605	5.991	7.378	9.210	10.597	13.816
3	0.352	0.584	1.213	2.366	4.108	6.251	7.815	9.348	11.345	12.838	16.266
4	0.711	1.064	1.923	3.357	5.385	7.779	9.488	11.143	13.277	14.860	18.467

(Continued)

Statistics in Nutrition and Dietetics, First Edition. Michael Nelson.
© 2020 John Wiley & Sons Ltd. Published 2020 by John Wiley & Sons Ltd.
Companion website: www.wiley.com/go/nelson/statistics

(Continued)

Percentage of the area under the curve in one tail	Probability (P) of greater value for χ^2 in one direction										
	0.95	0.9	0.75	0.5	0.25	0.1	0.05	0.025	0.01	0.005	0.001
	95.0%	90.0%	75.0%	50.0%	25.0%	10.0%	5.0%	2.5%	1.0%	0.5%	0.1%
5	1.145	1.610	2.675	4.351	6.626	9.236	11.070	12.833	15.086	16.750	20.515
6	1.635	2.204	3.455	5.348	7.841	10.645	12.592	14.449	16.812	18.548	22.458
7	2.167	2.833	4.255	6.346	9.037	12.017	14.067	16.013	18.475	20.278	24.322
8	2.733	3.490	5.071	7.344	10.219	13.362	15.507	17.535	20.090	21.955	26.124
9	3.325	4.168	5.899	8.343	11.389	14.684	16.919	19.023	21.666	23.589	27.877
10	3.940	4.865	6.737	9.342	12.549	15.987	18.307	20.483	23.209	25.188	29.588
11	4.575	5.578	7.584	10.341	13.701	17.275	19.675	21.920	24.725	26.757	31.264
12	5.226	6.304	8.438	11.340	14.845	18.549	21.026	23.337	26.217	28.300	32.909
13	5.892	7.042	9.299	12.340	15.984	19.812	22.362	24.736	27.688	29.819	34.528
14	6.571	7.790	10.165	13.339	17.117	21.064	23.685	26.119	29.141	31.319	36.123
15	7.261	8.547	11.037	14.339	18.245	22.307	24.996	27.488	30.578	32.801	37.697
16	7.962	9.312	11.912	15.338	19.369	23.542	26.296	28.845	32.000	34.267	39.252
17	8.672	10.085	12.792	16.338	20.489	24.769	27.587	30.191	33.409	35.718	40.790
18	9.390	10.865	13.675	17.338	21.605	25.989	28.869	31.526	34.805	37.156	42.312
19	10.117	11.651	14.562	18.338	22.718	27.204	30.144	32.852	36.191	38.582	43.820
20	10.851	12.443	15.452	19.337	23.828	28.412	31.410	34.170	37.566	39.997	45.315
21	11.591	13.240	16.344	20.337	24.935	29.615	32.671	35.479	38.932	41.401	46.797
22	12.338	14.041	17.240	21.337	26.039	30.813	33.924	36.781	40.289	42.796	48.268
23	13.091	14.848	18.137	22.337	27.141	32.007	35.172	38.076	41.638	44.181	49.728
24	13.848	15.659	19.037	23.337	28.241	33.196	36.415	39.364	42.980	45.559	51.179
25	14.611	16.473	19.939	24.337	29.339	34.382	37.652	40.646	44.314	46.928	52.620
26	15.379	17.292	20.843	25.336	30.435	35.563	38.885	41.923	45.642	48.290	54.052
27	16.151	18.114	21.749	26.336	31.528	36.741	40.113	43.195	46.963	49.645	55.476
28	16.928	18.939	22.657	27.336	32.620	37.916	41.337	44.461	48.278	50.993	56.892
29	17.708	19.768	23.567	28.336	33.711	39.087	42.557	45.722	49.588	52.336	58.301
30	18.493	20.599	24.478	29.336	34.800	40.256	43.773	46.979	50.892	53.672	59.703
40	26.509	29.051	33.660	39.335	45.616	51.805	55.758	59.342	63.691	66.766	73.402
50	34.764	37.689	42.942	49.335	56.334	63.167	67.505	71.420	76.154	79.490	86.661
60	43.188	46.459	52.294	59.335	66.981	74.397	79.082	83.298	88.379	91.952	99.607
70	51.739	55.329	61.698	69.334	77.577	85.527	90.531	95.023	100.425	104.215	112.317
80	60.391	64.278	71.145	79.334	88.130	96.578	101.879	106.629	112.329	116.321	124.839
90	69.126	73.291	80.625	89.334	98.650	107.565	113.145	118.136	124.116	128.299	137.208
100	77.929	82.358	90.133	99.334	109.141	118.498	124.342	129.561	135.807	140.169	149.449

APPENDIX A8

Quantiles of the Spearman Rank Correlation Coefficient

	P, one-tailed								
	0.25	0.1	0.05	0.025	0.01	0.005	0.0025	0.001	0.0005
	P, two-tailed								
n	0.5	0.2	0.1	0.05	0.02	0.01	0.005	0.002	0.001
3	1.000								
4	0.600	1.000	1.000						
5	0.500	0.800	0.900	1.000	1.000				
6	0.371	0.657	0.829	0.886	0.943	1.000	1.000		
7	0.321	0.571	0.714	0.786	0.893	0.929	0.964	1.000	1.000
8	0.310	0.524	0.643	0.738	0.833	0.881	0.905	0.952	0.976
9	0.267	0.483	0.600	0.700	0.783	0.833	0.867	0.917	0.933
10	0.248	0.455	0.564	0.648	0.745	0.794	0.830	0.879	0.903
11	0.236	0.427	0.536	0.618	0.709	0.755	0.800	0.845	0.873
12	0.217	0.406	0.503	0.587	0.678	0.727	0.769	0.818	0.846
13	0.209	0.385	0.484	0.560	0.648	0.703	0.747	0.791	0.824
14	0.200	0.367	0.464	0.538	0.626	0.679	0.723	0.771	0.802
15	0.189	0.354	0.446	0.521	0.604	0.654	0.700	0.750	0.779
16	0.182	0.341	0.429	0.503	0.582	0.635	0.679	0.729	0.762
17	0.176	0.328	0.414	0.488	0.566	0.618	0.659	0.711	0.743
18	0.170	0.317	0.401	0.472	0.550	0.600	0.643	0.692	0.725

(Continued)

Statistics in Nutrition and Dietetics, First Edition. Michael Nelson.
© 2020 John Wiley & Sons Ltd. Published 2020 by John Wiley & Sons Ltd.
Companion website: www.wiley.com/go/nelson/statistics

(Continued)

n	P, one-tailed								
	0.25	0.1	0.05	0.025	0.01	0.005	0.0025	0.001	0.0005
	P, two-tailed								
	0.5	0.2	0.1	0.05	0.02	0.01	0.005	0.002	0.001
19	0.165	0.309	0.391	0.460	0.535	0.584	0.628	0.675	0.709
20	0.161	0.299	0.380	0.447	0.522	0.570	0.612	0.662	0.693
21	0.156	0.292	0.370	0.436	0.509	0.556	0.599	0.647	0.678
22	0.152	0.284	0.361	0.425	0.497	0.544	0.586	0.633	0.665
23	0.148	0.278	0.353	0.416	0.486	0.532	0.573	0.621	0.652
24	0.144	0.271	0.344	0.407	0.476	0.521	0.562	0.609	0.640
25	0.142	0.265	0.337	0.398	0.466	0.511	0.551	0.597	0.628
26	0.138	0.259	0.331	0.390	0.457	0.501	0.541	0.586	0.618
27	0.136	0.255	0.324	0.383	0.449	0.492	0.531	0.576	0.607
28	0.133	0.250	0.318	0.375	0.441	0.483	0.522	0.567	0.597
29	0.130	0.245	0.312	0.368	0.433	0.475	0.513	0.558	0.588
30	0.128	0.240	0.306	0.362	0.425	0.467	0.504	0.549	0.579
31	0.125	0.236	0.301	0.356	0.419	0.459	0.496	0.540	0.570
32	0.124	0.232	0.296	0.350	0.412	0.452	0.489	0.532	0.562
33	0.121	0.229	0.291	0.345	0.405	0.446	0.482	0.525	0.554
34	0.119	0.225	0.287	0.340	0.400	0.439	0.475	0.517	0.546
35	0.118	0.222	0.283	0.335	0.394	0.433	0.468	0.510	0.539
36	0.116	0.219	0.279	0.330	0.388	0.427	0.462	0.503	0.532
37	0.114	0.215	0.275	0.325	0.383	0.421	0.456	0.497	0.525
38	0.113	0.212	0.271	0.321	0.378	0.415	0.450	0.491	0.519
39	0.111	0.210	0.267	0.317	0.373	0.410	0.444	0.485	0.512
40	0.110	0.207	0.264	0.313	0.368	0.405	0.439	0.479	0.506
41	0.108	0.204	0.261	0.309	0.364	0.400	0.433	0.473	0.501
42	0.107	0.202	0.257	0.305	0.359	0.396	0.428	0.468	0.495
43	0.105	0.199	0.254	0.301	0.355	0.391	0.423	0.462	0.489
44	0.104	0.197	0.251	0.298	0.351	0.386	0.419	0.457	0.484
45	0.103	0.194	0.248	0.294	0.347	0.382	0.414	0.452	0.479
46	0.102	0.192	0.246	0.291	0.343	0.378	0.410	0.448	0.474
47	0.101	0.190	0.243	0.288	0.340	0.374	0.405	0.443	0.469
48	0.100	0.188	0.240	0.285	0.336	0.370	0.401	0.439	0.465
49	0.098	0.186	0.238	0.282	0.333	0.366	0.397	0.434	0.460
50	0.097	0.184	0.235	0.279	0.329	0.363	0.393	0.430	0.456

For $n > 50$, compute $u = \rho\sqrt{n-1}$ and refer to Appendix A2 (areas in the tails of the normal distribution) to find $\frac{1}{2}P$.

Percentages in the Tail of the F Distribution

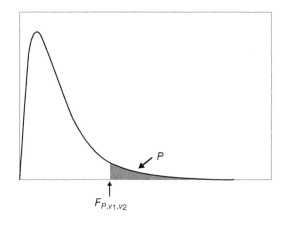

$$F_{P,v1,v2}$$

Values for F for given levels of:

- P (the shaded area in the right-hand tail)
- ν_1 (degrees of freedom for numerator)
- ν_2 (degrees of freedom for denominator)

Values of the F Statistic		Degrees of Freedom for Numerator (ν_1)							
Degrees of Freedom for Denominator (ν_2)	P	1	2	3	4	5	6	7	8
1	0.05	161.4	199.5	215.7	224.6	230.2	234.0	236.8	238.9
	0.02	1012.5	1249.5	1350.5	1405.8	1440.6	1464.5	1481.8	1495.0
	0.01	4052.2	4999.5	5403.4	5624.6	5763.6	5859.0	5928.4	5981.1
	0.005	16210.7	19999.5	21614.7	22499.6	23055.8	23437.1	23714.6	23925.4
2	0.05	18.51	19.00	19.16	19.25	19.30	19.33	19.35	19.37
	0.02	48.51	49.00	49.17	49.25	49.30	49.33	49.36	49.37
	0.01	98.50	99.00	99.17	99.25	99.30	99.33	99.36	99.37
	0.005	198.50	199.00	199.17	199.25	199.30	199.33	199.36	199.37
3	0.05	10.13	9.55	9.28	9.12	9.01	8.94	8.89	8.85
	0.02	20.62	18.86	18.11	17.69	17.43	17.25	17.11	17.01
	0.01	34.12	30.82	29.46	28.71	28.24	27.91	27.67	27.49
	0.005	55.55	49.80	47.47	46.19	45.39	44.84	44.43	44.13
4	0.05	7.71	6.94	6.59	6.39	6.26	6.16	6.09	6.04
	0.02	14.04	12.14	11.34	10.90	10.62	10.42	10.27	10.16
	0.01	21.20	18.00	16.69	15.98	15.52	15.21	14.98	14.80
	0.005	31.33	26.28	24.26	23.15	22.46	21.97	21.62	21.35
5	0.05	6.61	5.79	5.41	5.19	5.05	4.95	4.88	4.82
	0.02	11.32	9.45	8.67	8.23	7.95	7.76	7.61	7.50
	0.01	16.26	13.27	12.06	11.39	10.97	10.67	10.46	10.29
	0.005	22.78	18.31	16.53	15.56	14.94	14.51	14.20	13.96
6	0.05	5.99	5.14	4.76	4.53	4.39	4.28	4.21	4.15
	0.02	9.88	8.05	7.29	6.86	6.58	6.39	6.25	6.14
	0.01	13.75	10.92	9.78	9.15	8.75	8.47	8.26	8.10
	0.005	18.63	14.54	12.92	12.03	11.46	11.07	10.79	10.57
7	0.05	5.59	4.74	4.35	4.12	3.97	3.87	3.79	3.73
	0.02	8.99	7.20	6.45	6.03	5.76	5.58	5.44	5.33
	0.01	12.25	9.55	8.45	7.85	7.46	7.19	6.99	6.84
	0.005	16.24	12.40	10.88	10.05	9.52	9.16	8.89	8.68
8	0.05	5.32	4.46	4.07	3.84	3.69	3.58	3.50	3.44
	0.02	8.39	6.64	5.90	5.49	5.22	5.04	4.90	4.79
	0.01	11.26	8.65	7.59	7.01	6.63	6.37	6.18	6.03
	0.005	14.69	11.04	9.60	8.81	8.30	7.95	7.69	7.50
9	0.05	5.12	4.26	3.86	3.63	3.48	3.37	3.29	3.23
	0.02	7.96	6.23	5.51	5.10	4.84	4.65	4.52	4.41
	0.01	10.56	8.02	6.99	6.42	6.06	5.80	5.61	5.47
	0.005	13.61	10.11	8.72	7.96	7.47	7.13	6.88	6.69

Values of the F Statistic		Degrees of Freedom for Numerator (ν_1)							
Degrees of Freedom for Denominator (ν_2)	P	9	10	12	14	16	18	20	∞
1	0.05	240.5	241.9	243.9	245.4	246.5	247.3	248.0	254.3
	0.02	1 505.3	1 513.7	1 526.3	1 535.4	1 542.3	1 547.6	1 551.9	1 591.2
	0.01	6 022.5	6 055.8	6 106.3	6 142.7	6 170.1	6 191.5	6 208.7	6 365.9
	0.005	24 091.0	24 224.5	24 426.4	24 571.8	24 681.5	24 767.2	24 836.0	25 464.5
2	0.05	19.38	19.40	19.41	19.42	19.43	19.44	19.45	19.50
	0.02	49.39	49.40	49.42	49.43	49.44	49.44	49.45	49.50
	0.01	99.39	99.40	99.42	99.43	99.44	99.44	99.45	99.50
	0.005	199.39	199.40	199.42	199.43	199.44	199.44	199.45	199.50
3	0.05	8.81	8.79	8.74	8.71	8.69	8.67	8.66	8.53
	0.02	16.93	16.86	16.76	16.69	16.63	16.59	16.55	16.23
	0.01	27.35	27.23	27.05	26.92	26.83	26.75	26.69	26.13
	0.005	43.88	43.69	43.39	43.17	43.01	42.88	42.78	41.83
4	0.05	6.00	5.96	5.91	5.87	5.84	5.82	5.80	5.63
	0.02	10.07	10.00	9.89	9.81	9.75	9.71	9.67	9.32
	0.01	14.66	14.55	14.37	14.25	14.15	14.08	14.02	13.46
	0.005	21.14	20.97	20.70	20.51	20.37	20.26	20.17	19.32
5	0.05	4.77	4.74	4.68	4.64	4.60	4.58	4.56	4.36
	0.02	7.42	7.34	7.23	7.16	7.10	7.05	7.01	6.65
	0.01	10.16	10.05	9.89	9.77	9.68	9.61	9.55	9.02
	0.005	13.77	13.62	13.38	13.21	13.09	12.98	12.90	12.14
6	0.05	4.10	4.06	4.00	3.96	3.92	3.90	3.87	3.67
	0.02	6.05	5.98	5.88	5.80	5.74	5.69	5.65	5.29
	0.01	7.98	7.87	7.72	7.60	7.52	7.45	7.40	6.88
	0.005	10.39	10.25	10.03	9.88	9.76	9.66	9.59	8.88
7	0.05	3.68	3.64	3.57	3.53	3.49	3.47	3.44	3.23
	0.02	5.24	5.17	5.06	4.98	4.92	4.88	4.84	4.47
	0.01	6.72	6.62	6.47	6.36	6.28	6.21	6.16	5.65
	0.005	8.51	8.38	8.18	8.03	7.91	7.83	7.75	7.08
8	0.05	3.39	3.35	3.28	3.24	3.20	3.17	3.15	2.93
	0.02	4.70	4.63	4.53	4.45	4.39	4.34	4.30	3.94
	0.01	5.91	5.81	5.67	5.56	5.48	5.41	5.36	4.86
	0.005	7.34	7.21	7.01	6.87	6.76	6.68	6.61	5.95
9	0.05	3.18	3.14	3.07	3.03	2.99	2.96	2.94	2.71
	0.02	4.33	4.26	4.15	4.07	4.01	3.96	3.92	3.55
	0.01	5.35	5.26	5.11	5.01	4.92	4.86	4.81	4.31
	0.005	6.54	6.42	6.23	6.09	5.98	5.90	5.83	5.19

(Continued)

(Continued)

Values of the F Statistic		Degrees of Freedom for Numerator (ν_1)							
Degrees of Freedom for Denominator (ν_2)	P	1	2	3	4	5	6	7	8
10	0.05	4.96	4.10	3.71	3.48	3.33	3.22	3.14	3.07
	0.02	7.64	5.93	5.22	4.82	4.55	4.37	4.23	4.13
	0.01	10.04	7.56	6.55	5.99	5.64	5.39	5.20	5.06
	0.005	12.83	9.43	8.08	7.34	6.87	6.54	6.30	6.12
12	0.05	4.75	3.89	3.49	3.26	3.11	3.00	2.91	2.85
	0.02	7.19	5.52	4.81	4.42	4.16	3.98	3.85	3.74
	0.01	9.33	6.93	5.95	5.41	5.06	4.82	4.64	4.50
	0.005	11.75	8.51	7.23	6.52	6.07	5.76	5.52	5.35
14	0.05	4.60	3.74	3.34	3.11	2.96	2.85	2.76	2.70
	0.02	6.89	5.24	4.55	4.16	3.90	3.72	3.59	3.48
	0.01	8.86	6.51	5.56	5.04	4.69	4.46	4.28	4.14
	0.005	11.06	7.92	6.68	6.00	5.56	5.26	5.03	4.86
16	0.05	4.49	3.63	3.24	3.01	2.85	2.74	2.66	2.59
	0.02	6.67	5.05	4.36	3.97	3.72	3.54	3.41	3.30
	0.01	8.53	6.23	5.29	4.77	4.44	4.20	4.03	3.89
	0.005	10.58	7.51	6.30	5.64	5.21	4.91	4.69	4.52
18	0.05	4.41	3.55	3.16	2.93	2.77	2.66	2.58	2.51
	0.02	6.51	4.90	4.22	3.84	3.59	3.41	3.27	3.17
	0.01	8.29	6.01	5.09	4.58	4.25	4.01	3.84	3.71
	0.005	10.22	7.21	6.03	5.37	4.96	4.66	4.44	4.28
20	0.05	4.35	3.49	3.10	2.87	2.71	2.60	2.51	2.45
	0.02	6.39	4.79	4.11	3.73	3.48	3.30	3.17	3.07
	0.01	8.10	5.85	4.94	4.43	4.10	3.87	3.70	3.56
	0.005	9.94	6.99	5.82	5.17	4.76	4.47	4.26	4.09
25	0.05	4.24	3.39	2.99	2.76	2.60	2.49	2.40	2.34
	0.02	6.18	4.59	3.93	3.55	3.30	3.13	2.99	2.89
	0.01	7.77	5.57	4.68	4.18	3.85	3.63	3.46	3.32
	0.005	9.48	6.60	5.46	4.84	4.43	4.15	3.94	3.78
30	0.05	4.17	3.32	2.92	2.69	2.53	2.42	2.33	2.27
	0.02	6.04	4.47	3.81	3.43	3.19	3.01	2.88	2.78
	0.01	7.56	5.39	4.51	4.02	3.70	3.47	3.30	3.17
	0.005	9.18	6.35	5.24	4.62	4.23	3.95	3.74	3.58

Values of the F Statistic		Degrees of Freedom for Numerator (ν_1)							
Degrees of Freedom for Denominator (ν_2)	P	9	10	12	14	16	18	20	∞
10	0.05	3.02	2.98	2.91	2.86	2.83	2.80	2.77	2.54
	0.02	4.04	3.97	3.87	3.79	3.73	3.68	3.64	3.27
	0.01	4.94	4.85	4.71	4.60	4.52	4.46	4.41	3.91
	0.005	5.97	5.85	5.66	5.53	5.42	5.34	5.27	4.64
12	0.05	2.80	2.75	2.69	2.64	2.60	2.57	2.54	2.30
	0.02	3.66	3.59	3.48	3.40	3.34	3.29	3.25	2.87
	0.01	4.39	4.30	4.16	4.05	3.97	3.91	3.86	3.36
	0.005	5.20	5.09	4.91	4.77	4.67	4.59	4.53	3.90
14	0.05	2.65	2.60	2.53	2.48	2.44	2.41	2.39	2.13
	0.02	3.40	3.33	3.23	3.15	3.09	3.04	3.00	2.61
	0.01	4.03	3.94	3.80	3.70	3.62	3.56	3.51	3.00
	0.005	4.72	4.60	4.43	4.30	4.20	4.12	4.06	3.44
16	0.05	2.54	2.49	2.42	2.37	2.33	2.30	2.28	2.01
	0.02	3.22	3.15	3.05	2.97	2.90	2.86	2.82	2.42
	0.01	3.78	3.69	3.55	3.45	3.37	3.31	3.26	2.75
	0.005	4.38	4.27	4.10	3.97	3.87	3.80	3.73	3.11
18	0.05	2.46	2.41	2.34	2.29	2.25	2.22	2.19	1.92
	0.02	3.09	3.02	2.91	2.83	2.77	2.72	2.68	2.28
	0.01	3.60	3.51	3.37	3.27	3.19	3.13	3.08	2.57
	0.005	4.14	4.03	3.86	3.73	3.64	3.56	3.50	2.87
20	0.05	2.39	2.35	2.28	2.22	2.18	2.15	2.12	1.84
	0.02	2.98	2.91	2.81	2.73	2.67	2.62	2.58	2.17
	0.01	3.46	3.37	3.23	3.13	3.05	2.99	2.94	2.42
	0.005	3.96	3.85	3.68	3.55	3.46	3.38	3.32	2.69
25	0.05	2.28	2.24	2.16	2.11	2.07	2.04	2.01	1.71
	0.02	2.81	2.74	2.63	2.55	2.49	2.44	2.40	1.97
	0.01	3.22	3.13	2.99	2.89	2.81	2.75	2.70	2.17
	0.005	3.64	3.54	3.37	3.25	3.15	3.08	3.01	2.38
30	0.05	2.21	2.16	2.09	2.04	1.99	1.96	1.93	1.62
	0.02	2.69	2.62	2.52	2.44	2.37	2.32	2.28	1.84
	0.01	3.07	2.98	2.84	2.74	2.66	2.60	2.55	2.01
	0.005	3.45	3.34	3.18	3.06	2.96	2.89	2.82	2.18

(Continued)

(Continued)

Values of the F Statistic		Degrees of Freedom for Numerator (ν_1)							
Degrees of Freedom for Denominator (ν_2)	P	1	2	3	4	5	6	7	8
40	0.05	4.08	3.23	2.84	2.61	2.45	2.34	2.25	2.18
	0.02	5.87	4.32	3.67	3.30	3.05	2.88	2.74	2.64
	0.01	7.31	5.18	4.31	3.83	3.51	3.29	3.12	2.99
	0.005	8.83	6.07	4.98	4.37	3.99	3.71	3.51	3.35
60	0.05	4.00	3.15	2.76	2.53	2.37	2.25	2.17	2.10
	0.02	5.71	4.18	3.53	3.16	2.92	2.75	2.62	2.51
	0.01	7.08	4.98	4.13	3.65	3.34	3.12	2.95	2.82
	0.005	8.49	5.79	4.73	4.14	3.76	3.49	3.29	3.13
120	0.05	3.92	3.07	2.68	2.45	2.29	2.18	2.09	2.02
	0.02	5.56	4.04	3.40	3.04	2.80	2.62	2.49	2.39
	0.01	6.85	4.79	3.95	3.48	3.17	2.96	2.79	2.66
	0.005	8.18	5.54	4.50	3.92	3.55	3.28	3.09	2.93
∞	0.05	3.84	3.00	2.60	2.37	2.21	2.10	2.01	1.94
	0.02	5.41	3.91	3.28	2.92	2.68	2.51	2.37	2.27
	0.01	6.63	4.61	3.78	3.32	3.02	2.80	2.64	2.51
	0.005	7.88	5.30	4.28	3.72	3.35	3.09	2.90	2.74

Values of the F Statistic		Degrees of Freedom for Numerator (ν_1)							
Degrees of Freedom for Denominator (ν_2)	**P**	**9**	**10**	**12**	**14**	**16**	**18**	**20**	**∞**
40	0.05	2.12	2.08	2.00	1.95	1.90	1.87	1.84	1.51
	0.02	2.56	2.49	2.38	2.30	2.23	2.18	2.14	1.68
	0.01	2.89	2.80	2.66	2.56	2.48	2.42	2.37	1.80
	0.005	3.22	3.12	2.95	2.83	2.74	2.66	2.60	1.93
60	0.05	2.04	1.99	1.92	1.86	1.82	1.78	1.75	1.39
	0.02	2.43	2.36	2.25	2.17	2.10	2.05	2.01	1.51
	0.01	2.72	2.63	2.50	2.39	2.31	2.25	2.20	1.60
	0.005	3.01	2.90	2.74	2.62	2.53	2.45	2.39	1.69
120	0.05	1.96	1.91	1.83	1.78	1.73	1.69	1.66	1.25
	0.02	2.30	2.23	2.12	2.04	1.97	1.92	1.88	1.33
	0.01	2.56	2.47	2.34	2.23	2.15	2.09	2.03	1.38
	0.005	2.81	2.71	2.54	2.42	2.33	2.25	2.19	1.43
∞	0.05	1.88	1.83	1.75	1.69	1.64	1.60	1.57	1.00
	0.02	2.19	2.12	2.00	1.92	1.85	1.80	1.75	1.00
	0.01	2.41	2.32	2.18	2.08	2.00	1.93	1.88	1.00
	0.005	2.62	2.52	2.36	2.24	2.14	2.06	2.00	1.00

Flow Chart for Selecting Statistical Tests

Statistics in Nutrition and Dietetics, First Edition. Michael Nelson.
© 2020 John Wiley & Sons Ltd. Published 2020 by John Wiley & Sons Ltd.
Companion website: www.wiley.com/go/nelson/statistics

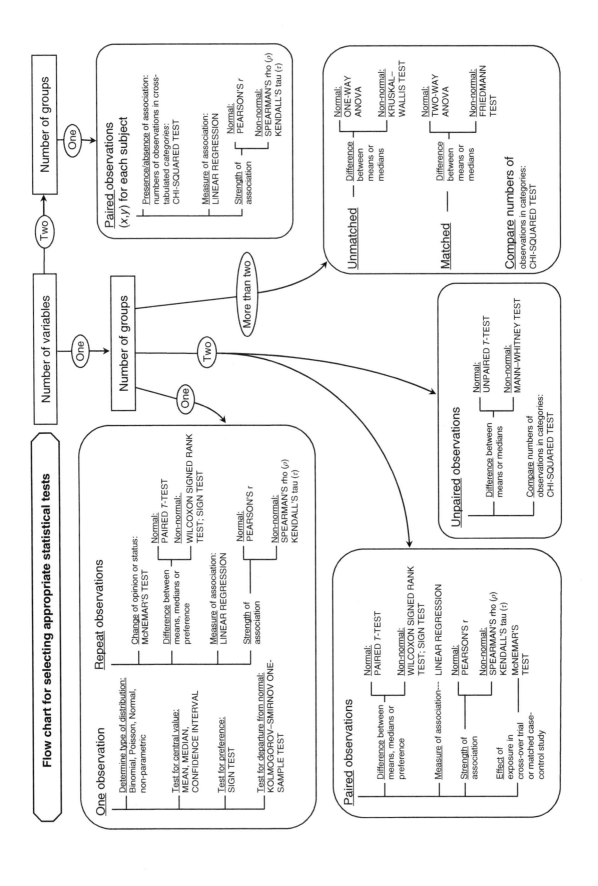

Flow chart for selecting appropriate statistical tests

Number of variables

One

Number of groups

Two

Paired observations (*x,y*) for each subject

Presence/absence of association: numbers of observations in cross-tabulated *categories*:
CHI-SQUARED TEST

Measure of association:
LINEAR REGRESSION

Strength of association

Normal:
PEARSON'S *r*

Non-normal:
SPEARMAN'S rho (*ρ*)
KENDALL'S tau (*τ*)

Number of groups

More than two

Unmatched — Difference between means or medians

Normal:
ONE-WAY ANOVA

Non-normal:
KRUSKAL–WALLIS TEST

Matched — Difference between means or medians

Normal:
TWO-WAY ANOVA

Non-normal:
FRIEDMANN TEST

Compare numbers of observations in categories:
CHI-SQUARED TEST

One

Two

Unpaired observations

Difference between means or medians

Normal:
UNPAIRED *T*-TEST

Non-normal:
MANN–WHITNEY TEST

Compare numbers of observations in categories:
CHI-SQUARED TEST

One observation

Determine type of distribution: Binomial, Poisson, Normal, non-parametric

Test for central value:
MEAN, MEDIAN, CONFIDENCE INTERVAL

Test for preference:
SIGN TEST

Test for departure from normal:
KOLMOGOROV–SMIRNOV ONE-SAMPLE TEST

Repeat observations

Change of opinion or status:
McNEMAR'S TEST

Difference between means, medians or preference

Normal:
PAIRED *T*-TEST

Non-normal:
WILCOXON SIGNED RANK TEST; SIGN TEST

Measure of association:
LINEAR REGRESSION

Strength of association

Normal:
PEARSON'S *r*

Non-normal:
SPEARMAN'S rho (*ρ*)
KENDALL'S tau (*τ*)

Paired observations

Difference between means, medians or preference

Normal:
PAIRED *T*-TEST

Non-normal:
WILCOXON SIGNED RANK TEST; SIGN TEST

Measure of association---LINEAR REGRESSION

Strength of association

Normal:
PEARSON'S *r*

Non-normal:
SPEARMAN'S rho (*ρ*)
KENDALL'S tau (*τ*)

Effect of exposure in cross-over trial or matched case-control study

McNEMAR'S TEST

Index

Page numbers in *italics* refer to illustrations; those in **bold** refer to tables

Statistics in Nutrition and Dietetics, First Edition. Michael Nelson.
© 2020 John Wiley & Sons Ltd. Published 2020 by John Wiley & Sons Ltd.
Companion website: www.wiley.com/go/nelson/statistics